Diagnosing Skin Disease in Skin of Color

Editor

SUSAN C. TAYLOR

DERMATOLOGIC CLINICS

www.derm.theclinics.com

Consulting Editor
BRUCE H. THIERS

July 2023 • Volume 41 • Number 3

ELSEVIER

1600 John F. Kennedy Boulevard • Suite 1800 • Philadelphia, Pennsylvania, 19103-2899

http://www.theclinics.com

DERMATOLOGIC CLINICS Volume 41, Number 3
July 2023 ISSN 0733-8635, ISBN-13: 978-0-323-94037-5

Editor: Stacy Eastman
Developmental Editor: Karen Justine S. Dino

Dermatologic Clinics (ISSN 0733-8635) is published quarterly by Elsevier Inc., 360 Park Avenue South, New York, NY 10010-1710. Months of publication are January, April, July, and October. Business and editorial offices: 1600 John F. Kennedy Blvd., Suite 1800, Philadelphia, PA 19103-2899. Customer service office: 11830 Westline Drive, St. Louis, MO 63146. Periodicals postage paid at New York, NY, and additional mailing offices. Subscription prices are USD 438.00 per year for US individuals, USD 899.00 per year for US institutions, USD 478.00 per year for Canadian individuals, USD 1,097.00 per year for Canadian institutions, USD 536.00 per year for international individuals, USD 1,097.00 per year for international institutions, USD 100.00 per year for US students/residents, USD 100.00 per year for Canadian students/residents, and USD 240 per year for international students/residents. International air speed delivery is included in all *Clinics* subscription prices. All prices are subject to change without notice. **POSTMASTER:** Send address changes to *Dermatologic Clinics*, Elsevier Health Sciences Division, Subscription Customer Service, 3251 Riverport Lane, Maryland Heights, MO 63043. **Customer Service: 1-800-654-2452 (U.S. and Canada); 314-447-8871 (outside U.S. and Canada). Fax: 314-447-8029. E-mail: journalscustomerservice-usa@elsevier.com (for print support); journalsonlinesupport-usa@elsevier.com (for online support).**

Reprints. For copies of 100 or more, of articles in this publication, please contact the Commercial Reprints Department, Elsevier Inc., 360 Park Avenue South, New York, New York 10010-1710. Tel.: 212-633-3874; Fax: 212-633-3820; Email: reprints@elsevier.com.

The *Dermatologic Clinics* is covered in *MEDLINE/PubMed (Index Medicus)*, *Current Contents/Clinical Medicine*, *Excerpta Medica*, *Chemical Abstracts*, and *ISI/BIOMED*.

Contributors

CONSULTING EDITOR

BRUCE H. THIERS, MD
Professor and Chairman Emeritus, Department
of Dermatology and Dermatologic Surgery,
Medical University of South Carolina,
Charleston, South Carolina, USA

EDITOR

SUSAN C. TAYLOR, MD, FAAD
Bernett L. Johnson Endowed Professor of
Dermatology, Vice Chair for Diversity, Equity
and Inclusion, Department of Dermatology,
University of Pennsylvania Perelman School of
Medicine, Philadelphia, Pennsylvania, USA

AUTHORS

WALEED ADAWI, MS
Department of Dermatology, Johns Hopkins
School of Medicine, Baltimore, Maryland, USA

VICTORIA BARBOSA, MD, MPH, MBA
University of Chicago Medicine Section of
Dermatology, Chicago, Illinois, USA

TIARA BRADLEY, BS
Meharry Medical College, Nashville,
Tennessee, USA

CHERYL BURGESS, MD, FAAD
Assistant Clinical Professor, The George
Washington School of Medicine and Health
Sciences, Washington, DC, USA

VALERIE D. CALLENDER, MD, FAAD
Professor of Dermatology, Howard University
College of Medicine, Washington, DC, USA;
Callender Dermatology & Cosmetic Center,
Glenn Dale, Maryland, USA

AVROM CAPLAN, MD
Assistant Professor, Ronald O. Perelman
Department of Dermatology, NYU School of
Medicine, New York, New York, USA

LESLIE CASTELO-SOCCIO, MD, PhD
Attending Physician, Dermatology
Branch, National Institute of Arthritis,
Musculoskeletal, and Skin Diseases, National
Institutes of Health, Bethesda, Maryland,
USA

MARISSA S. CERESNIE, DO
Department of Dermatology, Multicultural
Clinic, Henry Ford Health, Detroit, Michigan,
USA

HANNAH CORNMAN, BS
Department of Dermatology, Johns Hopkins
School of Medicine, Baltimore, Maryland,
USA

SEEMAL R. DESAI, MD
Innovative Dermatology, PA, Plano, Texas,
USA; Department of Dermatology, The
University of Texas Southwestern Medical
Center, Dallas, Texas, USA

ALICIA EDWARDS, MS
Howard University College of Medicine,
Washington, DC, USA

NADA ELBULUK, MD, MSc
Associate Professor, Director Skin of Color and Pigmentary Disorders Program, Director Diversity and Inclusion Program, Department of Dermatology, Keck School of Medicine of USC, University of Southern California, Los Angeles, California, USA

NNENNA EZEH, MD
Harvard Combined Medicine-Dermatology Residency, Massachusetts General Hospital, Boston, Massachusetts, USA

NKANYEZI FERGUSON, MD
Department of Dermatology, University of Missouri, Columbia, Missouri, USA

ELISABETH A. GEORGE, MD
Mount Sinai Hospital, New York, New York, USA

DONALD A. GLASS II, MD, PhD
Department of Dermatology, Eugene McDermott Center for Human Growth and Development, The University of Texas Southwestern Medical Center, Dallas, Texas, USA

SARAH GONZALEZ, BS
Wayne State University College of Medicine, Detroit, Michigan, USA

KARINA GRULLON, BS
University of Chicago Pritzker School of Medicine, Maywood, New Jersey, USA

ILTEFAT H. HAMZAVI, MD
Department of Dermatology, Multicultural Clinic, Henry Ford Health, Detroit, Michigan, USA

SHANAE HENRY, MS
Department of Dermatology, Johns Hopkins School of Medicine, Baltimore, Maryland, USA

ROBERT HIGHT, BS, MS
University of Chicago Pritzker School of Medicine, Maywood, New Jersey, USA

SOTONYE IMADOJEMU, MD, MBE
Assistant Professor, Department of Dermatology, Brigham and Women's Hospital, Harvard Medical School, Boston, Massachusetts, USA

JAHDONNA ISAAC, MS, MD
Department of Dermatology, Howard University College of Medicine, Washington, DC, USA

TONI JENKINS, MS
Howard University College of Medicine, Washington, DC, USA

ANUSHA KAMBALA, BS
Department of Dermatology, Johns Hopkins School of Medicine, Baltimore, Maryland, USA

RAMONA KHANNA, BA
Georgetown University School of Medicine, Washington, DC, USA

RAYVA KHANNA, MD
Department of Internal Medicine, MedStar Washington Hospital Center, Washington, DC, USA

ARIEL KNOWLES, MBBS
Department of Dermatology, The University of Texas Southwestern Medical Center, Dallas, Texas, USA

SHAWN G. KWATRA, MD
Department of Dermatology, Associate Professor of Dermatology and Oncology, Director, Johns Hopkins Itch Center, Johns Hopkins School of Medicine, Baltimore, Maryland, USA

JORGE LARRONDO, MD, MSC
Department of Dermatology, Wake Forest Baptist Health, Winston-Salem, North Carolina, USA; Department of Dermatology, Clínica Alemana-Universidad del Desarrollo, Santiago, Chile

VICTORIA LEE, MD, PhD
Resident, Section of Dermatology, University of Chicago, Chicago, Illinois, USA

AMY J. MCMICHAEL, MD
Department of Dermatology, Wake Forest Baptist Health, Winston-Salem, North Carolina, USA

ANANYA MUNJAL, MS
University of Iowa Carver College of Medicine, Iowa City, Iowa, USA

JANAYA NELSON, MS
Meharry Medical College, Nashville, Tennessee, USA

KAMARIA NELSON, MHS, MD
Department of Dermatology, The George Washington School of Medicine and Health Sciences, Washington, DC, USA

CHRISTY NWANKWO, BA
University of Missouri, Kansas City School of Medicine, Kansas City, Missouri, USA

MICHELLE OBOITE, MD
Assistant Professor of Clinical Dermatology and Pediatrics, University of Pennsylvania Perelman School of Medicine, Children's Hospital of Philadelphia, Philadelphia, Pennsylvania, USA

CHIAMAKA OHANENYE, BS
Lewis Katz School of Medicine at Temple University, Philadelphia, Pennsylvania, USA

GINETTE A. OKOYE, MD
Professor and Department Chair, Department of Dermatology, Howard University College of Medicine, Washington, DC, USA

OLUWAKEMI ONAJIN, MD
Assistant Professor, Section of Dermatology, University of Chicago, Chicago, Illinois, USA

CLAUDIA QUARSHIE, BS
Keck School of Medicine of USC, University of Southern California, Los Angeles, California, USA

MISHA ROSENBACH, MD
Associate Professor, Department of Dermatology, University of Pennsylvania, Philadelphia, Pennsylvania, USA

OLAYEMI SOKUMBI, MD
Associate Professor, Department of Dermatology and Laboratory Medicine Pathology, Mayo Clinic, Jacksonville, Florida, USA

NICOLE C. SYDER, BA
Keck School of Medicine of USC, University of Southern California, Los Angeles, California, USA

SUMAYAH TALIAFERRO, MD
Medical Director, Atlanta Dermatology & Aesthetics, PC, Atlanta, Georgia, USA

Contents

Diagnosing psoriasis in patients of color can pose both diagnostic and treatment challenges. It is important to keep psoriasis on the differential diagnosis with conditions such as lichen planus, tinea corporis, and subcutaneous lupus for patients of color. Biopsy can help delineate the causes and guide treatment. Although there is no documented difference in efficacy of certain treatments for psoriasis based on racial group, cultural norms, hair washing practices, health literacy, and attitudes toward certain treatment options should be elicited in all patients.

Collagen vascular diseases such as lupus erythematosus and dermatomyositis (DM) occur 2 to 3 times more often among patients with skin of color. In this article, the authors review DM and cutaneous lupus erythematosus, including acute cutaneous lupus erythematosus, subacute cutaneous lupus erythematosus, and discoid lupus erythematosus. They discuss the distinguishing features between these entities and highlight distinct presentations and management considerations in patients with skin of color to aid in prompt and correct diagnoses in this patient population.

Sarcoidosis is a chronic, multisystem, inflammatory disorder that is characterized by noncaseating granulomas that cause organ dysfunction with various clinical subphenotypes. The incidence and prevalence of sarcoidosis varies greatly by ethnic background. There are significant racial disparities in prevalence, severity, and outcomes; however, there is a dearth of studies investigating the impact of structural racism. The skin is often the presenting and second most frequently involved organ with significant implications on diagnosis and management in patients with darkly pigmented skin. Workup should be comprehensive given the multisystem involvement. There are many therapies for sarcoidosis, although none is universally effective.

Hidradenitis suppurativa (HS) is a chronic disease characterized by recurrent painful abscesses and chronic sinus tracts in intertriginous areas. In the United States, HS disproportionally affects adults of African-American heritage. Depending on the severity of disease, the consequences of HS can be far-reaching, significantly affecting mental health and quality of life. In recent years, concerted research efforts have been made to better understand the pathophysiology of the disease as well as identify emerging new treatment targets. Herein, we discuss the clinical presentation, diagnostic criteria, and treatment approach of HS with a focus on skin of color.

Skin cancer is often associated with greater morbidity and mortality in skin of color patients because most medical literature and research on skin cancer to date has been predominantly focused on lighter skin types. It is crucial that dermatologic providers be able to recognize different presentations of skin cancer in skin of color patients to optimize the early detection of these tumors and ensure equitable outcomes. This article details the epidemiology, risk factors, clinical features, and disparities in the treatment of melanoma, squamous cell carcinoma, basal cell carcinoma, and mycosis fungoides subtype of cutaneous T-cell lymphoma in skin of color patients.

Pediatric dermatoses can present at birth or develop over time. When managing dermatology conditions in children, caregiver involvement is important. Patients may have lesions that need to be monitored or need assistance with therapeutic administration. The following section provides a subset of pediatric dermatoses and notable points for presentation in skin of color patients. Providers need to be able to recognize dermatology conditions in patients of varying skin tones and provide therapies that address the condition and any associated pigmentary alterations.

Keloids are an exuberant response to skin wound healing in which abundant scar tissue grows beyond the boundaries of the inciting insult. Age, race, location, family history and personal history of keloids are relevant factors concerning the risk of developing keloids. Because keloids are prone to recurrence after surgical excision, post-operative management plays an important role in the treatment of keloids. There are many modalities that can be used to treat keloids or prevent their recurrence; a multimodal approach is often necessary in difficult cases.

African hair shaft and pigmented scalp have unique features that challenge diagnosis in scarring alopecia. In addition, Black patients may associate 2 or more types of hair disorders. Therefore, it is imperative to understand their findings thoroughly to establish a good diagnosis. Differential diagnosis on the frontal scalp includes traction alopecia and frontal fibrosing alopecia. Disorders such as central centrifugal cicatricial alopecia, fibrosing alopecia in a pattern distribution, discoid lupus erythematosus, and lichen planopilaris usually affect the middle scalp. Folliculitis decalvans, dissecting cellulitis, and acne keloidalis nuchae are the main differential diagnosis of the posterior scalp.

Tinea capitis, folliculitis, seborrheic dermatitis, and pediculosis capitis are four common scalp conditions. Although tinea capitis and seborrheic dermatitis are found more commonly in patients with skin of color and highly textured hair, all of these conditions have special diagnostic or management considerations in these populations. This article reviews the diagnosis and management of these common scalp conditions.

Skin of color in dermatology encompasses individuals of various ethnic backgrounds including Black or those of African descent, Hispanic or Latino, Asian,

Native American, Pacific Islander, and those of mixed ethnicities. Because these populations continue to expand, more patients of color (POC) are seeking out cosmetic enhancements and treatments. Aside from cosmeceuticals, nonsurgical cosmetic rejuvenation options, such laser and light-based treatments, neurotoxins, soft tissue augmentation, and more recently body contouring and skin tightening, are becoming increasingly popular worldwide. This article examines risks of cosmetic enhancement procedures in POC and best practices to prevent adverse events.

DERMATOLOGIC CLINICS

Preface
Diagnosing Skin Diseases in Skin of Color

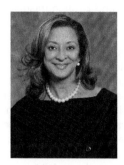

Susan C. Taylor, MD, FAAD
Editor

Skin of Color (SOC) is a broad term that has been used to refer to populations who identify as other than non-Hispanic white: Black/African, Hispanic/Latina/o/x/e, Asian/Pacific Islander, American Indian/Native Alaskan, Indigenous Australian, Middle Eastern, or biracial/multiracial. It is also commonly defined as including individuals with Fitzpatrick skin types IV to VI. Many gaps have emerged regarding knowledge related to disorders that occur in SOC populations. Among these is the unfamiliarity by dermatologists of phenotypic differences in some cutaneous diseases. Common diseases may appear quite different in individuals with darker skin tones compared with lighter skin tones with variations in color, location, morphology, and severity of disease. Incomplete or inadequate SOC education, which occurs along a continuum from medical school to dermatology residency, fellowship, and continuing medical education offerings for dermatologists, leads to missed and/or delayed diagnoses, adverse events, and patient dissatisfaction and may perpetuate health inequities.

This issue of *Dermatologic Clinics* entitled, "Diagnosing Skin Diseases in Skin of Color," has a laser focus on the diagnosis of a spectrum of diseases that occur in SOC populations. The issue begins by discussing diagnostic challenges associated with facial erythema and hyperpigmentation and elucidating key features that present in disorders located on facial skin. Cutaneous disorders

characterized by hypopigmentation and depigmentation in patients with darker skin tones are discussed and may require specific tools to distinguish them. Cutaneous diseases that may occur commonly or uniquely in SOC populations are then highlighted.

- "Diagnosing disorders of facial erythema" provides a guide to the identification of specific patterns, shades, and intensity of erythema in SOC patients to improve diagnostic accuracy of common dermatologic disorders. Erythema is often less noticeable in darker skin types, and the interplay of inflammation and variance of skin tone contributes to appreciable differences in the clinical appearance of cutaneous disease in darker complexions. This article discusses common disorders that present with facial erythema in SOC populations and offers distinguishing features of each disorder to assist the clinician with diagnosing these conditions in the presence of deeply pigmented skin.
- "Disorders of facial hyperpigmentation" are generally more common in SOC populations, and these challenging conditions can arise due to a myriad of etiologic factors. Cutaneous disorders causing facial hyperpigmentation include those that are acquired or hereditary, epidermal or dermal, or primary or secondary to underlying systemic diseases. These

Dermatol Clin 41 (2023) xiii–xv
https://doi.org/10.1016/j.det.2023.03.001
0733-8635/23/© 2023 Elsevier Inc. All rights reserved.

conditions involve unique diagnostic and therapeutic considerations. This article provides a comprehensive review of disorders of facial hyperpigmentation, including epidemiology, pathogenesis, diagnostic considerations, and treatment approaches of these conditions.

- "Disorders of hypopigmentation and depigmentation" are a top concern for patients with SOC seeking care from a dermatologist. The visual contrast between involved and uninvolved skin in these disorders makes them particularly burdensome for patients with SOC. These disorders may have a wide differential of diagnosis, as patients with SOC may present differently or more frequently than white patients for certain conditions. Clues from a comprehensive history and physical examination with standard lighting and a Wood light are essential for clinching the diagnosis.

- "Atopic dermatitis", a pruritic inflammatory skin disease that disproportionately affects African American, Asian, and Hispanic patients, has increased prevalence, disease severity, and health care utilization for some of these populations. Unique clinical presentations in SOC patients may include greater extensor involvement, dyspigmentation, as well as papular and lichenified presentations. In this disease, erythema is also more difficult to appreciate and can result in an underappreciation of disease severity in SOC patients.

- "Psoriasis", a chronic immune-mediated, genetic disease with diversity in presentation and manifestations, often poses a diagnostic challenge for dermatologists due to the lack of conspicuous "erythema" and overlap with features of other dermatologic disorders. Delayed diagnosis or inadequate treatment of psoriasis can precipitate severe systemic involvement, such as psoriatic arthritis and increased risk for cardiac disease.

- Lupus erythematosus and dermatomyositis are collagen vascular diseases that occur two to three times more often among patients with SOC. There are distinguishing features between these entities, although overlap can occur. This article highlights the intricacies of correct diagnoses of collagen vascular diseases in this patient population.

- "Sarcoidosis", a chronic, multisystem, inflammatory disorder that is characterized by noncaseating granulomas, has various clinical subphenotypes. The skin is often the presenting and second most frequently involved organ, with significant implications on diagnosis and management in patients with darkly pigmented skin.

- "Hidradenitis suppurativa", a chronic disease characterized by recurrent painful abscesses and chronic sinus tracts in intertriginous areas, disproportionally affects adults of African American heritage and is often misdiagnosed as folliculitis, epidermal inclusion cysts, or simply boils. The effects of HS may be far-reaching, significantly affecting mental health and quality of life.

- "Skin cancer", although less common in SOC patients, is often associated with greater morbidity and mortality in this population. With the rapidly evolving SOC demographic landscape, this article provides a roadmap for dermatologic providers to be able to recognize different presentations of skin cancer in SOC patients, in an effort to optimize early detection of these tumors and ensure equitable outcomes.

- Pediatric dermatoses can present at birth or develop over childhood. A subset of pediatric dermatoses with notable points for presentation and diagnosis in SOC patients is provided. Dermatologic providers must be equipped to recognize dermatology conditions in patients of varying skin tones and provide therapies that address the condition and any associated pigmentary alterations.

- Keloids, a fibroproliferative inflammatory disorder of the skin where scars grow excessively past the original borders of the inciting agent and invade into normal adjacent tissue, occur in the general population from 4.5% to 6.2% and up to 16% in those of African descent, while the incidence in the Taiwanese Chinese and whites is reported to be as low as less than 1%. It is important to be able to distinguish keloidal scars from hypertrophic scars and understand the principle of prevention and treatment.

- "Scarring alopecia" in populations with pigmented scalp and tightly coiled hair as found in many black populations has unique features that challenge diagnosis. Two or more types of hair disorders may further complicate diagnosis. A complete understanding of these findings is necessary to establish a correct diagnosis.

- "Scalp infections and inflammation" disorders, including tinea capitis, folliculitis, seborrheic dermatitis, and pediculosis capitis, have special diagnostic or management considerations in SOC populations. While tinea capitis and seborrheic dermatitis are found more commonly in patients with SOC and highly textured hair, folliculitis and pediculosis capitis also present unique diagnostic considerations.

- Cosmetic enhancements and treatments have become increasingly popular among SOC populations. Due to skin structural, functional, and biological differences, SOC populations have unique cosmetic concerns compared with individuals with lighter phenotypes as well as differences in the risks and benefits associated with treatments. A review of the risks of cosmetic enhancement procedures, including for pigmentary changes, antiaging remedies, and nonsurgical cosmetic rejuvenation, in SOC populations as well as best practices to prevent adverse events is highlighted.

It is our wish that this comprehensive issue, "Diagnosing Skin Diseases in Skin of Color," will assist you in caring for your patients with SOC.

Susan C. Taylor, MD, FAAD
Department of Dermatology
Perelman School of Medicine
University of Pennsylvania
3400 Civic Center Boulevard
South Tower, 7-768
Philadelphia, PA 19104, USA

E-mail address:
Susan.Taylor@pennmedicine.upenn.edu

Diagnosing Disorders of Facial Erythema

Chiamaka Ohanenye, BS[a], Sumayah Taliaferro, MD[b], Valerie D. Callender, MD[c],*

KEYWORDS

- Facial erythema • Erythema • Skin of color • Acne vulgaris • Rosacea • Lupus erythematosus
- Psoriasis • Seborrheic dermatitis

KEY POINTS

- Erythema in darker skin types is difficult to detect, especially in Fitzpatrick skin types V and VI
- A common sequela of acne vulgaris in patients with skin of color (SOC) is postinflammatory hyperpigmentation (PIH)
- Rosacea is not uncommon in the SOC population and is frequently misdiagnosed and underreported
- Dyschromia and violaceous erythema may be presenting signs of lupus and other autoimmune skin diseases
- Fitzpatrick skin types IV-VI have a higher minimal erythema dose than those with skin types I-III due to increased melanin in their skin which makes them less likely to burn

INTRODUCTION

How to Detect Erythema in Skin of Color

Facial skin erythema can be associated with various inflammatory cutaneous diseases and external stimuli that increase blood flow in superficial capillaries and induce a change in the skin (Box 1).[1] However, as noted, detecting erythema in darker skin tones, Fitzpatrick skin types (FST) V and VI are challenging and can be difficult and often cause misdiagnosis in patients with SOC. There are several techniques used to assess skin erythema. These include visual assessment scales, the use of colorimetry, and spectra-based and imaging-based assessment devices (Table 1).[1] Valid and reliable skin erythema assessment tools are crucial in clinical trials. For example, these methods of measurement are often used in rosacea clinical trials to assess the efficacy of medications and surgical techniques (Box 2). The most common visual assessment tool for erythema is the use of a 4-point scale, developed by the National Rosacea Society, however interrater reliability may exist (Box 3).[2,3] Utilizing advanced technologies, such as spectrophotometry, a tool that assesses optical properties of materials based on wavelength, is often useful in clinical trials, but not in clinical practice, to assess erythema and is commonly used along with the 4-point visual assessment scale. Both tools are used more often in clinical trials rather than computer analysis of digital photographs.

Although there are limited tools used to assess erythema in clinical practice and in clinical trials, detecting erythema in SOC, in particular FST VI, remains difficult. This can result in a delay of diagnosis for patients with deeper skin tones and further progression of disease. Certain diagnostic methods such as testing the skin for blanching, use of dermatoscopes, photographing the patient on a dark blue background, and ensuring there is adequate lighting in examination rooms may aid in diagnosing erythema in darker skin tones.[4]

Dermatology Clinics: Diagnosing Skin Disease in Skin of Color.

[a] Lewis Katz School of Medicine at Temple University, 3500 North Broad Street, Philadelphia, PA 19140, USA; [b] Atlanta Dermatology & Aesthetics, PC, 232 19th Street Northwest, Atlanta, GA 30363, USA; [c] Callender Dermatology & Cosmetic Center, 12200 Annapolis Road, Suite 315, Glenn Dale, MD 20769, USA

* Corresponding author. 12200 Annapolis Road, Suite 315, Glenn Dale, MD 20769, USA.

E-mail address: drcallender@CallenderSkin.com

Dermatol Clin 41 (2023) 377–392

https://doi.org/10.1016/j.det.2023.02.004

Box 1
Causes of facial skin erythema

Inflammatory Skin Diseases

Acne

Rosacea

Atopic dermatitis

Psoriasis

Seborrheic dermatitis

Sunburn from electromagnetic radiation (ultraviolet light)

Radiation therapy

Physical pressure

Skin ulceration

Application of medical and cosmetic topical agents

Electrical stimuli

However, erythema in SOC patients can still go unnoticed, despite those efforts. Therefore, a novel assessment methodology used in research to assess erythema in darker skin types is needed, which may enable SOC patients to be included in clinical trials that traditionally exclude them based on their skin type.

Acne Vulgaris

Acne vulgaris is a very common cause of facial erythema. It often presents in young adults and adolescents but may occur at any age. The pathogenesis of acne vulgaris is multifactorial and results in comedone formation and inflammation, which can present differently depending on skin tone. The pathophysiology of acne vulgaris does not seem to differ across different ethnicities or skin colors. However, acne in SOC patients is often complicated by postinflammatory hyperpigmentation (PIH).

Clinically, acne vulgaris presents as comedones, pustules, papules, and cysts most commonly on the face, chest, back, and upper extremities. In many patients, acne may predominate along the oily T-zone on the forehead, nose, and chin. In others, acne may predominate on the lower parts of the face, such as the cheeks and jaw, which is consistent with a hormonal distribution. The inflammation that occurs in acne manifests as erythema, which is easier to appreciate in lighter skin tones, such as in patients with FST IV and some patients with FST V (**Fig. 1**). In darker

---

Table 1
Assessment techniques—advantages versus disadvantages

	Advantages	Disadvantages
Visual assessment	• Requires no equipment • Rapid • Convenient • Simple • Useful in the clinical setting	• Subjective • Imprecise • Metamerism • Poor durability
Colorimetry Assessment: color charts, colorimeter devices	• Able to easily assess and quantify skin color changes • Allows for easy data communication and archiving • Simple	• Subjective • Unreliable
Spectra-based Assessment: narrow-band spectroscopic devices, diffuse reflectance spectroscopy, laser Doppler flowmetry	• Efficient • Objective • Accurate	• Low sensitivity • Can be costly • Cumbersome • Requires direct skin contact so cannot be used in sensitive regions • Limited ROI investigation
Imaging-based Assessment: digital color imaging, polarized light imaging, fluorescence imagine, spectral imaging	• Objective • Does not require skin contact • Can examine larger skin ROIs	• Complex • Expensive • UV damage with fluorescence imaging

Abbreviations: ROI, region of interest; UV, ultraviolet.
Data from Abdlaty R, Hayward J, Farrell T, Fang Q. Skin erythema and pigmentation: a review of optical assessment techniques. Photodiagnosis Photodyn Ther. 2021;33:102127.

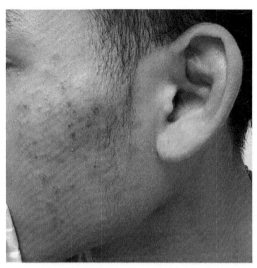

Fig. 1. Inflammatory acne in a Hispanic/Latino man. (*Courtesy of* V Callender, MD, FAAD, Glenn Dale, MD.)

In an examination performed by dermatologists at the Skin of Color Center, Black, Hispanic, and Asian patients were more likely to have papular lesions and acne hyperpigmented macules over pustular and cystic lesions.[6] Another form of acne commonly seen in Black Americans is "pomade acne," characterized by closed comedones along the hairline and on the forehead, caused by long-term use of comedogenic hair products. This more commonly occurs in African Americans due to less frequent hair washing according to hair type and increased use of thick, oily products on the scalp.

First-line treatments of acne vulgaris depend on the severity of the condition. Mild acne is treated with topical products such as benzoyl peroxide, topical retinoids, or topical antibiotics (erythromycin, clindamycin). Moderate acne is treated similarly to mild acne but often with the addition of oral antibiotics such as doxycycline and minocycline. Additional therapies indicated for the treatment of mild-to-moderate acne include topical dapsone, azelaic acid, and oral and topical androgen receptor inhibitors. Severe acne can be treated with all the previous treatments with the addition of oral isotretinoin.[7] Other treatments for acne vulgaris include oral contraceptive pills, topical dapsone, spironolactone, salicylic acid, and glycolic acid.

skin tones as seen in patients with FST VI, cutaneous inflammation can manifest as areas of hyperpigmentation, which may mask facial erythema.

The differential diagnosis of acne vulgaris includes acne conglobata, acne fulminans, folliculitis, perioral dermatitis, rosacea, tuberous sclerosis, and sebaceous hyperplasia.[5] The diagnosis of acne vulgaris is typically clinical. Diagnosing acne vulgaris in SOC is more nuanced due to increased skin pigmentation. Inflammation-induced erythema easily visualized in Caucasian patients is often missed in patients of darker skin tones and further masked by acne-induced hyperpigmentation in these patients.

When treating acne vulgaris in SOC, special consideration should be taken to minimize its possible sequelae of PIH and hypertrophic/keloid scarring. Both occur more commonly in darker skin patients than in those with lighter skin. In a study by Taylor and colleagues, 65.3% of Black patients and 52.7% of Hispanic patients developed PIH after the occurrence of acne.[8] Treatments such as azelaic acid and hydroquinone can be used to treat PIH by inhibiting tyrosinase and therefore, the production of melanin. Sunscreen use is also advised in patients with PIH to prevent the darkening of hyperpigmentation. Procedural treatments such as laser therapy (eg, 1064 nanometer ND:YAG laser, 1726 nanometer laser, or microsecond 1064 ND:YAG laser) or chemical peels can also be used to treat acne, PIH, and scarring, although these are not first-line therapies. Erythema from acne is a direct result of inflammation. Thus, the use of anti-inflammatory agents such as doxycycline and topicals containing aloe vera, green tea, niacinamide, and vitamin C are commonly used to soothe the skin and reduce inflammation. Cooling the skin is often important in procedural therapies such as laser and energy-based devices.

Rosacea

Rosacea is a chronic inflammatory facial dermatosis commonly reported in fair-skinned individuals with an increased incidence among Northern Europeans. It has a lower prevalence among those with darker skin but it is not uncommon in SOC.[4] The hallmark feature of rosacea is facial erythema, and it is also characterized by telangiectasia, flushing, papules, and pustules often centrally located on the face (**Fig. 2**). Recognition of erythema of rosacea is more difficult in darker skin. This may result in delayed diagnosis and underreporting of rosacea in SOC. The inflammation of rosacea may lead to PIH or hypopigmentation, further complicating the diagnosis. Rosacea may also present with thickening of the skin on and around the nose and with ocular manifestations. Other features include skin sensitivity, a reduced barrier function of the skin, and increased dryness of the skin.

Ultraviolet (UV) light is a contributing factor in rosacea. Climate and sun exposure have long been known to affect flares. Although the pathophysiology of rosacea remains incompletely understood, other etiologic mechanisms include aberrant immune processes, neuronal dysregulation, and certain microorganisms.[9,10] The 2 main microorganisms implicated in rosacea include *Demodex folliculorum*[11] and *Helicobacter pylori*. Rosacea has also been associated with gastrointestinal disease. Reports indicate higher rates of Crohn disease and ulcerative colitis in patients with rosacea.[12,13]

Rosacea has been classified into 4 main types: 1. erythematotelangiectatic, 2. papulopustular, 3. phymatous, and 4. ocular.[14] The erythematotelangiectatic and papulopustular types are more common. Rhinophyma often indicates more advanced disease and may cause disfigurement (**Fig. 3**). The prevalence of rhinophyma is higher in men than in women. Ocular rosacea is likely more common but possibly underreported due to clinician unfamiliarity. The most frequent presentation of ocular rosacea is chronically inflamed margins of the eyelids with scales and crust similar to seborrheic dermatitis (SD). Other signs include pain, photophobia, and foreign body sensation. Ophthalmic manifestations of rosacea may develop before cutaneous manifestations, and eye involvement may not correlate with the severity of rosacea.[15]

Although the clinical characteristics and pathophysiology of rosacea are the same across all ethnicities, diagnosis of rosacea in SOC is often delayed. Because it is more difficult to observe erythema on darkly pigmented skin and even more so when hyperpigmentation is superimposed, screening for other signs remains important in patient assessment.[4] Close inspection of the skin should be made for detecting telangiectasia and central distribution of papules and pustules.

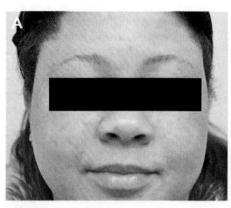
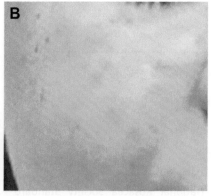

Fig. 2. (*A*) Rosacea in Fitzpatrick skin type IV. (*B*) Close-up of erythematous papules in rosacea. (*Courtesy of* V Callender, MD, FAAD, Glenn Dale, MD.)

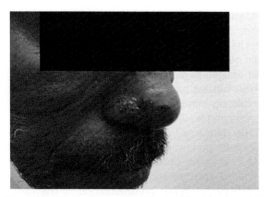

Fig. 3. Rosacea in a male Fitzpatrick skin type VI. (*Courtesy of* S Taliaferro, MD, Atlanta, GA.)

Careful attention should be provided to reports of sensitive skin with burning and stinging of the face with the use of skincare products. Other signs of rosacea include "flares" after eating spicy foods and consuming alcoholic beverages, occurrences with cold and hot weather, and episodes with timing corresponding to emotional upset or stress.

Granulomatous rosacea is considered to be a variant of rosacea. In this subtype, papules and pustules in a perioral and periocular distribution are dominant and erythema and flushing are less prominent. Perioral dermatitis and facial Afro-Caribbean eruption are thought to be related to rosacea.[16]

The differential diagnosis of facial erythema of rosacea includes acne vulgaris, SD, contact dermatitis (CD), lupus erythematosus, sarcoidosis, steroid acne, dermatomyositis (DM), and keratosis pilaris rubra.

Given its multifactorial cause, the treatment of rosacea often involves combined therapies. Topical Food and Drug Administration (FDA)-approved agents are azelaic acid, metronidazole, sodium sulfacetamide, ivermectin, and alpha-adrenergic agonists. Off-label topical treatments frequently used and are the mainstay of therapy include topical retinoids, topical clindamycin, topical erythromycin, benzoyl peroxide, calcineurin inhibitors, and permethrin. The tetracycline class of antibiotics is an FDA-approved systemic treatment of rosacea. A submicrobial dose of doxycycline is an effective FDA-approved treatment of rosacea. Other systemic treatments used are beta-blockers, isotretinoin, and ivermectin. Low-dose isotretinoin has been particularly useful in cases refractory to more common treatments.[17,18] Alpha-agonists such as brimonidine and oxymetazoline can also be used to reduce the facial erythema seen in rosacea.[19]

Attention to skin care is an important part of the treatment of rosacea. Gentle, nonsoap cleansers are recommended. Overall, products that are light, mild, fragrance-free, water-based, and containing fewer preservatives are best tolerated. The importance of sunscreen must be emphasized particularly among patients of color, who have a reduced use of photoprotection. Physical sunblocks, such as zinc oxide and titanium dioxide, are preferred over chemical sunscreens. Mineral-based foundations over cream-based are better suited for patients with rosacea. They should be counseled to avoid chemicals, exfoliants, and astringents that could further exacerbate the skin barrier. Thus, barrier repair skin care products are often helpful.

Systemic Lupus Erythematosus

Lupus erythematosus is a well-known cause of facial erythema. Images dating back to the 1800s displaying erythema over the cheeks and nose display the early presence of the disease. Although systemic lupus erythematosus (SLE) has a wide spectrum of clinical findings, the presentation of malar erythema is one of the most familiar expressions of acute cutaneous lupus erythematosus. Usually appearing after sun exposure, characteristically, the erythema spreads over the medial cheeks and nose without involving the nasolabial folds.[20] However, the classic malar rash may occur less frequently in African Americans. Erythema may also present with more brownish to violaceous discoloration in deeply pigmented skin. The malar rash is often accompanied by fatigue, arthralgia, as well as photosensitivity, although many patients of color may be unaware of the sensitivity to light. The manifold manifestations of lupus include alopecia, Raynaud phenomenon, panniculitis, cardiac disease, and renal disease. Some studies that analyzed the clinical presentations of lupus show trends of clinical manifestations by race. For example, African Americans with cutaneous lupus present more commonly with discoid lupus, nephritis, and anti-Sm and anti-ribonucleoprotein (RNP) antibodies.[21] Among the myriad cutaneous manifestations, dyschromia with variations of erythema, hyperpigmentation, and hypopigmentation is a frequent complaint in SOC patients with lupus. Rarely, a chronic form of cutaneous lupus may present with prominent widespread erythema over the face—erythema perstans faciei.

Discoid lupus is one of the most common forms of cutaneous lupus. Discoid lupus has a female predominance but the ratio (3:2–3:1) between men and women is not as large as that observed with systemic lupus (8:1). Only 5% to 10% of patients with chronic cutaneous lupus develop SLE.[21] Discoid lupus plaques are characterized by erythematous slightly scaly atrophic plaques with central hypopigmentation and hyperpigmented peripheral borders (**Fig. 4**). An increased risk of squamous cell carcinoma developing within long-standing plaques of discoid lupus has been reported.[22]

Subacute cutaneous lupus erythematosus (SCLE) is a variant of cutaneous lupus described in 1979 by Sontheimer, Thomas, and Gilliam. SCLE more frequently affects White women aged between 15 and 40 years but it is not uncommon in persons of color. Occurring in genetically predisposed individuals, most patients are positive for anti-Ro (SSA) antibodies. The pathophysiology is thought to involve the alteration of autoantibodies, epidermal cytokines, and adhesion molecules by ultraviolet light leading to keratinocyte apoptosis. Patients present clinically with erythematous patches, often in a psoriasiform pattern or polycyclic annular arrangement with light scale. SCLE skin eruptions favor sun-exposed areas—face, neck, upper back, and upper anterior chest (**Fig. 5**).[23,24]

Lupus profundus is a variant of chronic cutaneous lupus that primarily involves subcutaneous fat. It typically presents with painful erythematous nodules and indurated plaques that tend to heal with atrophy and scars. Another less common form of cutaneous lupus, lupus tumidus, is characterized by indurated erythematous plaques but in this subtype, the affected skin may lack scale and follicular plugging. Lupus tumidus occurs most commonly on sun-exposed areas—typically the head and neck region, and these patients are highly photosensitive. Usually, underlying systemic involvement is not present. Lupus tumidus is distinct histologically from other forms of cutaneous lupus by the absence of alterations of the dermal–epidermal junction and epidermis.[25]

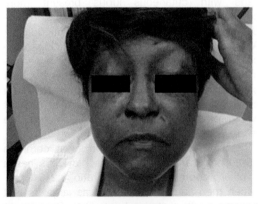

Fig. 4. Erythema and hyperpigmentation in discoid lupus Fitzpatrick skin type V. (*Courtesy of* S Taliaferro, MD, Atlanta, GA.)

Lupus, generally considered the prototypical autoimmune disease, is a polygenic disorder, and its cause cannot be tracked down to one specific gene. The cause involves cross-reactions to a self-antigen in genetically susceptible individuals, which initiates an autoimmune response involving circulating immune complexes that drive inflammation and lead to organ damage.

The differential diagnosis of facial erythema in the malar pattern includes rosacea, eczema, CD, DM, erysipelas, cellulitis, SD, lupus pernio, lupus vulgaris, and pellagra. Fifth disease, eczema, and tinea are other considerations.[26] The diagnosis of acute and chronic lupus is made based on clinical findings, and if necessary, confirmed with a skin biopsy. Laboratory tests as part of a workup of malar erythema include a complete blood count with differential, metabolic panel, urinalysis, sedimentation rate, antinuclear antibodies with titer plus reflex laboratories, anti-Ro (SSA) and anti-La (SSB) antibodies.

First-line treatments of cutaneous lupus erythematosus are daily photoprotection, topical and intralesional corticosteroids, and topical immunomodulators (tacrolimus and pimecrolimus). Systemic treatments include hydroxychloroquine, retinoids (acitretin, isotretinoin), and dapsone. Cytotoxic agents such as methotrexate and azathioprine are therapeutic options. Other treatments include interferon-alpha 2a and thalidomide.[26]

Contact Dermatitis

CD is an adverse skin reaction that occurs after the skin is in contact with an irritant such as a chemical or metal. The prevalence of CD does not differ between races. There are 2 main classes of CD: allergic and irritant. Both forms of CD involve disruption of the epidermal keratinocytes.[27] Allergic contact dermatitis (ACD) is an immune-modulated T-cell response to antigens. It is classified as a type 4 hypersensitivity reaction. Irritant contact dermatitis (ICD) is a result of a toxin disrupting the skin's protective barrier, which triggers a non–T-cell-mediated immune response. The face is a common site for CD to manifest due to its constant exposure to the environment and to consumer products. Facial CD is typically caused by skincare products such as chemical sunscreens, exfoliants, hair care products such as hair dye, or cosmetics, in particular makeup. Each is a potential cause of facial erythema from CD.

CD generally presents clinically as well-defined erythematous patches with scales, vesicles, or bullae that can itch or burn (**Fig. 6**). Acute cases of CD may involve bullae or vesicle formation,

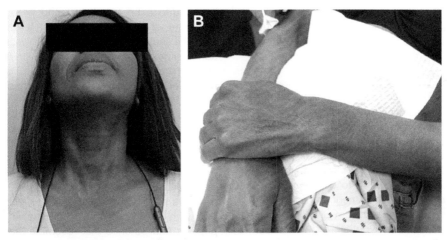

Fig. 5. SCLE in African American female. (*A*) Annular patches with PIH. (*B*) Similar patches on the hands in the same patient. (*Courtesy of* S Taliaferro, MD, Atlanta, GA.)

whereas chronic cases frequently involve lichenification with fissuring.[28] ICD usually presents primarily on areas of the skin directly exposed to the irritant. ACD, however, can cause a rash that spreads beyond where the allergen made contact. In fair-skinned patients, CD presents as itchy pink or red patches. In darker skinned patients, it can present as hyperpigmented patches with shades ranging from brown to purple. Studies have shown that vesicle formation and oozing are more commonly seen in those with lighter skin tones while hyperpigmentation, violaceous discoloration, and lichenification are more common in those with darker skin tones (**Fig. 7**).[29]

Patch testing is a method of identifying causative agents. It involves placing small amounts of allergens on the skin and leaving them on the skin for days to evaluate if the skin interacts with the allergens. Patch testing on dark skin can be more difficult due to the lack of pronounced visible erythema. Additionally, in SOC, lichenification and dyspigmentation are often manifestations of allergic or irritant reactions.[30] Because of this, a diagnosis of CD can be missed.

The differential diagnosis of CD includes urticaria, atopic dermatitis, nummular dermatitis, dyshidrotic dermatitis, SD, rosacea, psoriasis, and fixed drug eruption. CD is best managed by avoiding contact with the irritant or allergen. If treatment is pursued, CD is often treated with a topical

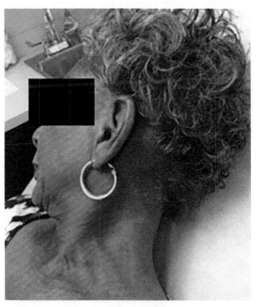

Fig. 7. Violaceous erythema and hyperpigmentation in an African-American female with an ACD. (*Courtesy of* S Taliaferro, MD, Atlanta, GA.)

Fig. 6. Prominent erythema caused by an ACD in skin type V. (*Courtesy of* S Taliaferro, MD, Atlanta, GA.)

steroid. If the skin eruption occurs in delicate areas, topical calcineurin inhibitors can be used. Antihistamines are also used to reduce pruritus.

Seborrheic Dermatitis

SD is a common inflammatory condition that can be chronic or relapsing in nature. It is a common cause of facial erythema in people of all skin colors. It is present in about 3% to 12% of the adult population (31) and has a trimodal incidence: in the first 3 months of life, during puberty, and in adulthood ranging from 40 to 60 years old (32). Studies show that African Americans and West Africans have an increased risk of SD (31).

The cause of SD is hypothesized to be from a diminished T-cell response to the fungus *Malassezia* species, a commensal lipophilic fungus that is part of the normal skin flora. SD is often associated with neurologic and psychiatric conditions, such as Parkinson disease, epilepsy, and tardive dyskinesia. It is also associated with states of immunosuppression. SD presents as well-delineated patches with yellow, greasy, flaky scales in areas rich with sebaceous glands such as the scalp, nasolabial folds, eyebrows, retroauricular area, cheeks, and upper back. It can present with intense pruritus, burning, skin sensitivity, or can be asymptomatic. In lighter skinned individuals, the greasy patches are erythematous. However, in darker skinned individuals, the patches can be erythematous or simply hypopigmented or hyperpigmented with little to no marked erythema (Fig. 8). An annular presentation is also common in African-American patients. The disparity in presentation between different skin tones can make this a challenging diagnosis in SOC and can delay treatment. After treating SD in patients of color, the dyspigmentation may remain despite treatment. This should be considered when treating patients with richly melanized skin.

Dandruff is a mild and common form of SD seen on the scalp. The inflammation caused by dandruff is thought to be subclinical and produces mild erythema of the affected areas. It can spread from the scalp to the hairline, eyebrows, and retroauricular area. Approximately 50 million Americans are estimated to have dandruff.[31] Dandruff is particularly prevalent in the African American community with an estimated 81% to 95% of African Americans with the condition.[31] In darker skinned patients, severe dandruff can cause hypopigmented areas on the scalp and forehead, which differs from patients with lighter complexions. Another form of SD that is usually seen in darker skinned patients is called petaloid SD. It initially presents as small follicular and perifollicular papules with greasy scales and progresses to form papules and patches that resemble the shape of flowers,[32,33] termed polycyclic coalescing rings. These papules and patches are classically pink or hypopigmented.

The differential diagnosis for SD includes rosacea, psoriasis, atopic dermatitis, tinea capitis, and SLE. Because SD can be chronic or relapsing, treatment is focused on calming flares and preventing recurrence. Treatments include antifungal shampoos, keratolytics such as salicylic acid, and anti-inflammatory agents such as corticosteroids or calcineurin inhibitors.

Psoriasis

Psoriasis is a chronic inflammatory skin disease that affects populations across the globe. Epidemiologic data report a lower incidence in non-White individuals compared with Caucasians: 3.6% in Caucasians versus 1.9% in African-Americans and 1.6% in Hispanics.[34] Although it is widely held that psoriasis is less common in many ethnic populations, the question of possible underreporting has recently been raised. There are appreciable differences in clinical appearance of psoriasis in SOC patients. Lack of inclusion of minority populations in several clinical trials on psoriasis has been acknowledged.

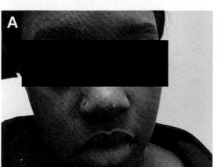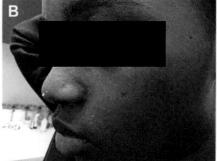

Fig. 8. (A, B) SD on the face in African American woman. (*Courtesy of* S Taliaferro, MD, Atlanta, GA.)

Psoriasis classically presents with erythematous plaques with overlying silvery scales that have a predilection for the scalp, trunk, gluteal cleft, and extensor surfaces, especially the knees and elbows. The plaques can be itchy or painful. On the face, psoriasis typically presents on the hairline, forehead, and cheeks, and it is a marker of more severe disease. The plaques are usually symmetric. In lighter skin, psoriasis plaques are characterized as pink to red hues with silvery-white scales. The erythematous plaques take on a violaceous and brown hue in darker skin, which makes them more difficult to appreciate. PIH is common in patients of color. Patients with richly melanized skin may also have thicker plaques, more scaling, and lichenification. Active inflammation of the plaques is less noticeable in SOC and is commonly perceived as PIH.[35] Nail changes often accompany the skin plaques of psoriasis and include yellowish discoloration, onycholysis, and pitting of the nails.

In comparison to Caucasian individuals, African-Americans report more dyspigmentation and less erythema with psoriasis.[36] Hyperpigmentation and hypopigmentation are common sequelae seen in SOC patients in comparison to Caucasian patients and can cause an increased burden on the patient. Dyspigmentation can take months to years to resolve. Additionally, African-Americans tend to have increased body surface area involvement than Caucasians: 3% to 10% in African-Americans versus 1% to 2% in Caucasians.[37]

There are 5 main types of psoriasis that differ in their presentation. These include plaque, guttate, pustular, inverse, and erythrodermic psoriasis. Plaque psoriasis is the most common type seen in all races. There is a higher incidence of pustular and erythrodermic psoriasis in non-Caucasians than in Caucasians. Inverse psoriasis has a lower incidence in SOC. Scalp psoriasis, which is commonly seen across all races, typically has a more severe presentation in African-Americans due to less frequent hair washing in this population.[38] This severe presentation often involves the skin of the forehead and causes erythema and scaling, which can progress to facial dyspigmentation in African-Americans.[39]

The differential diagnosis of facial erythema of psoriasis includes atopic dermatitis, CD, lichen planus, SD, tinea, cutaneous lupus erythematosus, sarcoidosis, and pityriasis rosea. Treatment of psoriasis includes managing active flares, as there is no curative treatment of the condition. Topical treatments are first-line for the treatment of psoriasis. These topical treatments include corticosteroids such as fluocinonide, clobetasol, and hydrocortisone. Additional therapies include ultraviolet light therapy and systemic therapies.

Dermatomyositis

DM is a rare cause of facial erythema. DM is an inflammatory myopathy that presents with progressive symmetric, proximal muscle weakness and skin rash. Some patients may solely have skin findings and no laboratory or clinical signs of myositis.[40] The rashes associated with DM are usually not alleviated with topical treatments or photoprotective measures.

The characteristic facial rash that presents with DM is the heliotrope rash (Fig. 9). This rash can be the first sign that patients with this condition notice. It can also present simultaneously or after the incidence of muscle weakness. It presents with a symmetric rash over the eyelids and periorbital skin, which may or may not have edema, scaling, or desquamation. The heliotrope rash is described to be erythematous or violaceous in color.[41] These findings are typically seen in patients with lighter skin tones where the rash is more

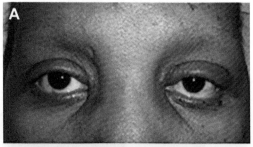

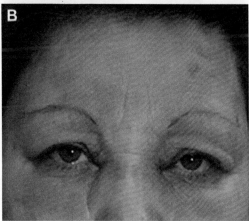

Fig. 9. DM—eyelid edema and heliotrope sign. (A) Inflammation of the upper eyelid can be more subtle in darkly pigmented skin. (B) The characteristic pink-violet color is seen with the involvement of the hairline, lower forehead, upper eyelids, and cheeks. (B, Courtesy, Jean L Bologna, MD.)

pronounced. However, in patients with darker skin tones, the rash is often less noticeable and can often present as hyperpigmentation along with the characteristic violaceous erythema (**Fig. 10**). Although heliotrope rashes are less pronounced in people with darker skin tones, studies have shown that African-Americans were more likely to have cutaneous findings at initial presentation than in Caucasian patients.[42]

Gottron papules are another cutaneous finding of DM, which is a hallmark of the disease. They classically present as violaceous papules with or without scaling seen over bony prominences, such as the dorsal metacarpophalangeal or interphalangeal joints. Other cutaneous manifestations of DM include the shawl sign, poikiloderma, and calcinosis cutis.

Studies have shown there is severe underrepresentation of images of the characteristic DM rashes in SOC in medical education literature.[43] This is a common trend seen in many dermatologic conditions. Some studies that compared

clinical characteristics of DM show trends that vary between races. For example, creatinine kinase, which is a marker of disease severity, tends to be significantly higher in African-American patients than in Caucasian patients. Additionally, the disease duration before the initial presentation was longer in African-Americans, which speaks to issues of delayed diagnosis in this population.[42]

DM may also present with diffuse alopecia and nail changes.[39] Patients with DM have a 6-fold increased risk of acquiring internal malignancy compared with the general population.[44] They are also at increased risk for interstitial lung diseases, cardiovascular diseases such as myocarditis, accelerated atherosclerosis of coronary arteries, heart failure, and so forth, and esophageal disease such as dysphagia. Detection of DM is imperative due to its debilitating symptoms and associated diseases. In patients of color, it is more difficult to appreciate clinical findings that can delay diagnosis.

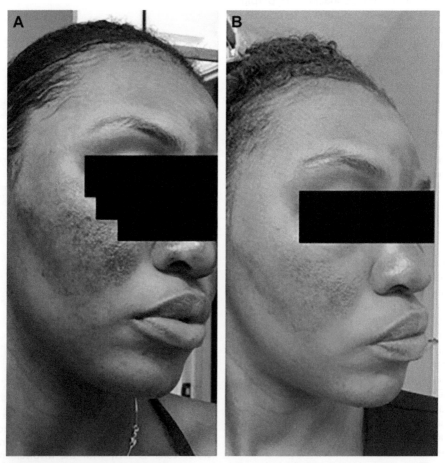

Fig. 10. (*A*) African American female with prominent PIH developed after DM. (*B*) Improvement after treatment. (*Courtesy of* S Taliaferro, MD, Atlanta, GA.)

The differential diagnosis of the heliotrope rash seen in DM includes SLE, eczema of the eyelid, discoid lupus, SCLE, rosacea, and sarcoidosis. Laboratory workup used to diagnose DM includes muscle biopsy, skin biopsy, creatinine kinase levels, antinuclear and anti-Mi-2 antibodies, and electromyography. The skin biopsy findings of DM are similar to those seen in SLE.[45] First-line treatments of DM include systemic glucocorticoids, immunosuppressive agents such as methotrexate or azathioprine, and antimalarials such as hydroxychloroquine. Rituximab and intravenous immunoglobulin are used in cases of resistant disease.

SUNBURN

Sunburn is the skin's natural response to having too much exposure to UV radiation from the sun or an artificial source such as tanning beds. It is an acute, self-limiting inflammatory response that commonly causes facial erythema. Sunburns are a result of UV-induced DNA damage that causes pyrimidine dimers, which induce apoptosis of cells and inflammation. This cascade of events produces vasodilation, erythema, pain, and swelling. There are 2 types of UV radiation: UVA and UVB. UVA radiation (315–400 nm) affects the dermis more than the epidermis while UVB radiation (280–315 nm) affects the epidermis more.[46] UVB rays have more energy than UVA rays and are the primary cause of sunburn. Certain medications can cause photosensitive reactions and increase the likelihood of one getting a sunburn (**Table 2**).

Erythema from sunburn becomes visible 3 to 6 hours after exposure, peaks at 12 to 24 hours

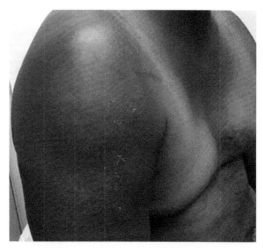

Fig. 11. Sunburn in SOC. (*Courtesy of* S Taliaferro, MD, Atlanta, GA.)

after exposure, and typically subsides around 3 to 7 days after being exposed depending on the severity of the burn.[47] Due to the constant exposure to the environment, the face is a common location to get sunburns and experience erythema.

Sunburns are stereotypically described as very red, painful, warm areas of skin that were exposed to UV rays. Edema, vesicle formation, blistering, and desquamation can accompany the pain and redness. In people with lighter skin, erythema

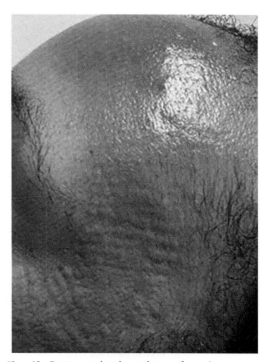

Fig. 12. Postprocedural erythema from laser treatment in an African American woman. (*Courtesy of* V Callender, MD, FAAD, Glenn Dale, MD.)

Table 2
Some medications that cause drug-induced photosensitivity

Antibiotics	Antidepressants
Tetracyclines	Tricyclics
(eg, doxycycline)	(eg, amitriptyline)
Fluoroquinolones	Diuretics
(eg, ciprofloxacin)	Thiazides (eg,
Dapsone	hydrochlorothiazide)
Trimethoprim	Loop diuretics
Antifungals	(eg, furosemide)
Griseofulvin	Antiarrhythmics
Acne Treatments	Amiodarone
Isotretinoin	Quinidine
Salicylic acid	Antihistamines
Benzoyl peroxide	Chlorpheniramine
NSAIDS	Promethazine
Ibuprofen	Sulfonylureas
Naproxen	Glyburide
Oral Contraceptives	Glipizide

Table 3
Differential diagnoses and distinguishing features of common causes of facial erythema

Condition	Differential Diagnosis	Distinguishing Features of the Condition	Features of Erythema
Acne vulgaris	Acne conglobata, acne fulminans, folliculitis, perioral dermatitis, rosacea, tuberous sclerosis, and sebaceous hyperplasia	The presence of open and closed comedones; lesions along the jawline in the adult women	Erythema clustered around the open and closed comedones Erythematous papules Postinflammatory erythematous macules
Rosacea	Acne vulgaris, SD, CD, lupus erythematosus, sarcoidosis, steroid acne, DM, and keratosis pilaris rubra	Central area of the face—glabellar area, nose, malar areas, and chin, the absence of open and closed comedones, telangiectasias, flushing, skin sensitivity, hypopigmentation; granulomatous-perioral and periocular papules	Macular erythema (flushing) along with telangiectasia Erythematous papules Persistent facial erythema
SLE	Rosacea, eczema, CD, DM, erysipelas, cellulitis, SD, lupus pernio, lupus vulgaris, and pellagra	Malar area of the face, spares the NLF, absence of scale, history of burning and flare when exposed to the sun, photosensitivity, Raynaud's, alopecia	Pink to violaceous macular erythema or erythematous patches
Discoid lupus	Sarcoidosis, cutaneous leishmaniasis, granuloma faciale	Atrophic scarring, seen on scalp, ear, face, nose	Erythema often an indicator of active disease, presenting alone or distributed centrally within plaques or along periphery of plaques. Can be violaceous
SCLE	Psoriasis, DM, mycosis fungioides, nummular eczema	Annular, polycylic lesions that favor sun exposed areas (face, neck, upper chest, upper back)	Erythematous plaques usually annular associated with scale Can be bright red to violaceous Hyperpigmentation common in darker skin
CD	Urticaria, atopic dermatitis, nummular dermatitis, dyshidrotic dermatitis, SD, rosacea, psoriasis, and fixed drug eruption	Itching, burning and stinging of the skin	Prominent pink-red patches (acute) Brown to violaceous with lichenification (chronic)
SD	Rosacea, psoriasis, atopic dermatitis, tinea capitis, and SLE	Scaling in the eyebrows, perinasal creases and ears, history of dandruff with scalp involvement, annular lesions hypopigmentation	Light erythema underneath scale and flaky skin Occurring with hypopigmentation, hyperpigmentation
Psoriasis	Atopic dermatitis, CD, lichen planus, SD, tinea, cutaneous lupus erythematosus, sarcoidosis, and pityriasis rosea	Involvement of the scalp, elbows and knees; thick silvery and violaceous plaques, nail changes, Koebner phenomenon	Light to dark brown erythematous to violaceous plaques covered with gray/white powdery and/or thick scale

(continued on next page)

Condition	Differential Diagnosis	Distinguishing Features of the Condition	Features of Erythema
Table 3 *(continued)*			
			Dark brownish erythema with lichenification Pink to white hypopigmentation with scale Bright pink-red or light pink-brown with overlying silvery scale (lighter skin)
DM rash	SLE, eczema of the eyelid, discoid lupus, SCLE, rosacea, and sarcoidosis	Violaceous heliotrope rash, muscle weakness	Light pink-red to brown to violaceous erythema
Sunburn	Photosensitive drug eruptions, photoallergic reactions, solar urticaria, phytophotodermatitis, porphyria, SLE	Burning and pain, occurrence immediately after long exposure to the sun	Brown with hints of erythema or bright pink to red erythema (fairer skin) with light desquamation and/or blistering
Postprocedure erythema	Sunburn, CD	Occurs immediately after a procedure—laser, light, and energy-based devices, chemical peels, electrodessication	Soft pink-red erythema or violaceous erythema

Abbreviation: NLF, nasolabial fold.

from sunburn is very pronounced and starkly different in appearance from unaffected skin. In those with deeper skin tones, erythema is more subtle or may not be visible at all. The affected skin may seem darker or remain the same shade. The typical course of the sunburn and other symptoms remain the same regardless of skin tone (**Fig. 11**).

Melanin is a component of the skin that protects against harmful UV rays. On average, those with Fitzpatrick skin types IV-VI have a higher minimal erythema dose than those with skin types I-III due to increased melanin in their skin, which makes them less likely to burn.[47] Because of this, there are common misconceptions that people with darker skin tones are unable to get sunburnt and do not need to wear sunscreen. However, more melanin does not provide immunity from the damaging effect of UV radiation. Sunburns can predispose individuals to skin cancers such as basal cell carcinoma, squamous cell carcinoma, and melanoma. Therefore, photoprotection is recommended for everyone, including people of color.

The differential diagnosis of sunburn includes photosensitive drug eruptions (see **Table 2**), photoallergic reactions, solar urticaria, phytophotodermatitis, porphyria, and SLE. Sunburns are self-limiting

with an average duration of 1 to 7 days depending on the severity of the burn. Common methods of ameliorating the pain include using aloe vera, taking cool baths, and using mild pain relievers such as NSAIDs. Rather than focusing on how to treat sunburns, more emphasis should be put on how to prevent their formation. Using sunscreen is imperative for everyone, regardless of skin tone. The use of sun-protective clothing such as hats and sunglasses is another way to protect the skin from UV radiation and to prevent facial erythema from sunburn.

Postinflammatory and Postprocedural Erythema

Postinflammatory erythema (PIE) refers to erythema of a localized skin area that is followed by preceding inflammation of the skin.[48] It may occur from an inflammatory skin condition such as acne, from trauma of the skin such as a burn, or after procedures such as laser resurfacing or chemical peels. The latter is generally referred to as postprocedural erythema (**Fig. 12**). PIE is important to recognize and address because it may persist and become cosmetically unacceptable and progress into PIH, one of the most common consequences of cutaneous inflammatory processes and procedures in SOC, which has a notable effect on quality of life.[49]

Techniques used to reduce postprocedural erythema include use of cold compresses, thermal spring water, and antioxidants, particularly vitamin C after or during procedures.[50,51] The use of niacinamide, azelaic acid, metronidazole, topical corticosteroids, topical tranexamic acid, and topical antihistamines and alpha-adrenergic blockers (oxymetazoline and brimonidine) are reported in the medical literature to improve PIE or postprocedural erythema. Emollients such as ceramide topicals and silicone gels are also reported to help.[52–55] When there is a major concern for ensuing hyperpigmentation, cautious pretreatment and posttreatment with hydroquinone are used and are helpful in some cases. After-care is often paramount to avoid PIE. Sunscreen use after treatments is crucial in preventing long-term erythema and hyperpigmentation.[56] Avoiding irritants must be practiced during and after procedures. Patients should be counseled verbally and sent home with specific instructions on skin care after laser treatments, chemical peels, microneedling, microdermabrasion, facials, and other procedures. Even under the best care, persistent erythema may develop. Many of the topicals mentioned above help improve persistent erythema when it occurs after treatments. Successful use of intense pulse light and vascular lasers to treat PIE is well documented but of limited use in darker skin types. However, laser treatments such as the 650-microsecond 1064 Nd:YAG and carefully selected fractional laser treatments may yield notable improvements in PIE in darker skin.[57,58]

SUMMARY

Facial erythema is a common sequela of many dermatologic conditions that people of all skin tones face. Although it may be more difficult to appreciate erythema in darker skin tones, dermatologists should make the effort to recognize erythema in skin with more melanin and link it to the clinical picture the patient presents with in order to make the correct diagnosis (Table 3).

Dermatology is a visual specialty that also has a lack of representation in the literature of conditions seen in SOC patients. In order to combat this, dermatologists should take pictures of diseases in patients with deeper skin tones in order to add to what is present in the literature. This will help increase the skill of dermatologists to diagnose diseases of facial erythema in SOC. Photographing and publishing skin diseases will also help patients

of color get proper and timely treatment of their conditions.

Further studies should be conducted to more objectively and reliably assess for erythema, particularly in darker skinned patients where it may be more challenging. Because hyperpigmentation is a common and unwanted consequence of facial erythema in SOC patients, clinical trials should be conducted to develop treatments that effectively prevent and treat hyperpigmentation when it occurs. Medical students and residents should train with an emphasis on detecting skin disease in all skin types and all skin tones. This may mitigate potential inequities in the diagnosis and treatment of skin disease in SOC.

CLINICS CARE POINTS

- Daily photoprotection is an essential component in the management of all skin disorders associated with facial erythema.
- Patients should be counseled verbally and sent home with specific instructions on skin care after aesthetic and surgical procedures to minimize postprocedure complications such as erythema and PIH.
- The differential diagnosis for malar erythema is SOC should include seborrheic dermatitis, rosacea, and lupus erythematosus.

CONFLICTS OF INTEREST DISCLOSURE

C. Ohanenye: None. Dr S. Taliaferro has served as a paid speaker and/or consultant for Pfizer, Galderma, Aerolase, and Dermavant outside of the submitted article. V.D. Callender: Clinical Investigator for Admiral, AbbVie/Allergan, Avava, Eli Lilly, Galderma, L'Oreal, Prollineum, Symatese. Consultant for Acne Store, Aerolase, Avita Medical, Beiersdorf, Cutera, Dermavant, Eli Lilly, Endo Aesthetics, EPI Health, Galderma, Incyte, Juenes Aesthetics, L'Oreal, Ortho Derm, Pfizer, Scientis, Sente Labs, SkinBetter Science, SkinCeuticals, UCB. Royalties: UpToDate.

REFERENCES

1. Abdlaty R, Hayward J, Farrell T, et al. Skin erythema and pigmentation: a review of optical assessment techniques. Photodiagnosis Photodyn Ther 2021; 33:102127.
2. Wilkins J, Dahl M, Detmar M, et al. Standard grading system for rosacea: report of the national Rosacea Society Expert Committee on the classification and

staging of rosacea. J Am Acad Dermatol 2004; 50(6):907–12.

3. Hopkinson D, Tuchayi SM, Alinia H, et al. Assessment of rosacea severity: a review of evaluation methods used in clinical trials. J Am Acad Dermatol 2015;73:138–43.

4. Alexis AF, Callender VD, Baldwin HE, et al. Global epidemiology and clinical spectrum of rosacea, highlighting skin of color: Review and clinical practice experience. J Am Acad Dermatol 2019;80(6):1722–9.e7.

5. Sutaria AH, Masood S, Schlessinger J. Acne Vulgaris. [Updated 2022 May 8]. In: StatPearls [Internet]. Treasure Island (FL): StatPearls Publishing. 2022. Available at: https://www.ncbi.nlm.nih.gov/books/NBK459173/.

6. Taylor Susan C, Cook-Bolden Fran, Rahman Zakia, et al. Acne vulgaris in skin of color. J Am Acad Dermatol 2002;46(2):S98–106. Supplement 2.

7. Hauk L. Acne Vulgaris: Treatment Guidelines from the AAD. Am Fam Physician 2017;95(11):740–1. PMID: 28671431.

8. Davis EC, Callender VD. A review of acne in ethnic skin: pathogenesis, clinical manifestations, and management strategies. J Clin Aesthet Dermatol 2010;3(4):24–38.

9. Sarkar R, Podder I, Jagadeesan S. Rosacea in skin of color: A comprehensive review. Indian J Dermatol Venereol Leprol 2020;86(6):611–21.

10. Scharschmidt TC, Yost JM, Truong SV, et al. Neurogenic rosacea: a distinct clinical subtype requiring a modified approach to treatment. Arch Dermatol 2011;147(1):123–6.

11. Chen W, Plewig G. Are Demodex mites principal, conspirator, accomplice, witness or bystander in the cause of rosacea? Am J Clin Dermatol 2015; 16(2):67–72.

12. Egeberg A, Weinstock LB, Thyssen EP, et al. Rosacea and gastrointestinal disorders: a population-based cohort study. Br J Dermatol 2017;176(1):100–6.

13. Lazaridou E, Korfitis C, Kemanetzi C, et al. Rosacea and Helicobacter pylori: links and risks. Clin Cosmet Investig Dermatol 2017;10:305–10.

14. Wilkin J, Dahl M, Detmar M, et al. Standard grading system for rosacea: report of the National Rosacea Society Expert Committee on the classification and staging of rosacea. J Am Acad Dermatol 2004; 50(6):907–12.

15. Stone DU, Chodosh J. Ocular rosacea: an update on pathogenesis and therapy. Curr Opin Ophthalmol 2004;15(6):499–502.

16. Khokhar O, Khachemoune A. A case of granulomatous rosacea: sorting granulomatous rosacea from other granulomatous diseases that affect the face. Dermatol Online J 2004;10(1):6.

17. Two AM, Wu W, Gallo RL, et al. Rosacea: part II. Topical and systemic therapies in the treatment of rosacea. J Am Acad Dermatol 2015;72(5):761–72.

18. van Zuuren EJ, Arents BWM, van der Linden MMD, et al. Rosacea: New Concepts in Classification and Treatment. Am J Clin Dermatol 2021;22(4):457–65.

19. Del Rosso JQ. What Is "PFE"? It May Just Be Time You Found Out. J Drugs Dermatol JDD 2019;18(6): 503.

20. Kazandjieva J, Tsankov N, Pramatarov K. The red face revisited: connective tissue disorders. Clin Dermatol 2014;32(1):153–8.

21. Cooper GS, Parks CG, Treadwell EL, et al. Differences by race, sex and age in the clinical and immunologic features of recently diagnosed systemic lupus erythematosus patients in the southeastern United States. Lupus 2002;11:161–7.

22. Caruso WR, Stewart ML, Nanda VK, et al. Squamous cell carcinoma of the skin in black patients with discoid lupus erythematosus. J Rheumatol 1987; 14:156–9.

23. Callen JP, Klein J. Subacute cutaneous lupus erythematosus: clinical, serologic, immunogenetic, and therapeutic considerations in seventy-two patients. Arthritis Rheum 1988;31:1007–13.

24. Lee LA, Werth VP. Bolognia JL Dermatology. 3rd edition. London: Elsevier Ltd; 2012. p. 601. Lupus Erythematosus.

25. Dreizen S. The butterfly rash and the malar flush. What diseases do these signs reflect? Postgrad Med 1991;89(1):233–4, 225–8.

26. Taliaferro S, Davis E, Callender V. Collagen Vascular Diseases. In: Taylor SC, Badreshia-Bansal S, Callender VD, editors, et al, editors. Treatments for Skin of Color. USA: Saunders; 2011.

27. Bains SN, Nash P, Fonacier L. Irritant Contact Dermatitis. Clinic Rev Allerg Immunol 2019;56:99–109.

28. Usatine RP, Riojas M. Diagnosis and management of contact dermatitis. Am Fam Physician 2010;82(3): 249–55.

29. Ruszczak Z, Abdelhadi S. Contact dermatitis in skin of color. In: Orfanos CZ, Assaf CC, editors. Pigmented ethnic skin and imported Dermatoses. Cham: Springer; 2018.

30. Stallings A, Sood A. Hair-care practices in African American women: potential for allergic contact dermatitis. Semin Cutan Med Surg 2016;35:207–10.

31. Elgash M, Dlova N, Ogunleye T, et al. Seborrheic Dermatitis in Skin of Color: Clinical Considerations. J Drugs Dermatol 2019;18(1):24–7.

32. Borda LJ, Wikramanayake TC. Seborrheic Dermatitis and Dandruff: A Comprehensive Review. J Clin Investig Dermatol 2015;3(2). https://doi.org/10.13188/2373-1044.1000019.

33. Schwartz RA, Janusz CA, Janniger CK. Seborrheic dermatitis: an overview. Am Fam Physician 2006; 74(1):125–30. PMID: 16848386.

34. Rachakonda TD, Schupp CW, Armstrong AW. Psoriasis prevalence among adults in the United States. J Am Acad Dermatol 2014;70(3):512–6.

35. Nicholas MN, Chan AR, Hessami-Booshehri M. Psoriasis in patients of color: differences in morphology, clinical presentation, and treatment. Cutis 2020; 106(2S):7–10. E10.

36. Oakley A. Psoriasis. DermNet. Available at. https://dermnetnz.org/topics/psoriasis.

37. Kaufman BP, Alexis AF. Psoriasis in Skin of Color: Insights into the Epidemiology, Clinical Presentation, Genetics, Quality-of-Life Impact, and Treatment of Psoriasis in Non-White Racial/Ethnic Groups. Am J Clin Dermatol 2018;19:405–23.

38. Alexis AF, Blackcloud P. Psoriasis in skin of color: epidemiology, genetics, clinical presentation, and treatment nuances. J Clin Aesthet Dermatol 2014; 7(11):16–24.

39. Schlager JG, Rosumeck S, Werner RN, et al. Topical treatments for scalp psoriasis. Cochrane Database Syst Rev 2016;2(2):CD009687.

40. Marvi U, Chung L, Fiorentino DF. Clinical presentation and evaluation of dermatomyositis. Indian J Dermatol 2012;57(5):375–81.

41. Callen Jeffrey P, Wortmann Robert L. Dermatomyositis. Clinics in Dermatology 2006;24(5):363–73.

42. Birbal Jain H, Liarki V, Ko K, et al. Comparison of Clinical Characteristics between African American and Caucasian Patients with Polymyositis and Dermatomyositis and Their Response to Conventional Treatment [abstract]. Arthritis Rheumatol 2017; 69(suppl 10).

43. Babool Sofia, Bhai Salman F, Sanderson Collin, et al. Racial disparities in skin tone representation of dermatomyositis rashes: a systematic review. Rheumatology 2022;61(6):2255–61.

44. Hu T, Vinik O. Dermatomyositis and malignancy. Can Fam Physician 2019;65(6):409–11.

45. Qudsiya Z, Waseem M. Dermatomyositis. [Updated 2022 Jun 12]. In: StatPearls [Internet]. Treasure Island (FL): StatPearls Publishing. 2022. Available at: https://www.ncbi.nlm.nih.gov/books/NBK558917/.

46. Soter NA. Acute effects of ultraviolet radiation on the skin. Semin Dermatol 1990;9(1):11–5.

47. Young A. and Tewari A., In: Dellavale R., Danzl D., Corona R. et al., UpToDate, 2022, Waltham, MA.

48. Bae-Harboe YS, Graber EM. Easy as PIE (Postinflammatory Erythema). J Clin Aesthet Dermatol 2013;6(9):46–7.

49. Huerth KA, Hassan S, Callender VD. Therapeutic Insights in Melasma and Hyperpigmentation Management. J Drugs Dermatol 2019;18(8):718–29.

50. Chen YT, Chang CC, Hsu CR, et al. Combined vitamin C sonophoresis and neodymium-doped yttrium aluminum garnet (NdYAG) laser for facial hyperpigmentation: An outcome observation study in Asian patients. Indian J Dermatol Venereol Leprol 2016;82(5):587. https://doi.org/10.4103/0378-6323.182806.

51. Dayal S, Sahu P, Yadav M, et al. Clinical Efficacy and Safety on Combining 20% Trichloroacetic Acid Peel with Topical 5% Ascorbic Acid for Melasma. J Clin Diagn Res 2017;11(9):WC08–11.

52. Jakhar D, Kaur I. Topical 5% tranexamic acid for acne-related postinflammatory erythema. J Am Acad Dermatol 2020;82(6):e187–8.

53. Agamia N, Essawy M, Kassem A. Successful treatment of the face post acne erythema using a topically applied selective alpha 1-Adrenergic receptor agonist, oxymetazoline 1.5%, a controlled left to right face comparative trial. J Dermatolog Treat 2022;33(2):904–9.

54. Lee SJ, Ahn GR, Seo SB, et al. Topical brimonidine-assisted laser treatment for the prevention of therapy-related erythema and hyperpigmentation. J Cosmet Laser Ther 2019;21(4):225–7.

55. Lueangarun S, Tempark T. Efficacy of MAS063DP lotion vs 0.02% triamcinolone acetonide lotion in improving post-ablative fractional CO_2 laser resurfacing wound healing: a split-face, triple-blinded, randomized, controlled trial. Int J Dermatol 2018; 57(4):480–7.

56. Wanitphakdeedecha R, Phuardchantuk R, Manuskiatti W. The use of sunscreen starting on the first day after ablative fractional skin resurfacing. J Eur Acad Dermatol Venereol 2014;28(11):1522–8.

57. Alam M, Voravutinon N, Warycha M, et al. Comparative effectiveness of nonpurpuragenic 595-nm pulsed dye laser and microsecond 1064-nm neodymium:yttrium-aluminum-garnet laser for treatment of diffuse facial erythema: A double-blind randomized controlled trial. J Am Acad Dermatol 2013; 69(3):438–43.

58. Alharbi MA. 1927 nm Thulium Laser Successfully Treats PostInflammatory Hyperpigmentation in Skin of Color. Dermatol Res Pract 2021;5560386.

Disorders of Facial Hyperpigmentation

Nicole C. Syder, BA, Claudia Quarshie, BS, Nada Elbuluk, MD, MSc*

KEYWORDS

- Facial pigmentation • Skin of color • Hyperpigmentation • Facial hyperpigmentation
- Hypermelanosis • Facial melanosis • Melasma • Periorbital hyperpigmentation • Ethnic skin

KEY POINTS

- Facial pigmentaton can be a diagnostic and therapeutic challenge.
- Detailed history and clinical examination should be performed to determine the correct diagnosis which will allow for accurate prognostic conversations and directed treatment.
- Treatment options for facial pigmentation vary depending on the cause of the pigmentation and can include topical, procedural, and combination therapies.

INTRODUCTION

Hyperpigmentation is the darkening of the skin which can occur due to a variety of factors. It is commonly seen from increased deposition of melanin in the epidermis and/or dermis.[1] Less frequently, it may be caused by the deposition of endogenous or exogenous pigments such as hemosiderin, iron, or heavy metals.[1] Carotenoids, vascularity and skin thickness are additional factors which can cause the skin to appear hyperpigmented.[2] Disorders of facial hyperpigmentation can affect individuals of all skin types but more commonly affect those with skin of color (Fitzpatrick skin type III–VI). For this latter population, dyspigmentation has been found to be one of the top dermatologic chief complaints.[3] Due to the visible nature of facial hyperpigmentation, it can also have profound effects on quality of life.[3] Diagnosing and adequately managing disorders of facial hyperpigmentation are essential to obtaining positive patient outcomes and helping to improve the quality of life for affected individuals.

Melasma

Melasma is a common disorder of hyperpigmentation with a complex pathogenesis that results in hyperfunctional melanocytes that deposit excess amounts of melanin in the skin.[3] This condition is more commonly seen in women of reproductive age and of color, particularly those from East and Southeast Asia, Africa, or Latin America.[3,4] Clinically, melasma presents with bilateral and symmetric hyperpigmented light to dark brown macules and patches in three predominant facial patterns: centrofacial, malar, and mandibular (Fig. 1).[3,5] The major clinical pattern is the centrofacial pattern, which affects the forehead, nose, and upper lip. Less commonly, extra-facial melasma can occur on non-facial body parts including the neck, sternum, forearms, and upper extremities.[5] Extra-facial melasma is more common in menopausal women, those with a personal history of facial melasma, and individuals with a family history of extra-facial melasma.[6,7]

The pathogenesis is complex and evolving. Extracellular matrix alterations, inflammation, hormonal influences, and angiogenesis all play a role in the development of melasma. Recent literature points to interactions between keratinocytes, mast cells, gene regulation abnormalities, neovascularization, impaired skin barrier, and disruption of the basement membrane.[8,9] Contributing factors involved in the pathogenesis include genetic influences, sun exposure, sensitivity to hormonal treatment/oral contraception, pregnancy, and cosmetics.[3,4] Histopathology can reveal increased melanin deposition in all layers of the epidermis,

Department of Dermatology, Keck School of Medicine of University of Southern California, Keck School of Medicine, University of Southern California, 830 South Flower Street, Suite 100, Los Angeles, CA 90017, USA
* Corresponding author.
E-mail address: nada.elbuluk@med.usc.edu

Dermatol Clin 41 (2023) 393–405
https://doi.org/10.1016/j.det.2023.02.005

Fig. 1. Reticulated light brown patches on the mid-forehead occurring in centrofacial melasma. *Courtesy of* N Elbuluk, MD, MSc, Los Angeles, CA.

hypertrophied melanocytes in normal quantities, and increased melanosomes.[3] Increases in mast cell numbers and increased vascularity in staining studies for angiogenesis have also been reported.[10] Additionally, features of increased solar elastosis and lymphohistiocytic infiltrates are also often seen. Dermal melanophages can also be present in those with dermal or mixed (epidermal and dermal) melasma.[5]

Topical treatments, including photoprotection, are typically the first-line therapies for melasma.[5,11] Visible light can induce persistent hyperpigmentation similar to ultraviolet (UV) radiation, therefore, mineral sunscreens which contain zinc oxide, titanium dioxide, or iron oxide are recommended for photoprotection from visible and UV light.[12,13] McKesey and colleagues reviewed all available melasma treatments and found that hydroquinone monotherapy and triple combination cream are the most effective and well-studied treatments for melasma compared with all other treatment options.[14] Topical non-hydroquinone skin lighteners including ingredients derived from botanic extracts, azelaic acid, kojic acid, and niacinamide are also commonly used with varying efficacy.[3,5,11] Oral treatments such as tranexamic acid, glutathione, and polypodium leucotomos are also used as monotherapy or adjunctive therapy.[5,11] Tranexamic acid inhibits the plasminogen/plasmin pathway to inhibit melanin synthesis and angiogenesis. Glutathione works as an antioxidant to decrease inflammation, and polypodium leucotomos provides additional photoprotection and inhibits reactive oxygen species.[5,8] Procedural melasma therapies including chemical peels, microneedling, microneedling radiofrequency, microdermabrasion, mesotherapy, and lasers can be used as adjuvant or second-line or third-line treatments in addition to topical therapies and photoprotection.[5] Glycolic acid (20%–50%), salicylic acid (SA, 20%–30%), mandelic acid (10%) combination, and trichloroacetic acid (10%–20%) chemical peels have shown efficacy in melasma treatment and can be used safely in darker skin. Lights and lasers used for treatment include Q-switched (QS) and picosecond lasers, non-ablative fractional lasers, intense pulsed light, and ablative carbon dioxide and erbium: yttrium aluminum garnet (YAG) lasers.[5,15] Ablative lasers should be avoided in skin of color (SOC) due to risk of dyspigmentation. The chronic nature of melasma can make it challenging to treat, so it is important for patients to understand the importance of treatment compliance to achieve remissions and to know that there is no cure for the condition.

Post-Inflammatory Hyperpigmentation

Post-inflammatory hyperpigmentation (PIH) is a reactive process resulting in darkening of the skin secondary to cutaneous injury or inflammation. This condition can occur at any age and has equal incidence in men and women. Although PIH may occur in any skin color, it is more common in skin of color (fitzpatrick skin type [FST] IV–VI). Individuals often present with macules or patches in areas of previous or ongoing inflammation. Epidermal PIH can appear tan to dark brown, whereas dermal PIH tends to appear darker brown or blue-gray (**Fig. 2**).[16]

The inflammatory process that leads to PIH can be endogenous or exogenous.[16,17] Common endogenous inflammatory causes include acne vulgaris, atopic dermatitis, psoriasis, and other cutaneous inflammatory disorders. Exogenous causes can include burns, nonionizing radiation therapy, phototoxicity as well as cosmetic and surgical procedures.[16,17]

Molecular pathogenesis of PIH is thought to be related to inflammatory mediators which include prostaglandins E2 and D2, leukotrienes B4, C4, D4, and E4, and thromboxane B2. In vitro, these metabolites have been found to increase the size of melanocytes and melanocyte dendritic proliferation leading to melanin production.[18,19] Following the production of melanin, it then deposits in the epidermis and/or dermis through the gaps in basal lamina or through macrophages that engulf melanin in the epidermis and then migrate to the dermis leading to dermal pigmentation.[18] The

Combination therapy is generally more effective than monotherapy. Oral tranexamic acid has recently been used successfully in several studies for PIH.[22] The use of fractionated non-ablative lasers can also be used safely with a low density and low fluence in darker skin types.[23] For treatment-resistant patients, QS ruby, alexandrite, and neodymium (Nd):YAG lasers have been used to expedite resolution with promising results.[20,23] Picosecond lasers have also been shown to be a safe and effective alternative to QS lasers.[24] Treatment therapies for PIH, especially lasers, should be used with caution and appropriate settings to avoid exacerbation of PIH.[17,23]

Maturational Hyperpigmentation

Maturational hyperpigmentation (MH) is an acquired darkening of the bilateral cheeks that has a propensity to extend superiorly to the temples and inferiorly to the melolabial folds.[25] It is a facial melanosis that was coined and described in 2006 by Dr Melvin Alexander.[26] MH primarily develops in the fourth to fifth decade in skin types V and VI.[3,27] Clinical presentation generally consists of dark brown to black patches with poorly defined borders on the lateral aspects of the face.[3] MH is often cosmetically bothersome, particularly in women.[28]

Etiology and pathogenesis are currently unclear but are likely associated with chronic sun exposure with obesity and diabetes being potential predisposing factors.[27,29] Histopathology shows mild to moderate proliferation of melanocytes and some reports of papillomatosis.[1,29,30] Differential diagnosis for this condition includes melasma, PIH, acanthosis nigricans, photoallergic dermatitis, and exogenous ochronosis.[1]

The first-line treatment of this condition is prevention with the proper use of broad-spectrum sunscreen.[3] Topical treatments include hydroquinone alone or in combination with tretinoin cream and/or a topical corticosteroid. Chemical peels with glycolic acid (20%–50%), salicylic acid (20%–30%), lactic acid (20%–30%), or Jessner solution have also been used.[25,31] A study by Quiñonez and colleagues recommend treating MH in SOC by chemoexfoliating with 30% salicylic acid at 2- to 6-week intervals along with topical 4% hydroquinone twice daily and tretinoin cream 0.05% three to five times per week.[25] Success following a 650-m pulse from a 1064-nm Nd:YAG laser in addition to topical therapy has also been reported.[25,31]

Facial Acanthosis Nigricans

Facial acanthosis nigricans (AN) is characterized by velvety, hyperpigmented patches and plaques

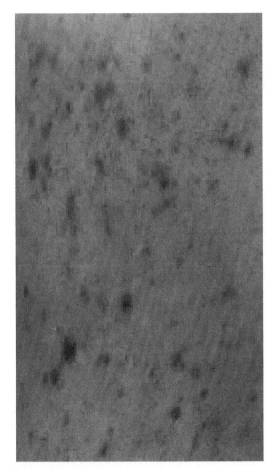

Fig. 2. Dark brown macules of varying sizes from prior dermatitis resulting in PIH. *Courtesy of* N Elbuluk, MD, MSc, Los Angeles, CA.

intensity of PIH is determined by the cause, degree, and depth of inflammation, degree of disruption at the dermoepidermal junction, and stability of melanocytes.[19] Depending on the extent of injury, PIH can be epidermal, dermal, or mixed. Histopathologic features can include increased epidermal melanin with variable amount of perivascular lymphohistiocytic infiltrate and presence of melanophages in the dermis.[16]

Treatment begins with prevention and active treatment of inflammation from endogenous causes. Therapeutic options are similar to those for melasma, with vigilant photoprotection and topical lightening agents being first line.[1] Patients with epidermal pigmentation tend to respond better to topical treatments which can include retinoids, hydroquinone, azelaic acid, kojic acid, deoxyarbutin, niacinamide, n-acetylglucosamine, ascorbic acid (vitamin C), licorice (*Glycyrrhiza glabra*) extract. Polypodium leucotomos, and/or peeling agents (eg, glycolic acid or salicylic acid) have also been used adjunctively.[20,21]

with ill-defined margins commonly seen on the zygomatic region of the face.[3,32,33] It can affect both men and women, as well as patients of any age. Overweight and diabetic patients with metabolic syndrome are more prone to developing facial AN. The prevalence of this condition appears to be more common among Native American, African, and Hispanic populations.[32,34]

Facial AN may be acquired or inherited through an autosomal dominance pattern with variable penetrance. Associations of this condition include obesity, endocrine and metabolic disorders associated with insulin resistance, certain genetic syndromes, malignancy, and drug reactions involving medications that promote hyperinsulinemia.[32,34]

Abnormalities involving tyrosine kinase receptors insulin-like growth factor receptor-1 (IGFR1), fibroblast growth factor receptor (FGFR), and epidermal growth factor receptor (EGFR) are thought to be potential contributing factors.[32] Elevated levels of insulin may stimulate keratinocyte and dermal fibroblast proliferation via interaction with IGFR1, resulting in the plaque-like lesions that characterize the condition. Mutations in certain FGFRs may also contribute to facial AN through the promotion of keratinocyte proliferation and survival. Excessive activation of EGFR may contribute to the development of malignancy-associated facial AN. Histologic findings show hyperkeratosis and papillomatosis of the epidermis as well as occasional detection of increased melanin in the basal layer of the epidermis.[32,33]

Treatment relies on addressing the underlying cause as well as the use of various topical and/or procedural treatments. These include oral and topical retinoids, keratolytic agents such as ammonium lactate, calcipotriol, chemical peels, non-ablative fractional lasers, and long-pulsed alexandrite lasers.[32] Weight loss has also been linked to improvements in ANs in obese patients.

Erythema Dyschromicum Perstans

Erythema dyschromicum perstans (EDP), also sometimes referred to as ashy dermatosis or dermatosis cenicienta, is a less common pigmentary condition characterized by ashy-gray or blue-brown macules, typically in individuals with Fitzpatrick skin types III–VI.[35] Those from Latin America are more commonly affected.[36,37] EDP is usually seen in adults, but it may also occur in children.[35,36] Early EDP presents with localized asymptomatic brown to gray macules, and patches with raised erythematous borders, whereas late lesions tend to be dark brown or blue-gray in color (**Fig. 3**).[3] Lesions are typically symmetric and gradually enlarge over time. EDP

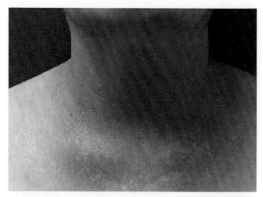

Fig. 3. Blue-gray macules coalescing into patches on the neck and upper chest of a Hispanic woman with EDP. *Courtesy of* N Elbuluk, MD, MSc, Los Angeles, CA.

can occur on the face though more commonly occurs on non-facial non-photoexposed body sites. EDP can share clinical and histologic similarities with lichen planus pigmentosus and the differential can also include pigmented contact dermatitis, drug-induced hyperpigmentation, PIH, hyperpigmented mycosis fungoides, syphilis, and mastocytosis.[35]

The etiology of EDP remains largely unknown, but it has been associated with various triggers including toxins (ammonium nitrite, cobalt, radiocontrast, and pesticides), drugs (ethambutol, penicillin, benzodiazepines, chlorothalonil), whipworm infection, and human immunodeficiency virus (HIV).[36,37] The HLA-DR4 allele may also be a risk factor in those of Mexican descent. Histopathology of early and active areas reveals increased epidermal melanin, vacuolar basal cell degeneration with pigment incontinence, dermal melanophages, and perivascular lymphohistiocytic infiltration.[35,37] In later stages histopathology may show pigment incontinence in the dermis without inflammation.[38] Based on these findings, it has been hypothesized that EDP may represent a cell-mediated immune reaction to an ingestant, contact allergen, or microorganism.

Although there is no gold standard treatment, EDP can wax and wane and has been reported to self-resolve in 50% of children.[36,37] Photoprotection is important to prevent worsening and recurrence of EDP after discontinuation of treatment can occur. Variable results have been reported with treatment. Topical treatments include corticosteroids, tretinoin, tacrolimus, dapsone, hydroquinone, and other topical non-hydroquinone lightening agents. Oral medications used include systemic corticosteroids, antibiotics, clofazimine, dapsone, isotretinoin, griseofulvin, and antimalarials. Procedural treatments used include phototherapy, fractionated non-ablative and ablative lasers, QS and picosecond lasers. Leung and colleagues report narrowband ultraviolet B (UVB) phototherapy with topical tacrolimus as a promising and effective treatment with significantly fewer side effects compared with clofazimine.[35]

Lichen Planus Pigmentosus

Lichen planus pigmentosus (LPP) is a rare variant of lichen planus that predominantly occurs in individuals with darker skin phototypes (Fitzpatrick III–VI).[39] Commonly affected individuals are young to middle-aged adults, particularly those from India, Latin America, and the Middle East. Patients tend to present with an asymptomatic diffuse and bilateral distribution of dark brown to gray macules and patches in sun-exposed areas, including the forehead, temples, and neck (Fig. 4).[40]

The exact pathogenesis of LPP is unknown. However, some studies point to the associated use of cosmetic fragrances, hair dyes, and certain oils (eg, mustard oil), that serve as potential photosensitizers.[39,40] Hepatitis C virus is a known association with LPP. In addition, frontal fibrosing alopecia and LPP occur concomitantly in up to 54% of patients, more commonly in patients with darker skin.[41,42] Facial papules are an additional association of LPP and the triad of LPP, frontal fibrosing alopecia, and facial papules are more common in women of color.[42] Histopathology of active disease reveals epidermal atrophy with interface dermatitis, dyskeratotic keratinocytes and colloid bodies, basal cell vacuolization, and superficial dermal melanophages.[39,40] Late-stage disease shows marked pigmentary incontinence,

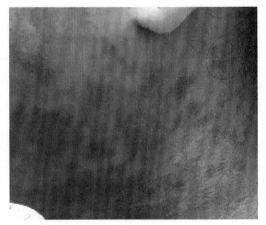

Fig. 4. Dark brown to brown-gray patches along the lateral cheeks and neck of an Asian woman with LPP. *Courtesy of* N Elbuluk, MD, MSc, Los Angeles, CA.

melanophages, decrease in vacuolar degeneration, and slight perivascular lymphocytic infiltrate.[39]

Limited data exist on the successful treatment of LPP; however, it can improve spontaneously over several months. Treatment methods include photoprotection, topical corticosteroids, topical calcineurin inhibitors, skin-lightening agents including hydroquinone and non-hydroquinone lightening agents. Phototherapy has also been utilized with varying success.[39] Oral treatments including antimalarials and isotretinoin, particularly at low doses, have also been used safely and effectively.[1,39] Procedural modalities have also been used often in combination with topical therapies. Lasers that have shown efficacy with LPP include QS and picosecond Nd:YAG lasers.[39,40,43,44] Chemical peels including glycolic acid, Jessner's, and modified phenol peels have also been used with varying success.[43,45]

Nevus of Ota

Nevus of Ota is a dermal melanocytosis that preferentially involves areas of the face in a trigeminal nerve distribution.[46] Affected individuals are most commonly of Asian or African American descent, and women are four times more likely to be affected than men. Clinically, patients present with blue-gray large unilateral pigmentation on the face consisting of macules coalescing into a patch following a trigeminal nerve distribution.[46,47] Oral mucosa or sclera may also be involved and approximately 10% of patients have bilateral involvement. The pigmentation may be present at birth or become apparent around puberty.

The pathogenesis of this condition may involve genetic factors, with up to 15% of lesions containing somatic activating mutations in the *GNAQ* and *GNA11* genes encoding G protein alpha subunits.[46] There have also been reports of familial cases of nevus of Ota as well as a rare association with melanoma. Histologic findings reveal numerous melanocytes diffusely distributed throughout the upper and lower dermis.[47]

Patients with nevus of Ota should be followed with yearly ophthalmologic examinations and educated regarding the clinical signs of ocular and cutaneous melanoma.[46] The cutaneous portion of nevus of Ota can be treated with various lasers including QS ruby laser, QS alexandrite laser, QS Nd:YAG laser, alexandrite picosecond, or ND:YAG picosecond lasers with usually good to excellent outcomes.[46] Potential side effects include hypo- or hyperpigmentation. Ge and colleagues report better clinical results and fewer adverse events with picosecond alexandrite lasers compared with the widely accepted QS alexandrite lasers for treatment of nevus of Ota.[48] Combinations of chemical peels with laser treatments have also shown success with the superficial peels being used as a priming agent to decrease the absorption of epidermal melanin by the laser.[49]

Hori's Nevi

Hori's nevi, also known as acquired bilateral nevus of Ota-like macules, is a dermal melanocytic hyperpigmentation seen in Asian populations, primarily in young and middle-aged Chinese and Japanese women aged 20 to 70 years.[50–52] Patients present with brown, gray, and blue-gray clusters of macules, most commonly involving the bilateral malar region, followed by the forehead, upper eyelids, temples, and the root and ala of the nose.[51] Hori's nevi may also present during adolescence and do not involve mucosal surfaces.

The pathogenesis is thought to involve ectopic placement of inactive poorly melanized dermal melanocytes at birth or soon after.[50] This is followed by the activation of these melanocytes in response to different factors such as sun exposure, pregnancy, hormones, stress, trauma, and/or cutaneous inflammatory conditions.[53] Histology reveals melanocytes dispersed in the upper and mid-dermis, in contrast to nevus of Ota, in which melanocytes are dispersed throughout the upper and lower dermis.[50,52] Perivascular distribution of melanocytes is also more noticeable in Hori nevi.

Combination laser therapy has shown to be a synergistic and effective treatment of Hori nevi. Methods such as dermabrasion and cryotherapy were previously used but have been largely replaced by laser treatment due to a higher risk of scar formation and hypopigmentation and depigmentation with the former.[50] QS lasers such as the QS ruby laser, QS ND:YAG laser, and QS alexandrite laser have all been used for the treatment of Hori's nevi since the first report by Hori and colleagues.[50,52] Use of the longer wavelength Nd:YAG is safest in individuals with skin of color.[3] The picosecond 755-nm and 1064 ND:YAG laser and laser combinations with fractionated ablative and non-ablative lasers have also been used safely and effectively.[54,55]

Lentigines/Ephelides

Ephelides and solar lentigines are common pigmented lesions which can occur on the face. Ephelides (or freckles) are promoted by sun exposure and fade during the winter months, whereas solar lentigines (or sun spots) occur in sun-exposed areas and increase in prevalence and number with higher age.[56] Affected individuals are typically patients with lighter skin phototypes.[57] Ephelides typically present in childhood whereas lentigines are seen more in adults.[58] Ephelides and lentigines present on sun-exposed areas of the face, upper trunk, and upper extremities.[58] Lentigines are numerous light to dark brown macules measuring a few millimeters to around 2 cm in diameter, whereas ephelides tend to be well-demarcated 1- to 3-mm light- or medium-brown macules.[3]

Variants of melanocortin-1 receptor (MC1R) genes play a role in the development of ephelides, whereas lentigines stem from sun-related UV radiation, which induces epidermal hyperplasia as well as proliferation and activity of melanocytes.[57,58] Histopathologically, ephelides present with a normal epidermis and increased melanocytic activity without increased melanocyte counts. Increased melanin in the basal epidermal layer is also seen. Lentigines may show epidermal hyperplasia with an increased number of melanocytes and basal layer pigmentation.[3,57]

Treatment options for ephelides and lentigines include topical and procedural therapies. In addition to photoprotection, topical therapy includes the use of topical lightening agents, alpha hydroxy acids, and antioxidants such as cysteamine and ascorbic acid (vitamin C). Procedural therapies include cryotherapy, chemical peels, laser therapy, and intense pulsed-light therapy.[59,60] Laser used includes pulsed dye, copper vapor, krypton, frequency-doubled Nd:YAG, QS, picosecond, CO_2, and argon diode lasers.[55,60] Chemical peels used include alpha-hydroxy acids (glycolic acid 20%–70%), beta hydroxy acids (salicylic acid 10%–30%), and Jessner's solution.[61,62] Medium and deep peels used effectively in the treatment of patients with fair skin include trichloroacetic acid (TCA) (30%–70%) and phenol (80%), however, these peel strengths are not safe in the treatment of darker skin types due to risk of burns and dyspigmentation.[59] Cryotherapy with liquid nitrogen can lead to significant lightening but must also be used with caution in those with darker skin types due to the risk of dyspigmentation.[62]

Photolichenoid Dermatoses

Photolichenoid dermatitis is considered a rare, lichen planus-like, eruption often occurring following exposure to a photosensitizing drug.[63] Affected individuals are typically middle-aged or older and men and women are equally affected. This condition has also been found to occur without exposure to photosensitizing medications more frequently in patients of African and Native American descent with HIV.[64]

A total of 22 agents have appeared in the dermatologic literature in relation to these reactions.[63,65] Reported photolichenoid drug reactions include quinidine, quinine, hydrochlorothiazide, sulfamethoxazole/trimethoprim, and democlocycline.[66] Lichen planus can present very similarly clinically histologically and should be included in the differential for this condition.

The pathogenesis of photolichenoid dermatitis is thought to be secondary to cell-mediated cytotoxicity. Antigen presentation by keratinocytes may induce T-cell accumulation, basement membrane disruption, and keratinocyte apoptosis.[67] Histopathologic features include a dense lymphocytic infiltrate at the dermal-epidermal junction, dyskeratotic keratinocytes, melanin incontinence, and dermal melanophages.[63]

Commonly affected areas are photo-exposed sites including the face, forearms, and chest. Individuals often present with erythematous to violaceous macules, patches and plaques which can be pruritic. Skin findings typically appear within 1 month of beginning the offending agent, but there have been accounts of presentations as early as 2 weeks. Affected individuals with HIV typically have advanced disease with CD4 counts of < 0.05 x 10(9)L.[66]

Treatment consists of immediately discontinuing the use of the offending medication. Topical steroids and tacrolimus 0.1% ointment have demonstrated efficacy.[68] Phototherapy can be used as adjunctive therapy.[69] Systemic steroids such as hydroxychloroquine can be used in recalcitrant cases. Most cases resolve following drug discontinuation, but PIH may occur, and therefore, diligent photoprotection should be employed to prevent worsening of hyperpigmentation.

Drug-Induced Facial Pigmentation

Drug-induced facial pigmentation can affect anyone following exposure to a myriad of drugs. These include amiodarone, antimalarials, anti-convulsive agents, cytotoxic drugs, anti-psychotics, minocycline, tetracyclines, non-steroidal anti-inflammatory drugs (NSAIDs), and tricyclic antidepressants.[70] These drugs can lead to cutaneous inflammation, thus triggering the increased production of melanin by epidermal melanocytes. They are also capable of impairing the clearance of melanin from dermal macrophages and this melanin can accumulate either freely in the dermis or sequestered in dermal melanophages.[71] On histology, findings can be very variable depending on the culprit. Pigment

incontinence, interface change, and lichenoid dermatitis can be seen.[72]

For making a diagnosis, there must be clinical history showing a temporal correlation between the onset of the pigmentation and beginning of this offending drug.[73] Of note, this condition can have a very slow onset and progress over months to years. The pigmentation is highly sensitive to sun exposure, and thus is often seen in sun-exposed areas and mucous membranes.[71] This increased sun sensitivity is postulated to be due to the reaction between certain drugs and melanin leading to the formation of drug–pigment complexes.[74] Treatment options begin with discontinuing the offending drug and the hyperpigmentation typically fades with time. However, in the case of persistent pigmentation, topical therapy with HQ has been highlighted as an effective modality for treatment. Non-hydroquinone lightening agents including retinoids can also be used.[75] Procedural therapies have also been used with notable benefits.[76,77] In particular, the 755-nm QS alexandrite laser has demonstrated favorable outcomes in the treatment of drug-induced facial hyperpigmentation.[78]

Periorbital Melanosis

Periorbital melanosis (PM), also known as periorbital hyperpigmentation, is a common condition that can affect individuals of all ages and racial/ethnic backgrounds, but is more common in those with darker skin phototypes.[79] There are very limited data on the pathogenesis of the condition, but the etiology seems to stem from various factors including genetics, sun exposure, allergies, facial anatomy, specifically orbital hollowing, and vasculature. Lack of sleep, use of contact lenses, alcohol overuse, excessive consumption of soda or caffeine, and smoking are lifestyle factors that can also contribute to the development of this condition. Periorbital inflammatory conditions including atopic dermatitis and allergic contact dermatitis may lead to post-inflammatory changes around the eye, typically as a sequelae of chronic rubbing leading to thickening of the skin. Allergic rhinitis can also lead to periorbital hyperpigmentation called "allergic shiners".[80]

There are two clinical types of PM differentiated by etiology. PM not associated with systemic or local disease is considered primary or idiopathic PM, whereas the second type of PM is related to a known systemic or local insult.[81] Patients will typically present with bilateral periocular light to dark brown patches and may believe they look more tired than usual. In cases related to those with atopy, lichenification of the skin can also be present.

Treatments of PM can be challenging and should be directed at the underlying cause. Soft tissue fillers and fat grafting are the most effective options when the PM is due to volume loss. Topical creams containing vitamin C, HQ, retinol, caffeine, or vitamin E can be effective when the PM is pigment-based. Additionally, trichloroacetic acid (TCA), salicylic acid, lactic acid, or glycolic acid chemical peels can also be beneficial when this is the etiology.[82] Laser therapies such as 1064 nm Nd:YAG (QS and long-pulsed), CO_2, QS ruby laser, and Er:YAG can be effective in treating pigment-based as well as PM with a vascular etiology. When there is excessive skin laxity, blepharoplasty can be used.[83] A combination of microneedling and 10% TCA has been shown to achieve significant esthetic improvement in treated patients.[84] Additionally, vitamin C mesotherapy or carboxy therapy has also been shown to be effective in reducing periorbital pigmentation.[85]

Exogenous Ochronosis

Exogenous ochronosis (EO) is an uncommon disorder that can occur as a complication of the overuse of hydroquinone-containing products or contact with phenol or resorcinol.[86] Black women are most commonly affected and the highest prevalence is among users of skin-lightening products.[87] There are two types of ochronosis, endogenous ochronosis or alkaptonuric ochronosis and EO, which will be discussed in this section. On histology, EO will present as yellow-brown curvilinear banana-shaped ochronotic pigment fibers comprised of collagen bundles bound to homogentisic acid in the dermis, and with more severe cases, there may be degradation of the collagen fibers. Inflammatory cells such as plasma cells, histiocytes, and multinucleated giant cells may also be present in the dermis.[88]

Patients with facial EO often present with asymptomatic, bilateral, blue-black, gray-blue, or dark brown-gray macules and/or papules typically on the temples and malar cheeks. There are three clinical grades of EO: stage I is characterized by erythema and mild pigmentation of the face and neck; stage II consists of more pronounced hyperpigmentation with black colloidal milia and atrophy with "caviar-like" papules; stage III consists of papulonodules that may or may not have surrounding inflammation.[88]

Treatment is extremely difficult and variable, but always begins with eliminating the offending agent. Topical retinoic acid as a stand-alone treatment has demonstrated mild benefits. A combination of retinoic acid, benzoyl peroxide, and

hydrocortisone has been helpful in achieving minimal lightening.[88] Topical acid peels including glycolic acid and tricarboxylic acid have demonstrated some improvement in pigmentation.[86] Procedural therapies such as dermabrasion,[89] the QS and picosecond 1064 nm Nd:YAG, and fractional CO_2 have all shown varying levels of efficacy as monotherapy and combination therapy.[90–92]

Riehl's Melanosis (Pigmented Contact Dermatitis)

Riehl's melanosis (RM), also widely known as pigmented contact dermatitis, is thought to be an acquired form of allergic contact dermatitis. The condition is most commonly seen in young to middle-aged women of Asian descent with darker skin.[93] The etiology of RM largely stems from direct contact with exogenous factors which serve as allergens including fragrances, dyes, red and yellow pigment, henna, lavender oil, lemon oil, and other cosmeceutical ingredients.[93]

Histopathology often reveals interface dermatitis consisting of vacuolar basal layer degeneration, lymphohistiocytic infiltrate, and pigmentary incontinence.[94] On physical exam, patients present with localized to diffuse scaly macules and patches ranging from black to gray-brown as well as satellite-pigmented follicular-based macules. The macules will often have a distinct reticular, network-like, pattern at the center. The sites of involvement are often the forehead, zygomatic, and temple regions where cosmeceutical products are typically applied, but various areas of the body can be affected. Of note, when the allergens are photosensitizers, the sun-exposed areas are most affected.[93]

There is no universal standardized treatment regimen for RM, but many modalities have been tried with varying results. It is imperative that the causative agent be discontinued. Following this, topical agents such as hydroquinone, retinoids, and topical corticosteroids may be employed as monotherapy or combination therapy. These topical creams can be used in addition to light to medium trichloroacetic acid or glycolic acid chemical peels.[93] Light and laser-based therapies such as intense pulsed-light therapy and low-fluence QS Nd: YAG lasers have also achieved therapeutic success.[93] For more recalcitrant cases, a study looking at the combination of oral glycyrrhizin compound, vitamin C, and salicylic acid peels once every 2 weeks demonstrated significant improvement.[95] An additional study found the combination of low-fluence 1064 nm QS Nd:YAG laser, hydroquinone cream, and oral tranexamic acid over 10 to 18 sessions to be effective for recalcitrant RM in eight Asian patients.[96]

Actinic Lichen Planus

Actinic lichen planus, also referred to as lichen planus subtropicus/tropicus or lichenoid melanodermatitis, is an uncommon variant of lichen planus mainly affecting the face.[97] It is most commonly seen in individuals of Middle Eastern, Indian, or African descent in the third decade of life, however, there have been cases reported in children.

There are three distinct subtypes of actinic lichen planus, the most common being annular and presenting as hyperpigmented atrophic plaques on the face surrounded by a hypopigmented halo. Other subtypes are pigmented/melasma-like and dyschromic.[98] The pigmented variant presents as gray to brown or black patches between 0.5 and 5 cm in diameter.[99] Dyschromic type is the least common and classically presents with white pin-point, coalescing papules primarily in photo-exposed regions.[98]

The pathogenesis of this condition has not been entirely elucidated, but sunlight exposure is theorized to trigger photo-koebernization of the disease.[98] Sunlight is considered the main precipitating factor with genetics, hormonal, toxic, and infectious factors also playing a role.[100] In terms of etiology, UV exposure coupled with the intake of photosensitizing drugs such as acitretin and hydrochlorothiazide has been indicated. Histopathology typically demonstrates interface dermatitis consisting of basal layer vacuolar changes, apoptotic bodies, and pigment incontinence. This condition can be self-limiting and resolves with time and diligent photoprotection, but other therapeutic options can include topical steroids, topical calcineurin inhibitors, oral dapsone, oral antimalarials, oral hydroxychloroquine, acitretin, and cyclosporine. Some improvement has been demonstrated with acitretin combined with topical steroids or cyclosporine.[101] Pigmented actinic LP has also been shown to respond favorably to intense pulsed light.[102]

Post-Chikungunya Hyperpigmentation

Post-chikungunya fever (CF) hyperpigmentation or "Chik sign" is facial hyperpigmentation following the acute febrile illness associated with having CF. CF is endemic to the Indian subcontinent, Southeast Asia, Africa, and the Pacific and subtropical areas of the Americas.

It typically presents with fever, joint pain, and various constitutional symptoms including but not limited to headache, muscle pain, and swelling.[103] Facial hyperpigmentation is considered to be the most common cutaneous manifestation of the infection.

The "Chik sign", also known as "brownie nose sign" consists of centrofacial hyperpigmented macules over the nose and cheeks. The sign develops a few weeks following the febrile illness, but may persist for a prolonged period after. It has been theorized that this hyperpigmentation is likely due to increased intradermal melanin retention and dispersion that is triggered by the virus.[104] On histology, dermal melanophages with perivascular infiltrate and increased basilar pigmentation may be seen.

The Chik sign is typically helpful in making a retrospective clinical diagnosis of CF. In the absence of disease, the hyperpigmentation is expected to gradually fade; however, sun protection should be emphasized. Hydroquinone and non-hydroquinone lightening agents can also be used to aid in lightening of dark patches.[103]

SUMMARY

Diseases of facial hyperpigmentation are common, particularly in skin of color populations, and can present diagnostic and therapeutic challenges. Furthermore, they can have profound effects on the quality of life for those affected. It is important that appropriate workup is done to first determine the correct diagnosis. This can help set prognostic expectations and clarify treatment options. For many of these conditions, no gold standard therapy exists. Often topical, oral, and/or procedural treatments are employed in combination. Procedural treatments continue to advance in their ability to safely and effectively improve pigmentation, including in those with darker skin types; however, caution should still be taken to avoid worsening of the underlying condition or irritation that could lead to new dyspigmentation. Treatment of disorders of facial hyperpigmentation is typically slow and patients must be counseled prognostically on the time course for treatment, and that in some severe cases, full resolution may be challenging to achieve. In all cases, photoprotection is a critical component of the overall treatment regimen and necessary for the prevention of disease progression. As the pathogenesis of these conditions becomes better understood, more treatment options are on the horizon to help improve clinical outcomes and quality of life for affected individuals.

FUNDING SOURCES

None.

CLINICS CARE POINTS

- Use of a woods lamp, dermoscopy, and biopsy if needed can be helpful tools in the diagnostic workup of facial pigmentation.
- Photoprotection is an important part of the prevention and treatment algorithm for most disorders of facial pigmentation.
- Facial photographs can be helpful to monitor progress of the condition and response to treatment.

DISCLOSURE

Dr N. Elbuluk is the director of Diversity and Inclusion as well as the Director of the Skin of Color and Pigmentary Disorders Program at the USC Department of Dermatology, Keck School of Medicine. She has served as a paid consultant, advisory board member and/or speaker for Allergan, Beiersdorf, La Roche Posay, VisualDx, Scientis, Galderma Laboratories LP, Zosano, Incyte, Estee Lauder, Avita, and L'Oreal. She has received royalties from McGraw Hill and serves on their editorial board.

REPRINT REQUESTS

Nada Elbuluk.

REFERENCES

1. Vashi N, Kundu RV. Acquired hyperpigmentation disorders. 2022. Available at: https://www-uptodate-com.libproxy1.usc.edu/contents/acquired-hyperpigmentation-disorders. Accessed March 7, 2022.
2. Atef A, El-Rashidy MA, Abdel Azeem A, et al. The Role of Stem Cell Factor in Hyperpigmented Skin Lesions. Asian Pac J Cancer Prev 2019;20(12):3723–8.
3. Vashi NA, Wirya SA, Inyang M, et al. Facial Hyperpigmentation in Skin of Color: Special Considerations and Treatment. Am J Clin Dermatol 2017;18(2):215–30.
4. Grimes PE. Melasma: Epidemiology, pathogenesis, clinical presentation, and diagnosis. UpToDate. Published online March 2022. Available at: https://www-uptodate-com.libproxy1.usc.edu/contents/melasma-epidemiology-pathogenesis-clinical-presentation-and-diagnosis. Accessed February 21, 2022.
5. Ogbechie-Godec OA, Elbuluk N. Melasma: an Up-to-Date Comprehensive Review. Dermatol Ther 2017;7(3):305–18.
6. Hexsel D, Lacerda DA, Cavalcante AS, et al. Epidemiology of melasma in Brazilian patients: a multicenter study. Int J Dermatol 2014;53(4):440–4.
7. Ritter CG, Fiss DVC, Borges da Costa JAT, et al. Extra-facial melasma: clinical, histopathological, and immunohistochemical case-control study. J Eur Acad Dermatol Venereol 2013;27(9):1088–94.
8. Rajanala S, Maymone MB de C, Vashi NA. Melasma pathogenesis: a review of the latest research, pathological findings, and investigational therapies. Dermatol Online J 2019;25(10). 13030/qt47b7r28c.
9. Gao YL, Jia XX, Wang M, et al. Melanocyte activation and skin barrier disruption induced in melasma patients after 1064 nm Nd:YAG laser treatment. Lasers Med Sci 2019;34(4):767–71.
10. Kwon SH, Park KC. Clues to the Pathogenesis of Melasma from its Histologic Findings. Journal of Pigmentary Disorders 2014;1(5):141.
11. Melasma. Management - UpToDate. Available at: https://www-uptodate-com.libproxy1.usc.edu/contents/melasma-management. Accessed May 9, 2022.
12. Castanedo-Cazares JP, Hernandez-Blanco D, Carlos-Ortega B, et al. Near-visible light and UV photoprotection in the treatment of melasma: a double-blind randomized trial. Photodermatol Photoimmunol Photomed 2014;30(1):35–42.
13. Dumbuya H, Grimes PE, Lynch S, et al. Impact of Iron-Oxide Containing Formulations Against Visible Light-Induced Skin Pigmentation in Skin of Color Individuals. J Drugs Dermatol 2020;19(7):712–7.
14. McKesey J, Tovar-Garza A, Pandya AG. Melasma Treatment: An Evidence-Based Review. Am J Clin Dermatol 2020;21(2):173–225.
15. Trivedi MK, Yang FC, Cho BK. A review of laser and light therapy in melasma. Int J Womens Dermatol 2017;3(1):11–20.
16. Davis EC, Callender VD. Postinflammatory hyperpigmentation: a review of the epidemiology, clinical features, and treatment options in skin of color. J Clin Aesthet Dermatol 2010;3(7):20–31.
17. Saedi N. Postinflammatory hyperpigmentation. UpToDate. Published online April 2, 2022. Available at: https://www-uptodate-com.libproxy1.usc.edu/contents/postinflammatory-hyperpigmentation. Accessed February 26, 2022.
18. Maghfour J, Olayinka J, Hamzavi IH, et al. A Focused review on the pathophysiology of post-inflammatory hyperpigmentation. Pigment Cell & Melanoma Research. 2022;1–8.
19. Silpa-archa N, Kohli I, Chaowattanapanit S, et al. Postinflammatory hyperpigmentation: A comprehensive overview: Epidemiology, pathogenesis, clinical presentation, and noninvasive assessment technique. J Am Acad Dermatol 2017;77(4):591–605.

20. Paller AS, Mancini AJ. Disorders of pigmentation. In: Paller and Mancini – hurwitz clinical pediatric Dermatology11, 6th edition; 2022. p. 287–325.e12.

21. Kaufman BP, Aman T, Alexis AF. Postinflammatory Hyperpigmentation: Epidemiology, Clinical Presentation, Pathogenesis and Treatment. Am J Clin Dermatol 2018;19(4):489–503.

22. Lindgren AL, Austin AH, Welsh KM. The Use of Tranexamic Acid to Prevent and Treat Post-Inflammatory Hyperpigmentation. J Drugs Dermatol 2021;20(3):344–5.

23. Zachary CB, Kelly KM. Lasers and Other Energy-Based Therapies. In: Dermatology: 2-Volume Set137. Elsevier; 2018. p. 2364–84.

24. Levin MK, Ng E, Bae YSC, et al. Treatment of pigmentary disorders in patients with skin of color with a novel 755 nm picosecond, Q-switched ruby, and Q-switched Nd:YAG nanosecond lasers: A retrospective photographic review. Lasers Surg Med 2016;48(2):181–7.

25. Quiñonez RL, Agbai ON, Burgess CM, et al. An update on cosmetic procedures in people of color. Part 2: Neuromodulators, soft tissue augmentation, chemexfoliating agents, and laser hair reduction. J Am Acad Dermatol 2022;86(4):729–39.

26. Verma S, Vasani R, Joshi R, et al. A descriptive study of facial acanthosis nigricans and its association with body mass index, waist circumference and insulin resistance using HOMA2 IR. Indian Dermatol Online J 2016;7(6):498–503.

27. Larocca CA, Kundu RV, Vashi NA. Physiologic pigmentation: Molecular mechanisms and clinical diversity. Available at: https://www.pigmentinternational.com/article.asp?issn=2349-5847;year=2014;volume=1;issue=2;spage=44;epage=51;aulast=Larocca. Accessed April 13, 2022.

28. Sonthalia S, Sarkar R, Neema S. Maturational hyperpigmentation: Clinico-dermoscopic and histopathological profile of a new cutaneous marker of metabolic syndrome. Pigment Int 2018;5(1):54–6.

29. Sonthalia S, Agrawal M, Sharma P, et al. Maturational Hyperpigmentation: Cutaneous Marker of Metabolic Syndrome. Dermatol Pract Concept 2020;10(2):e2020046.

30. Larocca. Physiologic pigmentation: Molecular mechanisms and clinical diversity. Available at: https://www.pigmentinternational.com/article.asp?issn=2349-5847;year=2014;volume=1;issue=2;spage=44;epage=51;aulast=Larocca. Accessed May 9, 2022.

31. Wong V, Burgin S. Maturational hyperpigmentation. In: Goldsmith LA, editor. VisualDX. 2022.

32. Maderal AD. Acanthosis nigricans. 2021. Available at: https://www-uptodate-com.libproxy1.usc.edu/contents/acanthosis-nigricans. Accessed March 1, 2022.

33. Shah VH, Rambhia KD, Mukhi JI, et al. Clinico-investigative Study of Facial Acanthosis Nigricans. Indian Dermatol Online J 2022;13(2):221–8.

34. Phiske MM. An approach to acanthosis nigricans. Indian Dermatol Online J 2014;5(3):239–49.

35. Leung N, Oliveira M, Selim MA, et al. Erythema dyschromicum perstans: A case report and systematic review of histologic presentation and treatment. Int J Womens Dermatol 2018;4(4):216–22.

36. Torrelo A, Zaballos P, Colmenero I, et al. Erythema dyschromicum perstans in children: a report of 14 cases. J Eur Acad Dermatol Venereol 2005;19(4):422–6.

37. Tlougan BE, Gonzalez ME, Mandal RV, et al. Erythema dyschromicum perstans. Dermatol Online J 2010;16(11):17.

38. Chang SE, Kim HW, Shin JM, et al. Clinical and histological aspect of erythema dyschromicum perstans in Korea: A review of 68 cases. J Dermatol 2015;42(11):1053–7.

39. Robles-Méndez JC, Rizo-Frías P, Herz-Ruelas ME, et al. Lichen planus pigmentosus and its variants: review and update. Int J Dermatol 2018;57(5):505–14.

40. Rieder E, Kaplan J, Kamino H, et al. Lichen planus pigmentosus. Dermatol Online J 2013;19(12):20713.

41. Dlova NC. Frontal fibrosing alopecia and lichen planus pigmentosus: is there a link? Br J Dermatol 2013;168(2):439–42.

42. Krueger L, Svigos K, Brinster N, et al. Frontal fibrosing alopecia: cutaneous associations in women with skin of color. Cutis 2018;102(5):335–8.

43. Wolff M, Sabzevari N, Gropper C, et al. A Case of Lichen Planus Pigmentosus with Facial Dyspigmentation Responsive to Combination Therapy with Chemical Peels and Topical Retinoids. J Clin Aesthet Dermatol 2016;9(11):44–50.

44. Wu CY, Lin FL. A successful combination therapy of tacrolimus, hydroxychloroquine and picosecond laser for lichen planus pigmentosus. Australas J Dermatol 2019;60(4):e336–7.

45. Sonthalia S, Vedamurthy M, Thomas M, et al. Modified phenol peels for treatment-refractory hyperpigmentation of lichen planus pigmentosus: A retrospective clinico-dermoscopic analysis. J Cosmet Dermatol 2019. https://doi.org/10.1111/jocd.12862.

46. Schaffer JV, Bolognia JL, Hunt R. Benign pigmented skin lesions other than melanocytic nevi (moles). 2021. Available at: https://www-uptodate-com.libproxy1.usc.edu/contents/benign-pigmented-skin-lesions-other-than-melanocytic-nevi-moles. Accessed March 7, 2022.

47. Mohan RPS, Verma S, Singh AK, et al. Nevi of Ota: the unusual birthmarks": a case review. BMJ Case Rep 2013;2013. https://doi.org/10.1136/bcr-2013-008648.

48. Ge Y, Yang Y, Guo L, et al. Comparison of a pico-second alexandrite laser versus a Q-switched alexandrite laser for the treatment of nevus of Ota: A randomized, split-lesion, controlled trial. J Am Acad Dermatol 2020;83(2):397–403.

49. Raj C, Dixit N, Debata I, et al. Combination of 1064-nm Q-switched neodymium-doped yttrium-aluminum-garnet laser with Modified Jessner's peel for the treatment of Nevus of Ota: A case series of seven patients. Dermatol Ther 2020;33(6): e14384.

50. Park JM, Tsao H, Tsao S. Acquired bilateral nevus of Ota-like macules (Hori nevus): etiologic and therapeutic considerations. J Am Acad Dermatol 2009; 61(1):88–93.

51. Ee HL, Wong HC, Goh CL, et al. Characteristics of Hori naevus: a prospective analysis. Br J Dermatol 2006;154(1):50–3.

52. Hori Y, Kawashima M, Oohara K, et al. Acquired, bilateral nevus of Ota-like macules. J Am Acad Dermatol 1984;10(6):961–4.

53. Murakami F, Soma Y, Mizoguchi M. Acquired symmetrical dermal melanocytosis (naevus of Hori) developing after aggravated atopic dermatitis. Br J Dermatol 2005;152(5):903–8.

54. Tian B. Novel treatment of Hori's nevus: A combination of fractional nonablative 2,940-nm Er:YAG and low-fluence 1,064-nm Q-switched Nd:YAG laser. J Cutan Aesthet Surg 2015;8(4):227–9.

55. Koh YP, Tan AWM, Chua SH. Treatment of Laser-Responsive Dermal Pigmentary Conditions in Type III-IV Asian Skin With a 755-nm Picosecond Pulse Duration Laser: A Retrospective Review of Its Efficacy and Safety. Dermatol Surg 2020; 46(11):e82–7.

56. Dinulos JGH. Light-Related Diseases and Disorders of Pigmentation. In: Habif's clinical Dermatology. 7th edition; 2021. p. 748–86. Chapter 19.

57. Praetorius C, Sturm RA, Steingrimsson E. Sun-induced freckling: ephelides and solar lentigines. Pigment Cell Melanoma Res 2014;27(3): 339–50.

58. Bastiaens M, ter Huurne J, Gruis N, et al. The melanocortin-1-receptor gene is the major freckle gene. Hum Mol Genet 2001;10(16):1701–8.

59. Mradula PR, Sacchidanand S. A split-face comparative study of 70% trichloroacetic acid and 80% phenol spot peel in the treatment of freckles. J Cutan Aesthet Surg 2012;5(4):261–5.

60. Ortonne JP, Pandya AG, Lui H, et al. Treatment of solar lentigines. J Am Acad Dermatol 2006;54(5 Suppl 2):S262–71.

61. O'Connor AA, Lowe PM, Shumack S, et al. Chemical peels: A review of current practice. Australas J Dermatol 2018;59(3):171–81.

62. Plensdorf S, Livieratos M, Dada N. Pigmentation Disorders: Diagnosis and Management. Am Fam Physician 2017;96(12):797–804.

63. Collazo MH, Sánchez JL, Figueroa LD. Defining lichenoid photodermatitis. Int J Dermatol 2009; 48(3):239–42.

64. Curtiss P, Riley K, Meehan SA, et al. Photolichenoid dermatitis: a presenting sign of human immunodeficiency virus. Cutis 2019;104(4):242–4.

65. Jones HE, Lewis CW, Reisner JE. Photosensitive lichenoid eruption associated with demeclocycline. Arch Dermatol 1972;106(1):58–63.

66. Berger TG, Dhar A. Lichenoid photoeruptions in human immunodeficiency virus infection. Arch Dermatol 1994;130(5):609–13.

67. Lichenoid tissue reaction/interface dermatitis: Recognition, classification, etiology, and clinicopathological overtones. Indian J Dermatol, Venereol Leprol 2011. Available at: https://ijdvl.com/lichenoid-tissue-reaction-interface-dermatitis-recognition-classification-etiology-and-clinicopathological-overtones/. Accessed February 9, 2022.

68. Tambe SA, Zambare US, Nayak CS, et al. Clinical and histopathological aspects of lichenoid dermatitis in patients of retroviral diseases. Indian J Sex Transm Dis AIDS 2022;43(1):59–63.

69. Rathod DG, Muneer H, Masood S. Phototherapy. In: StatPearls. StatPearls Publishing; 2022. Available at: http://www.ncbi.nlm.nih.gov/books/NBK563140/. Accessed August 31, 2022.

70. Hassan S, Zhou X. Drug Induced Pigmentation. In: StatPearls. StatPearls Publishing; 2022. Available at: http://www.ncbi.nlm.nih.gov/books/NBK542253/. Accessed September 12, 2022.

71. Nicolaidou E, Katsambas AD. Pigmentation disorders: hyperpigmentation and hypopigmentation. Clin Dermatol 2014;32(1):66–72.

72. Desai N, Alexis AF, DeLeo VA. Facial Hyperpigmentation Caused by Diltiazem Hydrochloride. :3.

73. Gerson D, Sriganeshan V, Alexis JB. Cutaneous drug eruptions: a 5-year experience. J Am Acad Dermatol 2008;59(6):995–9.

74. Drug-induced skin pigmentation | DermNet. Available at: https://dermnetnz.org/topics/drug-induced-hyperpigmentation. Accessed August 31, 2022.

75. Syder NC, Elbuluk N. Going Beyond Hydroquinone: Alternative Skin Lightning Agents. Cutis 2022;109(6):302–4.

76. Stratigos AJ, Katsambas AD. Optimal Management of Recalcitrant Disorders of Hyperpigmentation in Dark-Skinned Patients. Am J Clin Dermatol 2004;5(3):161–8.

77. Crowson AN, Brown TJ, Magro CM. Progress in the understanding of the pathology and pathogenesis

of cutaneous drug eruptions : implications for management. Am J Clin Dermatol 2003;4(6):407–28.

78. Wee SA, Dover JS. Effective treatment of psychotropic drug-induced facial hyperpigmentation with a 755-nm Q-switched alexandrite laser. Dermatol Surg 2008;34(11):1609–12.

79. Noble A, Greenstein J, Husain A, et al. Periorbital melanosis. Am J Emerg Med 2017;35(2):380.e1–2.

80. Kelso JM. How allergic are "allergic shiners". J Allergy Clin Immunol 2010;125(1):276.

81. Thappa DM, Chandrashekar L, Rajappa M, et al. Assessment of Patients with Periorbital Melanosis for Hyperinsulinemia and Insulin Resistance. Indian Dermatol Online J 2021;12(2):244–9.

82. Samaan CB, Cartee TV. Treatment of Periorbital Vascularity, Erythema, and Hyperpigmentation. Facial Plast Surg Clin North Am 2022;30(3):309–19.

83. Michelle L, Pouldar Foulad D, Ekelem C, et al. Treatments of Periorbital Hyperpigmentation: A Systematic Review. Dermatol Surg 2021;47(1): 70–4.

84. Kontochristopoulos G, Kouris A, Platsidaki E, et al. Combination of microneedling and 10% trichloroacetic acid peels in the management of infraorbital dark circles. J Cosmet Laser Ther 2016;18(5): 289–92.

85. Ahmed NA, Mohammed SS, Fatani MI. Treatment of periorbital dark circles: Comparative study of carboxy therapy vs chemical peeling vs mesotherapy. J Cosmet Dermatol 2019;18(1):169–75.

86. Bhattar PA, Zawar VP, Godse KV, et al. Exogenous Ochronosis. Indian J Dermatol 2015;60(6):537–43.

87. Hardwick N, Van Gelder LW, Van der Merwe CA, et al. Exogenous ochronosis: an epidemiological study. Br J Dermatol 1989;120(2):229–38.

88. Simmons BJ, Griffith RD, Bray FN, et al. Exogenous ochronosis: a comprehensive review of the diagnosis, epidemiology, causes, and treatments. Am J Clin Dermatol 2015;16(3):205–12.

89. Diven DG, Smith EB, Pupo RA, et al. Hydroquinone-induced localized exogenous ochronosis treated with dermabrasion and CO2 laser. J Dermatol Surg Oncol 1990;16(11):1018–22.

90. Kanechorn-Na-Ayuthaya P, Niumphradit N, Aunhachoke K, et al. Effect of combination of 1064 nm Q-switched Nd:YAG and fractional carbon dioxide lasers for treating exogenous ochronosis. J Cosmet Laser Ther 2013;15(1):42–5.

91. Tan SKS. Exogenous ochronosis - successful outcome after treatment with Q-switched Nd:YAG laser. J Cosmet Laser Ther 2013;15(5):274–8.

92. Méndez Baca I, Al-Niaimi F, Colina C, et al. A case of ochronosis successfully treated with the picosecond laser. J Cosmet Dermatol 2018. https://doi.org/10.1111/jocd.12834.

93. Daadaa N, Ben Tanfous A. Riehl Melanosis. In: StatPearls. StatPearls publishing. 2022. Available at: http://www.ncbi.nlm.nih.gov/books/NBK557437/ 2022. Accessed February 19, 2022.

94. Kim SM, Lee ES, Sohn S, et al. Histopathological Features of Riehl Melanosis. Am J Dermatopathol 2020;42(2):117–21.

95. Wang L, Wen X, Hao D, et al. Combination therapy with salicylic acid chemical peels, glycyrrhizin compound, and vitamin C for Riehl's melanosis. J Cosmet Dermatol 2020;19(6):1377–80.

96. Kwon HH, Ohn J, Suh DH, et al. A pilot study for triple combination therapy with a low-fluence 1064 nm Q-switched Nd:YAG laser, hydroquinone cream and oral tranexamic acid for recalcitrant Riehl's Melanosis. J Dermatolog Treat 2017;28(2):155–9.

97. Tiwary AK. Actinic Lichen Planus. Indian Pediatr 2018;55(8):715.

98. Ashraf R, Aggarwal D, Bhattacharjee R, et al. Dyschromic actinic lichen planus. Int J Dermatol 2021. https://doi.org/10.1111/ijd.15932.

99. Venturini M, Manganoni AM, Zanca A, et al. Pigmented actinic lichen planus (PALP) mimicking lentigo maligna melanoma: Usefulness of in vivo reflectance confocal microscopy in diagnosis and follow-up. JAAD Case Rep 2018;4(6):568–72.

100. Mebazaa A, Denguezli M, Ghariani N, et al. Actinic lichen planus of unusual presentation. Acta Dermatovenerol Alp Pannonica Adriat 2010;19(2):31–3.

101. Gallo L, Ayala F, Ayala F. Relapsing lichen actinicus successfully treated with cyclosporin. J Eur Acad Dermatol Venereol 2008;22(3):370–1.

102. Santos-Juanes J, Mas-Vidal A, Coto-Segura P, et al. Pigmented actinic lichen planus successfully treated with intense pulsed light. Br J Dermatol 2010;163(3):662–3.

103. Sil A, Biswas SK, Bhanja DB, et al. Post-chikungunya hyperpigmentation. Postgrad Med J 2021; 97(1143):60.

104. Bhatia SS, Shenoi SD, Hebbar SA, et al. The chik sign in dengue. Pediatr Dermatol 2019;36(5): 737–8.

Diagnosing Disorders of Hypopigmentation and Depigmentation in Patients with Skin of Color

Marissa S. Ceresnie, DO[a], Sarah Gonzalez, BS[b], Iltefat H. Hamzavi, MD[a],*

KEYWORDS

- Depigmentation • Hypopigmentation • Skin of color • Medical dermatology

KEY POINTS

- People with skin of color have unique and increased rates of depigmentation and hypopigmentation disorders than White patients.
- Stratifying the features of hypopigmented and depigmented skin disorders may be helpful for forming diagnoses. In cases of uncertainty, a biopsy can be obtained.
- Depending on the severity and underlying cause, depigmentation and hypopigmentation can be permanent or may last weeks, months, or years.

INTRODUCTION

Hypopigmented and depigmented skin disorders, where the melanin pigment in the skin is reduced or completely lost, significantly affect patients with skin of color and are the third most common reason patients with skin of color seek dermatologic care.[1] Although spotting hypopigmentation or depigmentation on darker skin tones is straightforward, underlying disorders are frequently misdiagnosed. Several of these conditions appear more frequently or differently in patients with skin of color. In addition, patients with skin of color have a disproportionally higher psychosocial burden of disease than patients who have lighter skin tones because of the inherent noticeability of hypopigmentation and depigmentation on darker skin tones.[2] Thus, the ability of dermatologists to recognize these distinctions is essential for ensuring patient satisfaction, an accurate diagnosis, and reduction of disparities in health care.[3] In this review, the authors focus on the key elements of diagnosis for the most common hypopigmentation and depigmentation disorders in patients with skin of color.

CLINICAL FINDINGS

Because of the wide range of conditions that can lead to skin hypopigmentation and depigmentation, extensive heterogeneity in lesion distribution, size, shape, and morphologic features can be seen. Thus, skin color is the main feature distinguishing hypopigmented and depigmented disorders. Under standard lighting, the contrast between involved and uninvolved skin allows for easy identification of hypopigmented and depigmented lesions. Although depigmented lesions contain no pigment and are sharply demarcated against darker skin, hypopigmented lesions may present with less distinct borders and appear in various shades.

a Department of Dermatology, Multicultural Clinic, Henry Ford Health, 3031 West Grand Boulevard, Suite 700, Detroit, MI 48202, USA; b Wayne State University College of Medicine, 540 East Canfield Avenue, Detroit, MI 48201, USA
* Corresponding author.
E-mail address: ihamzavi@hamzavi.com

Dermatol Clin 41 (2023) 407–416
https://doi.org/10.1016/j.det.2023.02.006
0733-8635/23/© 2023 Elsevier Inc. All rights reserved.

DIAGNOSIS

Most hypopigmentation and depigmentation disorders can be accurately diagnosed by obtaining a detailed patient history and performing a thorough physical examination. Identifying key clinical features using a systematic approach is critical to distinguish between disorders of hypopigmentation and depigmentation (**Figs. 1** and **2**). The degree of pigment loss, body distribution, pattern, and morphologic features of skin lesions are essential clues needed for diagnosis. If the diagnosis is uncertain, obtaining a skin biopsy and performing laboratory tests may be helpful.

Obtaining a complete medical history is essential, as certain disorders, such as vitiligo and postinflammatory hypopigmentation, may be triggered by a traumatic incident, occupational or household exposure to a chemical, or an underlying skin condition. A relapsing and remitting disease course is typical of acquired disorders, whereas stable disorders are associated with congenital disorders. Some of these disorders may have a genetic component; therefore, inquiring about family history of skin disorders and autoimmune disorders is essential.

A physical examination should be performed with normal lighting and a Wood's lamp for all patients presenting with a disorder of hypopigmentation or depigmentation. Ideally, a Wood's lamp examination should occur in a dark room with the light placed within a few inches of the patient's clean skin, as clothing lint and topical products such as makeup, deodorant, and cream can produce false-positive fluorescence. Depigmented lesions exhibit sharply demarcated and bright blue-white fluorescence under a Wood's lamp, whereas hypopigmented lesions show less vibrant fluorescence and less distinct borders. A Wood's lamp examination can also assist in differentiating certain hypopigmented conditions from each other. For example, skin will show orange fluorescence in areas with pityriasis versicolor but red fluorescence of hair follicles in progressive macular hypomelanosis.

Careful consideration of the distribution of lesions during the physical examination is essential. The characteristic regional distributions of dermatologic conditions may vary in different populations with skin of color. For example, extensor atopic dermatitis is more commonly observed in Black patients, and truncal atopic dermatitis is

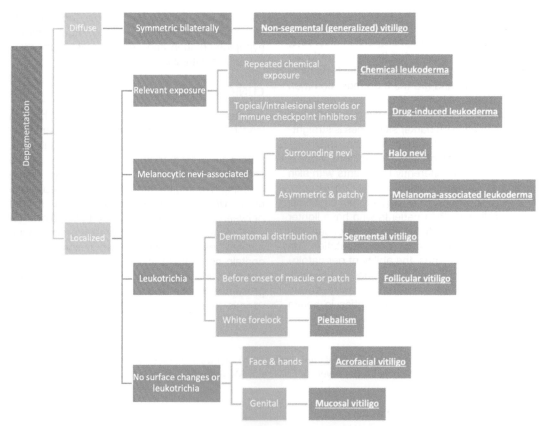

Fig. 1. Algorithm for diagnosing disorders of depigmentation in patients with skin of color.

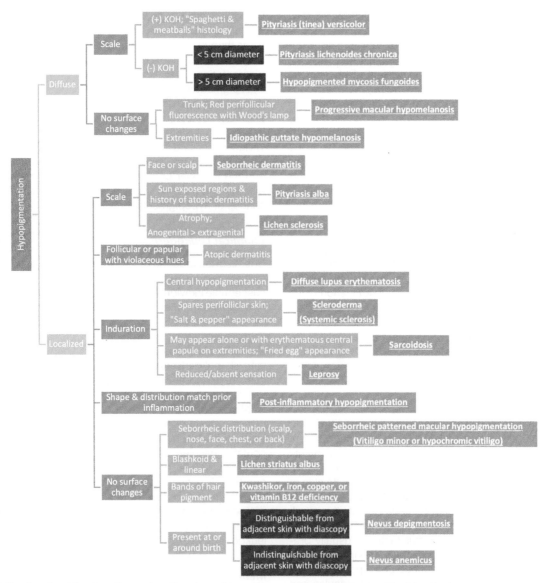

Fig. 2. Algorithm for diagnosing disorders of hypopigmentation in patients with skin of color.

more commonly detected in Black and Hispanic/Latinx patients.[4] For patients with skin depigmentation who are older than 50 years, examining the mucosal membranes and performing a focused ocular examination are essential because leukoderma may be associated with melanoma in this age group.[5] Vogt-Koyanagi-Harada disease should be suspected when adult patients with skin of color present with visual disturbances and progressive depigmentation; notably, the incidence of this disorder is highest in Asian, Indian, American Indian, Middle Eastern, and Mexican women.[5] For children, vaginal and perirectal examination is necessary to assess for skin atrophy with follicular plugging characteristic of lichen sclerosis et atrophicus, as a vitiligoid variant of lichen sclerosus that primarily affects pediatric patients with darker skin may be seen.[6]

Determining specific lesion patterns and morphology is essential not only for determining the correct diagnosis but also for assessing disease activity. Trichrome lesions, characterized by depigmented, light brown zones and typical skin colors, are a sign of active vitiligo, which are most often seen in patients with darker skin tones. Confetti-like lesions, appearing as depigmented speckles, and Koebnerization, which presents as depigmentation in areas of mechanical trauma to the skin, also indicate active vitiligo. Dermoscopy can differentiate active vitiligo from other disorders by revealing leukotrichia, or white hair, associated with segmental vitiligo.[7]

A biopsy can be considered if a diagnosis is uncertain or if features of hypopigmented mycosis fungoides or leprosy are present. Obtaining an excisional or large shave biopsy that includes both involved and uninvolved skin is important to histopathologically distinguish the diseased lesion from normal skin. The amount and location of melanocytes and melanin in the epidermis can be identified using the Fontana-Masson stain and melanoma antigen recognized by T cells 1 (MART1) or Melan-A immunohistochemistry.[8]

DIFFERENTIAL DIAGNOSIS

The differential diagnosis for disorders of hypopigmentation and depigmentation is wide. After determining if the lesion is hypopigmented or depigmented through physical examination using a Wood's lamp, the next step in the diagnostic algorithm is to consider body distribution and morphology along with relevant patient history to identify specific disorders (see **Figs. 1** and **2**).

DEPIGMENTED SKIN CONDITIONS
Vitiligo

The most common cause of depigmentation is vitiligo, which has an estimated prevalence of about 1% in the United States.[5,9] Many diseases mimic the appearance of vitiligo, which poses challenges in diagnosing this disorder. In patients with skin of color, vitiligo is more noticeable than in patients with lighter skin tones because of the stark contrast between involved and uninvolved skin. The cause of vitiligo is multifactorial, usually preceded by a trigger event, stress, pregnancy, cytotoxic compounds, or genetic predisposition.[10]

Vitiligo manifests as depigmented macules and patches distributed throughout the body and can be organized into several subtypes, with segmental and nonsegmental vitiligo identified as the most common types. Segmental vitiligo has unilateral involvement that follows Blaschko lines and is associated with leukotrichia. Nonsegmental vitiligo has a symmetric distribution usually without leukotrichia. Mucosal vitiligo affects the mucous membranes of the mouth and genitals, and acrofacial vitiligo involves the head and bilateral distal extremities. Patients with skin of color may also experience unique patterns of vitiligo, such as follicular vitiligo, seborrheic patterned macular hypopigmentation (also known as vitiligo minor or hypochromic vitiligo), and trichrome vitiligo at greater rates than White patients.[11–14] Follicular vitiligo, which manifests primarily with leukotrichia

preceding the appearance of depigmentation (**Fig. 3**), is easier to detect in patients with skin of color than in White patients, who may be underdiagnosed.[12] Seborrheic patterned macular hypopigmentation, first coined in 2022, describes hypopigmented macules distributed in a seborrheic pattern affecting the scalp, nose, face, chest, and back detected in a small cohort of middle-aged Black patients, similar to those observed in vitiligo minor and hypochromic vitiligo (**Fig. 4**).[14] Trichrome vitiligo, similar to confetti-like lesions and the Koebner phenomenon, is a sign of rapid disease progression and appears as at least 3 shades of hypopigmentation (**Fig. 5**).[15]

Chemical Leukoderma

Chemical leukoderma results from repeated exposure to melanocytotoxic compounds in genetically susceptible individuals.[5] In particular, patients with existing vitiligo may develop large-scale depigmentation following exposure to these agents.[10] Factory workers, cosmetologists, and handlers of pesticides are also at risk from regular contact with phenol derivatives, catechol derivatives, and sulfhydryls.[5] Manifestations of chemical leukoderma may begin in as early as 1 month and up to 24 years after the repeated insult. Differentiating chemical leukoderma from vitiligo is quite challenging, as most patients develop depigmented confetti macules that coalesce into patches at the primary site of exposure, and about one-quarter of patients develop depigmentation at distant sites.[5] Progressive depigmentation, a lack of Koebnerization, and a history of repeated exposure to a chemical favor a diagnosis of chemical leukoderma over vitiligo.[5]

Melanoma-Associated Leukoderma

Melanoma-associated leukoderma is a T cell–mediated autoimmune disorder that is distinct from vitiligo and that arises in 2% to 16% of patients with melanoma.[5] It can present with melanoma that is primary, recurrent, and metastatic or during immunotherapy with programmed cell death 1 or cytotoxic T lymphocyte antigen-4 inhibitors.[5] Melanoma-associated leukoderma may be suspected in adults older than 55 years who have depigmented macules and patches localized to photo-exposed regions.[5] Patients may also lack Koebnerization and may have no family history of vitiligo or serum antibodies against MART1. A thorough skin examination that includes evaluation of mucosal membranes, as well as a focused eye examination must be performed to identify the primary site of the melanoma.[5] Melanoma-associated

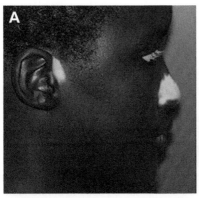
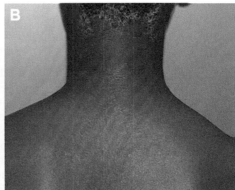

Fig. 3. Follicular vitiligo, manifesting as leukotrichia of the eyelashes (*A*), scalp, and body hairs (*B*) in a boy with skin of color. (Ezzedine, K., Amazan, E., Séneschal, J., Cario-André, M., Léauté-Labrèze, C., Vergier, B., Boralevi, F. and Taieb, A. (2012), Follicular vitiligo: a new form of vitiligo. Pigment Cell & Melanoma Research, 25: 527-529. https://doi.org/10.1111/j.1755-148X.2012.00999.x.)

leukoderma triggered by immunotherapy has a good prognosis.[5]

Postinflammatory Depigmentation

Postinflammatory depigmentation is a concern for people with skin of color. It can occur following skin trauma or inflammation.[15] Iatrogenic causes of skin trauma that may lead to depigmentation include corticosteroid injections and burns from cryotherapy or lasers with high fluences.[5] Severe scratching, which may be due to chronic atopic or contact dermatitis, may also result in depigmentation.[15]

Localized depigmentation may present with induration and atrophy of the epidermis and hair follicles, indicating an inflammatory scarring process, such as discoid lupus erythematosus, lichen sclerosis, and scleroderma.[15] Patients with systemic

sclerosis may present with a "salt and pepper" pattern of depigmented patches containing perifollicular pigmentation similar to vitiligo repigmentation.[15] Long-standing lesions of discoid lupus can progress to plaques with central depigmentation and hyperpigmented borders, which are sometimes confused with inflammatory vitiligo or marginal vitiligo repigmentation.[5] It is important to recognize discoid lupus in patients with skin of color, as non-Latino Black patients were found to have the highest incidence and prevalence compared with all other groups.[16]

HYPOPIGMENTED SKIN CONDITIONS—LOCALIZED DISTRIBUTION
Postinflammatory Hypopigmentation

Postinflammatory hypopigmentation can be caused by many dermatoses (Table 1). It is frequently seen

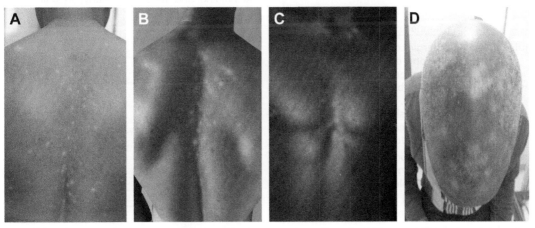

Fig. 4. Seborrheic macular hypopigmentation, also known as hypochromic vitiligo or vitiligo minor, in a patient with skin of color appearing as hypopigmented patches on the trunk (*A-C*) and scalp (*D*) in a seborrheic distribution. (*From* Krueger L, Saizan AL, Meehan SA, Ezzedine K, Hamzavi I, Elbuluk N. Seborrheic macular hypopigmentation: a case series proposing a new pigmentary disorder. *J Eur Acad Dermatol Venereol*. May 2022;36(5):e361-e362.)

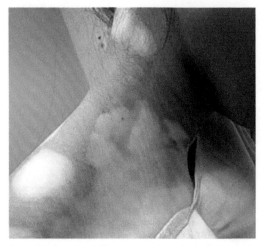

Fig. 5. Trichrome vitiligo, appearing clinically as multiple shades of hypopigmentation on the neck and shoulder in a patient with skin of color. (*From* Rodrigues M, Ezzedine K, Hamzavi I, Pandya AG, Harris JE. New discoveries in the pathogenesis and classification of vitiligo. *J Am Acad Dermatol.* Jul 2017;77(1):1-13.)

in patients with skin of color because of its increased noticeability on darker skin.[17–19] Although postinflammatory hypopigmentation is localized to areas of previous inflammation, low-grade inflammation may be clinically undetectable in patients with darker skin tones.[20] Pityriasis alba, pityriasis versicolor, seborrheic dermatitis, and atopic dermatitis (**Fig. 6**) are common causes of postinflammatory hypopigmentation and can be differentiated based on their distribution, associated morphologic features, and epidemiology.[20]

Pityriasis Alba

Pityriasis alba typically arises in patients by puberty and manifests as hypopigmented patches with ill-defined borders and minimal scale. This disorder normally occurs in patients with a personal or family history of atopy.[15] Lesions often appear after tanning, and areas of skin involvement frequently include sun-exposed regions such as the face and upper extremities.[15] The Wood's lamp can be used to differentiate pityriasis alba from early vitiligo, where patches of pityriasis alba do not fluoresce.[15]

Seborrheic Dermatitis

Seborrheic dermatitis is among the top 5 most common cutaneous diagnoses in patients with skin of color.[21] The incidence is marginally higher in African American patients. Evidence indicates that women with skin color have a disproportionately higher rate of seborrheic dermatitis, likely attributed to the frequent use of hair oils, pomades, and infrequent hair washing.[21] Seborrheic dermatitis is diagnosed by the presence of erythematous patches with a greasy scale in sebaceous body regions, such as the glabella, eyebrows, nasolabial folds, paranasal skin, bearded areas, upper chest, back, and skin flexures.[21] Erythema is not as noticeable in patients with darker skin, and this disorder may instead manifest as hypopigmentation. Petaloid seborrheic dermatitis is a subtype unique to adult patients with skin of color that appears as pink or hypopigmented polycyclic coalescing rings with minimal scale distributed along the hairline and face.[21] Similarly, in children of

Table 1 Common causes of postinflammatory hypopigmentation	
Cause	**Diagnoses**
Inflammatory	Allergic contact dermatitis, atopic dermatitis, discoid lupus erythematosus, insect-bite reaction, lichen planus, lichen striatus, pityriasis lichenoides chronica, psoriasis, sarcoidosis, scleroderma
Infectious	Chickenpox, herpes zoster, impetigo, pityriasis (tinea) versicolor, syphilis
Iatrogenic	Chemical peels, cryotherapy, dermabrasion, laser
Miscellaneous	Burns

Adapted from Vachiramon V, Thadanipon K. Postinflammatory hypopigmentation. *Clin Exp Dermatol.* Oct 2011;36(7):708-14.

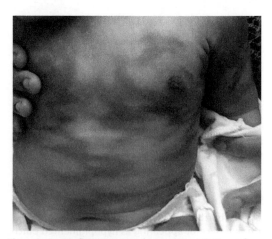

Fig. 6. Postinflammatory hypopigmentation from atopic dermatitis in an infant with skin of color.

color, seborrheic dermatitis is more likely to manifest with hypopigmentation, erythema, flaking, and overlying atopic dermatitis, rather than the conventional "cradle cap" appearance.[21]

Atopic Dermatitis

Although data show that atopic dermatitis is more common in children who are Black, Asian, and Pacific Islander than in White children, disease persistence and severity are much higher in Black children[18]; this is attributed to underrecognition, leading to delayed treatment.[18] In patients with skin of color, atopic dermatitis has a follicular or papular appearance with violaceous hues and is more likely to result in dyschromia.[18] The characteristic distribution of atopic dermatitis in infants and children is on the face or scalp and on the neck and flexural surfaces.[18] In patients with skin of color, extensor surfaces may also be involved.[18]

Leprosy

Leprosy is an infectious disease caused by *Mycobacterium leprae,* which is acquired from infected humans or armadillos. *M leprae* preferentially infects Schwann cells that are located in distal body sites with cooler temperatures, such as the nose, ears, elbows, knees, distal extremities, and testes.[20] Because of this, comparing pain sensations between the lesion and adjacent uninvolved skin is essential during diagnosis.[15,22] Numbness or hyperalgesia often develops before any cutaneous findings, which usually manifests as homogenous hypopigmented patches, erythema, and induration.[20] Progression of the disease destroys sweat glands and hair follicles, which leads to xerosis, scaliness, and atrichia.[22] The presence of any of these unique features warrants a biopsy.

Sarcoidosis

Compared with White patients, Black patients are diagnosed with sarcoidosis more frequently and often present with a more advanced systemic disease, leading to a poor prognosis.[23] Erythema nodosum is the most common nonspecific skin finding in sarcoidosis overall, and it is seen much less often in patients who are Black or Asian than in patients who are European, Puerto Rican, and Mexican.[23] Although a papular presentation predominates in Black patients, hypopigmented macules may be seen alone or in combination with brownish-red or violaceous papules, nodules, or plaques on the extremities.[23] The diagnostic granuloma may not be easily seen on histopathology in hypopigmented sarcoidosis, so a biopsy should be obtained from a location that exhibits induration or a papule, as well as hypopigmentation.[23]

Nevus Depigmentosus

Naevus depigmentosus is a benign lesion that manifests primarily in childhood. Despite its name, it appears as a unilateral hypopigmented patch with jagged borders.[15] Although it can be mistaken for vitiligo, naevus depigmentosus characteristically retains the hair pigment and maintains the same size and shape over time.[15]

Nevus Anemicus

Naevus anemicus is a benign congenital lesion that is often mistaken for vitiligo.[15] Rather than depigmentation, the patch appears paler than the surrounding skin due to sustained vasoconstriction from local catecholamine hypersensitivity. Diascopy is diagnostic, as blanching the lesion makes it indistinguishable from adjacent skin.[15]

HYPOPIGMENTED SKIN CONDITIONS— DIFFUSE DISTRIBUTION
Pityriasis (Tinea) Versicolor

Pityriasis versicolor is caused by overgrowth of the commensal yeast *Malassezia furfur* that normally resides as a commensal organism on human skin.[24] Characteristically, it manifests as multiple round or oval macules with a fine scale ranging from 3 to 5 mm.[25] Although pityriasis versicolor macules can be hypopigmented or hyperpigmented, most patients with darker skin will have macules with a hypopigmented appearance.[25] Characteristically, the shoulders and trunk are the most commonly affected body regions, but patients with skin of color may also have facial and neck involvement.[25] Under microscopy prepped with potassium hydroxide, skin scrapings will show characteristic spores and hyphae, distinguishing pityriasis versicolor from other hypopigmentation disorders.[15]

Hypopigmented Mycosis Fungoides

Hypopigmented mycosis fungoides is a subtype of cutaneous T-cell lymphoma with a higher incidence and mortality rate among patients with skin of color.[26] Typically, it spares the face and has a predilection for sun-protected body sites, especially the trunk, proximal extremities, and buttocks.[26] Patients with skin of color present with significant variability in pigmentation, infiltration, and scale in lesions of hypopigmented mycosis fungoides, which are usually larger than 5 cm in diameter with alopecia.[27] Clinical and histopathological findings must be correlated to diagnose all cases of mycosis fungoides. However, the clinical and histopathologic presentation of hypopigmented mycosis fungoides can mimic inflammatory dermatoses. If histologic evidence is inadequate for diagnosis, the patient should be monitored closely if clinical findings are suspicious for hypopigmented mycosis fungoides, as subsequent biopsies may be necessary to confirm the diagnosis.[28] Hypopigmented lesions are targeted by phototherapy and monitored closely, as pigmentation returns with remission, and hypopigmentation is the first sign of relapse.[27]

Pityriasis Lichenoides Chronica

Although pityriasis lichenoides chronica characteristically manifests as scaly or crusty papules in a pediatric patient, there is a hypopigmented variant that may be seen in patients with skin of color. The hypopigmented variant of pityriasis lichenoides chronica can be distinguished clinically from hypopigmented mycosis fungoides based on the smaller diameter of lesions (<5 cm), as well as the absence of erythema and atrophy. Although both diagnoses can occur in pediatric patients, those with pityriasis lichenoides chronica are typically younger than those with hypopigmented mycosis fungoides.[27]

Idiopathic Guttate Hypomelanosis

Idiopathic guttate hypomelanosis (IGH) manifests as asymptomatic, hypopigmented, 1- to 3-mm distinct macules on the limbs of middle-aged to older adults.[15,19] The confetti-like presentation of IGH can be mistaken for the confetti lesions in vitiligo.[15] Unlike with vitiligo, IGH lesions remain stable over time, rarely changing in size or coalescing.[29] Hypopigmentation is exaggerated in those with Fitzpatrick skin types IV to VI.[19]

Progressive Macular Hypomelanosis

Progressive macular hypomelanosis (PMH) is another common idiopathic condition with associated hypopigmentation.[15] All skin types can experience PMH. However, women of color from tropical climates are most commonly affected.[19] Macules are hypopigmented, asymptomatic, and symmetric, with ill-defined borders that develop into confluent patches on the trunk. Previously *Propionibacterium acnes* was thought to be involved, but more recently *Cutibacterium acnes* has been implicated in the cause of this disorder.[1] *C acnes* produces porphyrin, which under Wood lamp appears as a follicular red fluorescence.[1,18,19] Histologic analysis shows decreased epidermal melanin, uncharacteristic lymphocyte infiltration of the dermis, and no change to the total number of melanocytes.[19] Dermoscopic findings of PMH demonstrate a brownish-white background, scaling

confined to skin cleavage lines, and mild reticular pigment.[24]

TREATMENT

Disorders of hypopigmentation and depigmentation can be challenging to treat and may be a significant source of stress for many patients with skin of color. Identifying the source of hypopigmentation or depigmentation is the first step in treatment, as the underlying cause can be targeted with therapy or the offending agent can be terminated.[21,30] However, in some cases of chemical leukoderma, acquired vitiligo may continue progressing even after the causative substance has been removed.[5] Patients with acquired vitiligo from chemical leukoderma, along with several other disorders of hypopigmentation and depigmentation, can be treated with the same modalities as for vitiligo, namely narrow-band ultraviolet B and excimer laser phototherapy.[5] Although phototherapy helps promote repigmentation, patients should be aware that it may also transiently darken their overall skin tone.[31] Ruxolitinib, a topical JAK1 inhibitor, is the first Food and Drug Administration–approved treatment of vitiligo, and it is also approved to treat atopic dermatitis, a disorder that may also lead to depigmentation in patients with skin of color.

CLINICAL OUTCOMES/LONG-TERM RECOMMENDATIONS

Most hypopigmentation and depigmentation disorders of the skin do not have life-threatening systemic manifestations, and depending on the severity and diagnosis, repigmentation can occur from 3 to 6 months to 2 years; however, depigmentation or hypopigmentation may be permanent.[17,32] Accurate recognition of these disorders in skin of all colors is essential to identify the correct treatment modality. Precautions should be made when using certain treatment modalities, such as energy-based devices, cryotherapy, and intralesional corticosteroids, to avoid the development of iatrogenic postinflammatory hypopigmentation.[32]

SUMMARY

Although hypopigmentation and depigmentation disorders of the skin occur in patients with all skin colors, they manifest differently and at different rates in people with skin of color. The stark contrast between involved and uninvolved skin in patients with darker skin tones contributes to a higher psychosocial disease burden in this patient population. Physicians have a responsibility to diagnose these disorders accurately by obtaining a comprehensive medical history and performing a detailed physical examination with a Wood's lamp, dermoscopy, and biopsy when indicated. Treatment should be based on the underlying cause of the disorder, and an alternative diagnosis may be made if repigmentation does not occur after treatment with particular therapeutic agents.

CLINICS CARE POINTS

- Physicians must be aware of the different manifestations of depigmentation and hypopigmentation disorders in patients with skin of color.
- The use of a Wood's lamp is essential for differentiating hypopigmented and depigmented skin disorders, even in patients with skin of color who have a stark contrast between involved and uninvolved skin.
- Inflammation is associated with hypopigmentation in patients with skin of color and may be challenging to detect if mild in severity.

DISCLOSURE

M.S. Ceresnie is a subinvestigator for Avita Medical, Incyte Corporation, Clinuvel Pharmaceuticals, and The Immune Tolerance Network. I.H. Hamzavi helped develop the vitiligo area scoring index but does not have a proprietary interest in the score and has served as an advisory board member for AbbVie; a consultant for Incyte Corporation, Pfizer, and UCB; a principal investigator for AbbVie, Bayer, Clinuvel Pharmaceuticals, Estée Lauder, Ferndale Laboratories, Galderma Laboratories LP, GE Healthcare, Incyte Corporation, Janssen, Janssen Biotech, Johnson & Johnson, Lenicura, LEO Pharma, Pfizer, and Unigen; a subinvestigator for Amgen, Bristol Myers Squibb, Foamix Pharmaceuticals, and Janssen; past-president of the Hidradenitis Suppurativa Foundation; and co-chair of the Global Vitiligo Foundation. The authors have no other relevant disclosures.

REFERENCES

1. Rodney IJPJ, Hexsel D, Halder RM. Disorders of Hypopigmentation. In: Kelly A, Taylor SC, Lim HW, et al, editors. Taylor and Kelly's Dermatology for skin of color, 2nd edition. McGraw Hill; 2016. chap Chapter 48: Disorders of Hypopigmentation.
2. Ezzedine K, Eleftheriadou V, Jones H, et al. Psychosocial Effects of Vitiligo: A Systematic Literature Review. Am J Clin Dermatol 2021;22(6):757–74.
3. Gorbatenko-Roth K, Prose N, Kundu RV, et al. Assessment of Black Patients' Perception of Their Dermatology Care. JAMA Dermatol 2019;155(10): 1129–34.
4. McKenzie S, Brown-Korsah JB, Syder NC, et al. Variations in Genetics, Biology, and Phenotype of Cutaneous Disorders in Skin of Color. Part II: Differences in Clinical Presentation and Disparities in Cutaneous Disorders in Skin of Color. J Am Acad Dermatol 2022. https://doi.org/10.1016/j.jaad.2022.03.067.
5. Saleem MD, Oussedik E, Schoch JJ, et al. Acquired disorders with depigmentation: A systematic approach to vitiliginoid conditions. J Am Acad Dermatol 2019;80(5):1215–31.e6.
6. Dennin MH, Stein SL, Rosenblatt AE. Vitiligoid variant of lichen sclerosus in young girls with darker skin types. Pediatr Dermatol 2018;35(2):198–201.
7. Chatterjee M, Neema S. Dermoscopy of Pigmentary Disorders in Brown Skin. Dermatol Clin 2018;36(4): 473–85.
8. Kim YC, Kim YJ, Kang HY, et al. Histopathologic features in vitiligo. Am J Dermatopathol 2008;30(2): 112–6.
9. Gandhi K, Ezzedine K, Anastassopoulos KP, et al. Prevalence of Vitiligo Among Adults in the United States. JAMA Dermatol 2022;158(1):43–50.
10. Boissy RE, Manga P. On the etiology of contact/occupational vitiligo. Pigment Cell Res 2004;17(3):208–14.
11. Hann SK, Kim YS, Yoo JH, et al. Clinical and histopathologic characteristics of trichrome vitiligo. J Am Acad Dermatol 2000;42(4):589–96.
12. Gan EY, Cario-André M, Pain C, et al. Follicular vitiligo: A report of 8 cases. J Am Acad Dermatol 2016;74(6):1178–84.
13. Ezzedine K, Mahé A, van Geel N, et al. Hypochromic vitiligo: delineation of a new entity. Br J Dermatol 2015;172(3):716–21.
14. Krueger L, Saizan AL, Meehan SA, et al. Seborrheic macular hypopigmentation: a case series proposing a new pigmentary disorder. J Eur Acad Dermatol Venereol 2022;36(5):e361–2.
15. Goh BK, Pandya AG. Presentations, Signs of Activity, and Differential Diagnosis of Vitiligo. Dermatol Clin 2017;35(2):135–44.
16. Izmirly P, Buyon J, Belmont HM, et al. Population-based prevalence and incidence estimates of primary discoid lupus erythematosus from the Manhattan Lupus Surveillance Program. Lupus Science & Medicine 2019;6(1):e000344. https://doi.org/10.1136/lupus-2019-000344.
17. Vachiramon V, Thadanipon K. Postinflammatory hypopigmentation. Clin Exp Dermatol 2011;36(7):708–14.
18. Okoji UK, Agim NG, Heath CR. Features of Common Skin Disorders in Pediatric Patients with Skin of Color. Dermatol Clin 2022;40(1):83–93.
19. Hadi A, Elbuluk N. Common conditions in skin of color. Semin Cutan Med Surg 2016;35(4):184–90.

20. Saleem MD, Oussedik E, Picardo M, et al. Acquired disorders with hypopigmentation: A clinical approach to diagnosis and treatment. J Am Acad Dermatol 2019;80(5):1233–50.e10.

21. Elgash M, Dlova N, Ogunleye T, et al. Seborrheic Dermatitis in Skin of Color: Clinical Considerations. J Drugs Dermatol 2019;18(1):24–7.

22. Tey HL. Approach to hypopigmentation disorders in adults. Clin Exp Dermatol 2010;35(8):829–34.

23. Heath CR, David J, Taylor SC. Sarcoidosis: Are there differences in your skin of color patients? J Am Acad Dermatol 2012;66(1). 121.e1-14.

24. Ankad BS, Koti VR. Dermoscopic approach to hypopigmentary or depigmentary lesions in skin of color. Clinical Dermatology Review 2020;4(2):79.

25. Kallini JR, Riaz F, Khachemoune A. Tinea versicolor in dark-skinned individuals. Int J Dermatol 2014; 53(2):137–41.

26. Rodney IJ, Kindred C, Angra K, et al. Hypopigmented mycosis fungoides: a retrospective clinico-histopathologic study. J Eur Acad Dermatol Venereol 2017;31(5):808–14.

27. Hinds GA, Heald P. Cutaneous T-cell lymphoma in skin of color. J Am Acad Dermatol 2009;60(3): 359–75. quiz 376-8.

28. Furlan FC, Sanches JA. Hypopigmented mycosis fungoides: a review of its clinical features and pathophysiology. An Bras Dermatol 2013;88(6):954–60.

29. Ayoade KO, Pandya AG. Idiopathic guttate hypomelanosis. Dermatology Atlas for Skin of Color 2014; 17–20.

30. Alexis A, Woolery-Lloyd H, Andriessen A, et al. Insights in Skin of Color Patients With Atopic Dermatitis and the Role of Skincare in Improving Outcomes. J Drugs Dermatol 2022;21(5):462–70.

31. Syed ZU, Hamzavi IH. Photomedicine and phototherapy considerations for patients with skin of color. Photodermatol Photoimmunol Photomed 2011;27(1): 10–6.

32. Adotama P, Papac N, Alexis A, et al. Common Dermatologic Procedures and the Associated Complications Unique to Skin of Color. Dermatol Surg 2021;47(3):355–9.

Diagnosing Atopic Dermatitis in Skin of Color

Waleed Adawi, MS[a], Hannah Cornman, BS[a], Anusha Kambala, BS[a], Shanae Henry, MS[a], Shawn G. Kwatra, MD[a],*

KEYWORDS

- Atopic dermatitis • Skin of color • Diagnosis • Erythema • African American • Asian • Itch
- Eczema

KEY POINTS

- Skin of color patients are disproportionately affected by atopic dermatitis (AD) and carry a heightened disease burden with greater disease severity and health care utilization.
- Unique features of AD in skin of color patients include greater papular and extensor involvement in African Americans and greater psoriasiform presentations in Asian AD patients.
- Erythema in dark skin can appear violaceous and brown; scoring tools reliant on erythema may delay diagnosis and underpredict severity of AD.
- Dyspigmentation is a common sequalae of AD in skin of color patients that carries a significant disease burden.

INTRODUCTION

Atopic Dermatitis (AD) is an extremely pruritic inflammatory skin disease that has a worldwide prevalence of approximately 2.69%, with significant variability by country.[1] In the United States, AD affects approximately 10% to 12% of children and 7% to 8% of adults.[2–4] Stratifying by age, AD is most prevalent among African American children and Asian adults.[5,6] As a chronic disease characterized by recurrent pruritus, AD adversely affects quality of life and is associated with sleep disturbance, many systemic disease comorbidities, and increased health care utilization.[7–11] AD disproportionately impacts Black patients, who incur greater disease severity and AD-related medical expenses compared with non-Black patients.[12–14] Given the disproportionate prevalence and burden placed on skin of color patients, it is important that clinicians are able to diagnose and treat AD in patients of all skin types to help reduce disparities in care. Here we highlight important differences in the pathogenesis, clinical presentation, and treatment options for AD in skin of color patients.

PATHOGENESIS

AD has a complex pathogenesis that involves interactions between the innate and adaptive immune system with various cell types in the skin and sensory nerves.[15] Early steps in the disease process involve dysfunction of the skin barrier, allowing entry of allergens and microbes, and initiating an abnormal innate immune response (Fig. 1).[16] Aberrant adaptive immune pathways are activated leading to degradation of the skin barrier, followed by immune activation and sensitization of sensory neurons (see Fig. 1).[15,17] Subsequent scratching further damages the skin, allowing for additional susceptibility to microbes, creating a positive feedback loop (Fig. 2). The degree of cutaneous immune activation can vary between patients, creating distinct AD endotypes.[13]

The authors have nothing to disclose.
[a] Department of Dermatology, Johns Hopkins University School of Medicine
* Corresponding author. Johns Hopkins Itch Center, Johns Hopkins University School of Medicine, 206, Koch CRBII, 1550 Orleans Street, Baltimore, MD 21231.
E-mail address: skwatra1@jhmi.edu
Twitter: @drshawnkwatra (S.G.K.)

Dermatol Clin 41 (2023) 417–429
https://doi.org/10.1016/j.det.2023.02.003

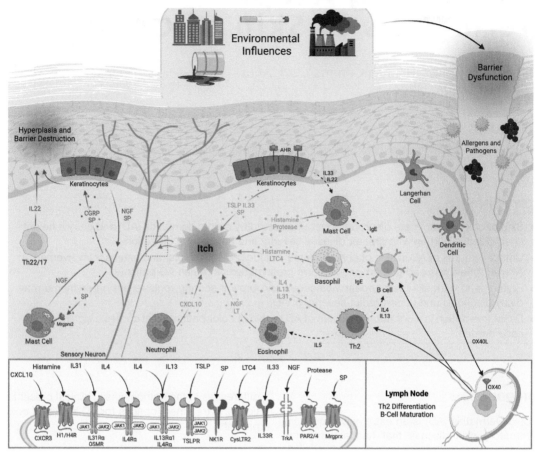

Fig. 1. Atopic dermatitis pathogenesis. AHR, aryl hydrocarbon receptor; CGRP, calcitonin gene-related peptide; CXCL10, CXC Motif Chemokine Ligand 10; CXCR3, CXC Motif Chemokine receptor; CysLTR2, cysteinyl leukotriene receptor 2; H1/4R, histamine receptor types 1 and 4; IgE, immunoglobulin E; IL13, interleukin 13; IL22, interleukin 22; IL31, interleukin 31; IL31R, interleukin 31 receptor; IL33, interleukin 33; IL4, interleukin 4; IL4R, interleukin 4 receptor; IL5, interleukin 5; LTC4, leukotriene C4; Mrgprx, mas-related G protein-coupled receptor; NGF, nerve growth factor; NK1R, neurokinin 1 receptor; OSMR, Oncostatin M Receptor; SP, substance P; Th17, Type 17 helper T-cell; Th2, Type 2 helper T-cell; Th22, Type 22 helper T-cell; TSLP, thymic stromal lymphopoietin; TSLPR, thymic stromal lymphopoietin receptor.

Skin Barrier Dysfunction

Skin barrier dysfunction is a hallmark component of AD. In AD-affected skin, stratum corneum barrier impairment is correlated with lower levels of ceramides and increased transepidermal water loss (TEWL) (see **Fig. 2**).[18,19] At baseline, normal African American skin has been found to have lower levels of ceramide, lower pH in the stratum corneum, and higher TEWL compared with normal Caucasian skin (see **Fig. 2**).[20] These findings likely contribute to the increased degree of xerosis experienced by Black patients.

The strongest genetic risk factor for barrier dysfunction in AD is a loss-of-function mutation in filaggrin (FLG), a stratum corneum structural protein. Patients with mutations in FLG are more likely to have an earlier onset and greater severity

of AD, compared with those without the mutation.[21] Interestingly, FLG mutations are observed significantly less frequently in African Americans with AD than in Caucasians with AD.[22] However, low levels of FLG2, a protein important for epidermal differentiation, are correlated with active skin inflammation in AD.[23] FLG2 mutations are associated with more persistent AD in African American children.[24] No association has been reported with FLG2 mutations in Europeans with AD.[23,24] Claudin 1, a tight junction gene, is also associated with barrier dysfunction and early-onset AD in Ethiopian patients.[25]

Immune Dysregulation

Dysregulation of the innate and adaptive immune response plays a crucial role in the development

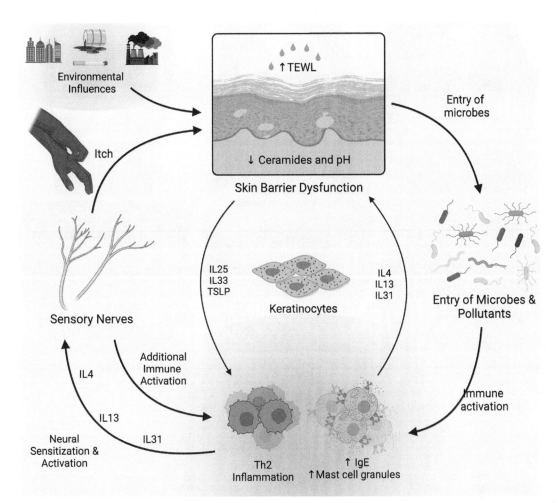

Fig. 2. Inflammatory cycle of AD. IL13, interleukin 13; IL25, interleukin 25; IL31, interleukin 31; IL33, interleukin 33; IL4, interleukin 4; Th2, Type 2 helper T-cell; TSLP, thymic stromal lymphopoietin; TWEL, transepidermal water loss.

of AD. Deficiencies in the immune system increase susceptibility to infection and trigger the inflammatory response. When activated, keratinocytes secrete cytokines that recruit mast cells, T-cells, dendritic cells, and eosinophils, several of which demonstrate racial differences.[26] Mast cells in African American skin contain larger granules, with variation in enzymes and cell structure.[27] In addition, African American AD lesions have greater infiltration of dendritic cells marked by high-affinity immunoglobulin E (IgE) receptors compared with European AD lesions.[28] African Americans also have higher serum IgE levels.[29]

AD is primarily driven by Th2 inflammation. Mutations in interleukin (IL) 4, IL13, IL31, and their appropriate receptors (IL4Rα, IL13Rα, and IL31Rα) are significantly associated with AD. IL4 and IL4Rα in particular are associated with an increased risk of AD in Egyptian children.[30] Recent advances indicate there are various AD disease

subtypes, partially attributed to the modulation of different immune pathways.[31] African Americans, for example, have broad immune pathway activation with increases in Th2-related and Th22-related pathways.[13] Increased expression of Th1 and Th17 cytokines has also been observed in sub-Saharan Africans compared with Central Europeans with AD.[32]

Environmental Triggers

The etiology of racial disparities in AD prevalence and severity reaches beyond genetics, highlighting the importance of environmental influence. Living in a metropolitan area is associated with a high risk of AD, likely due to environmental pollution and exposure to infectious diseases (see **Fig. 1**).[33] Urban living is also associated with alterations to the skin microbiome, with increased pathogenic microorganisms such as *Staphylococcal aureus*.[34]

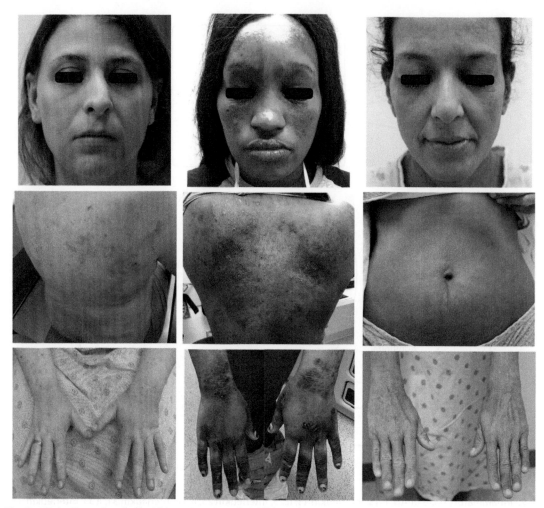

Fig. 3. AD in Caucasian (*left*), African American (*middle*), and Asian (*right*) skin.

Because African Americans are more likely than Caucasians to live in densely populated areas, they may have an increased risk for AD.[35]

Additionally, Black children have increased odds of being exposed to tobacco smoke and traffic-related air pollution, having a caregiver with lower educational attainment, and coming from a lower-income family (<$30,000/year).[36,37] Longitudinal exposure to the aforementioned environmental pollution is associated with the development of asthma and AD, particularly among Black children.[37]

CLINICAL PRESENTATION

Classically, AD presents as recurrent pruritic, inflammatory, and excoriated papules and plaques, classically in flexural areas. However, defining AD only by this classical clinical presentation is not adequate for diverse patient populations, as there are numerous racial and ethnic differences in AD morphology, distributions, texture, and pigmentation that make diagnosing AD challenging across skin types (**Fig. 3**).

Morphology

In skin of color patients, AD can have a heterogenous distribution and morphology compared with traditional, classical criteria for AD. For example, in both the Hanifin and Rajka and the UK Working Party, flexural involvement is listed as a major criterion for diagnosing AD.[38] Although exceedingly common in Caucasians, African Americans also often present with lesions on the extensor or truncal surfaces (**Fig. 4**).[39,40] Additionally skin lesions in skin of color patients commonly present with lichenification (**Figs. 5** and **6**) and with greater papular involvement of lesions with perifollicular accentuation (see **Fig. 4**; **Fig. 7**).[41,42] Psoriasiform thickening and scaling often manifest in Asian patients with AD (see **Fig. 5**E). Severe xerosis and concurrent prurigo

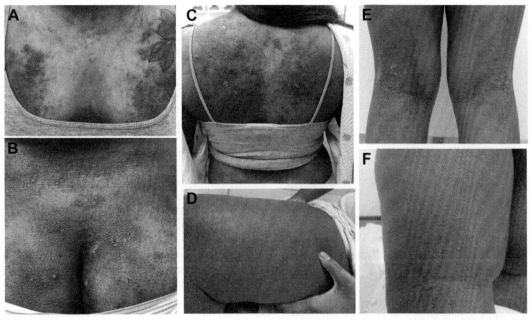

Fig. 4. AD in Black patients. Hyperpigmented perifollicular accentuation coalescing into plaques on the chest (*A*) and buttocks (*B*), with nodular development on the back (*C*). Erythema on the extensor lower extremity (*D*). Flexural plaques with skin fissuring on the popliteal fossa (*E*). Erythema and papules on the upper extremity (*F*).

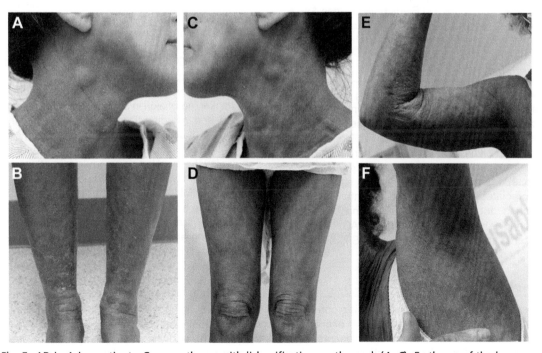

Fig. 5. AD in Asian patients. Gross erythema with lichenification on the neck (*A, C*). Erythema of the lower extremities with exfoliation (*B, D*). Erythematous papules and plaques in addition to psoriasiform scaling on the upper extremity (*E, F*).

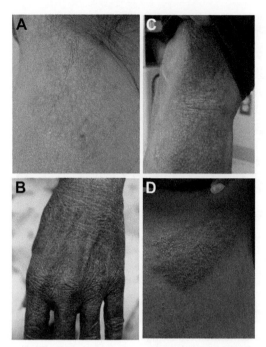

Fig. 6. Lichenification in skin of color patients. Lichenification of the forearm (*A*) and popliteal fossa (*C*) on an Asian patient with AD. Lichenification and xerosis of the extensor wrist (*B*) and trunk (*D*) on a Black patient with AD.

nodules in addition to eczematous lesions are also observed more often in Black patients (see **Fig. 6**; **Fig. 8**).[13] Finally, African Americans also have increased lichenification of lesions.[43]

Erythema

Erythema is a common skin finding in AD and is incorporated into several AD clinical scoring tools. Because of baseline differences in pigmentation, erythema can appear violaceous and brown in skin of color, thus it is harder to distinguish in darker skin tones (see **Figs. 4** and **5**; **Fig. 9**). For this reason, erythema is easily underappreciated in skin of color patients and using scoring tools reliant on erythema, such as scoring atopic dermatitis (SCORAD) and the eczema area and scoring index (EASI), may delay diagnosis and treatment.[44]

Dyspigmentation

Post-inflammatory dyspigmentation is a complication of AD that is more common in skin of color patients.[45] It most often presents as hypopigmentation, which persists after resolution of the disease. This can pose a significant burden as hypopigmentation contrasts more in darker skin

tones (**Fig. 10**).[46] Dyspigmentation can also occur with longer-term topical corticosteroid utilization, highlighting the importance of non-steroidal treatment options in skin of color patients.

Disease Severity

Skin of color patients are more likely to present with greater disease severity compared with other patients, both within adult and pediatric populations.[42,44] Significant health care disparities that impact health status and access to care are likely related to decreased socioeconomic status, systemic racism, and several additional contributing factors.[35,47] Black patients with poorly controlled AD are less likely to visit a dermatologist, while more likely to visit primary care or an emergency department compared with white patients.[48] Black children are also 1.5 times more likely to miss school because of AD compared with their White peers.[49]

DIAGNOSIS

The wide range of dermatological manifestations and variability across various races and ethnicities make AD challenging to diagnose. There are a few sets of validated diagnostic criteria that clinicians use when diagnosing AD; however, these may not account for the heterogeneity of AD in skin of color patients. Updates to diagnostic tools are needed to account for the differences in AD clinical presentation between races. We provide an example with an adopted Hanifin and Rajka criteria for AD in skin of color populations (**Fig. 11**)[50]; expanding it to include "extensor papular involvement, lichenification, or psoriasiform thickening of skin in skin of color" as a major criterion, and including "Dyspigmentation (post-inflammatory hypopigmentation and hyperpigmentation)", "Psoriasiform scaling", and "Secondary papular involvement/prurigo nodule formation" as minor criteria. By broadening the criteria to diagnose AD, clinicians can be better equipped to diagnose AD in a variety of patient populations.

There are many limitations with current diagnostic criteria and clinical bedside tools to accurately assess disease severity in skin of color patients with AD. When assessing disease severity in skin of color patients with AD, a patient's self-reported itch severity is a helpful adjunctive assessment as a surrogate marker of disease severity. Monitoring the itch numeric rating scale, from 0 to 10, and worst itch rating scale or peak pruritus scale, in skin of color patients is a real-time indicator of disease progression and treatment response.

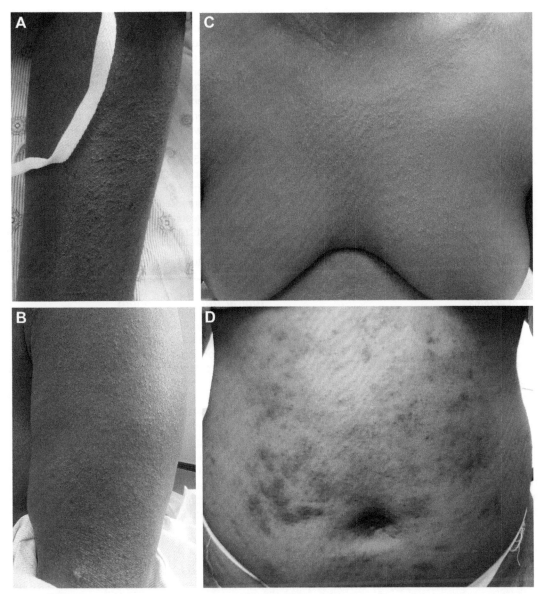

Fig. 7. Perifollicular accentuation on the lower extremity (*A*), upper extremity (*B*), chest (*C*), and trunk (*D*) in Black patients with AD.

DIFFERENTIAL DIAGNOSIS

The diagnosis of AD is made based on clinical presentation and patient history. Important differential diagnoses include seborrheic dermatitis, lichen planus, contact dermatitis, psoriasis, and cutaneous T-cell lymphoma. Especially in Asian patients, AD may present similar to psoriasis, with scaling lesions on extensor surfaces. Lichen planus appears violaceous and papular, which can be difficult to distinguish from erythema in Black patients. Mycosis fungoides, which also suffers from significant racial disparities in its clinical presentation and prognosis, also may mimic AD, often featuring a hypopigmented variant in Black patients.[51] Prurigo nodularis (PN) is another disease in the differential diagnosis for AD.[52] In skin of color patients, AD often has secondary prurigo nodules as well as papular variants.[53] As long as eczematous lesions are also present, this is still the chief diagnosis.[54] PN that is not associated with AD often develops in middle age and can be associated with type 2 diabetes, chronic kidney disease, and HIV.[55–58] Of note, PN disproportionately affects skin of color patients and is associated with several health disparities.[59–62]

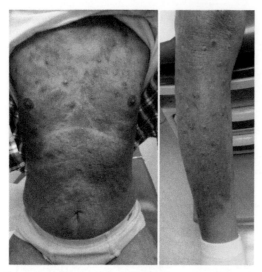

Fig. 8. Concurrent AD and PN. These represent secondary prurigo nodules appearing in the midst of areas of eczema.

TREATMENT

Across all races and ethnic groups, the treatment goals of AD include the prevention of flares to help decrease pain and itch and the repair and maintenance of a functional skin barrier. Initial management begins with moisturizers, the avoidance of irritants, and a variety of topical therapies. Topical agents include topical steroids, calcineurin inhibitors, phosphodiesterase-4 inhibitors, janus kinase (JAK)-signal transducer and activator of transcription (STAT) inhibitors, and wet wrap therapy. In recalcitrant AD, phototherapy and systemic

options that target key cytokines can offer more effective control of symptoms.

Despite the numerous treatment options available and the greater disease severity affecting patients of color, skin of color patients are less likely to receive novel therapies for AD than White patients.[63] Even when prescribed, the efficacy of common therapies in non-White ethnic groups is often unknown. This is likely due to the underrepresentation of non-White races in clinical trials, as only 59.5% of studies between 2000 and 2009 included race and ethnicity within the demographic information.[64] Additionally, only 10% of studies commented on race or ethnicity when interpreting results, making it difficult to extrapolate the results to other racial groups. The inclusion of race and ethnicity in future clinical trials is necessary to determine the best treatment regimen for all racial groups.

Topical Treatment Options

Until recently, initial therapy for AD relied greatly on emollients, non-specific topical anti-inflammatory agents, including topical corticosteroids and calcineurin inhibitors. For skin of color patients, colloidal oatmeal can protect the skin barrier and increase skin pH.[20] Long-term use of potent topical corticosteroids can cause hypopigmentation in darker skin tones that may persist after the resolution of AD. Non-steroidal agents are therefore of increased importance in skin of color patients with AD. Of the therapeutic studies that stratified treatment outcomes by race, pimecrolimus 1% cream showed similar efficacy between all racial groups.[65] Crisaborole, a PDE-4 inhibitor,

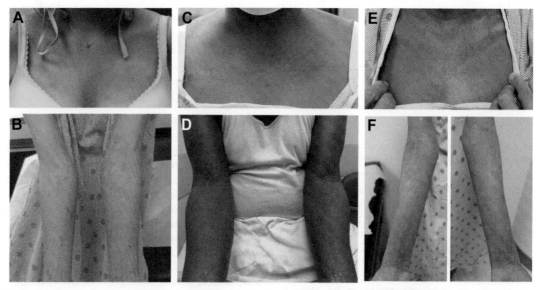

Fig. 9. AD on the chest and forearms of White (A, B), Black (C, D), and Asian (E, F) patients.

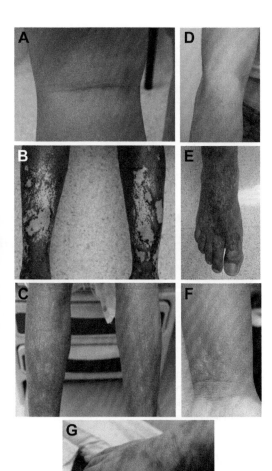

Fig. 10. Post-inflammatory hypopigmentation on Caucasian, Asian, and Black skin. Post-inflammatory hypopigmentation of the popliteal fossa (*A*) and lateral forearm (*D*) on a Caucasian patient. Asian patient with severe depigmentation of the shin (*B*) and dorsal foot (*E*). Black patient with hypopigmentation of the shin (*C*), distal forearm (*F*), and hand and wrist (*G*).

also demonstrated similar treatment outcomes across racial groups.[66] The topical JAK inhibitor roxulitinib, approved for the treatment of mild-to-moderate AD, significantly improves itch, sleep, and quality of life across various races and ethnicities in AD patients.[67] Roxulitinib provides greater itch reduction than triamcinolone, while not having the associated risk of hypopigmentation.[68] Several emerging topical therapies for AD such as the phosphodiesterase-4 (PDE-4) inhibitor, roflumilast, an aryl hydrocarbon receptor modulator, tapinarof, and a pan-JAK inhibitor, delgocitinib, have also shown promising outcomes in clinical trials.[69–71]

Systemic Treatment Options

Currently, there are four systemic agents available for the treatment of AD: dupilumab, tralokinumab, upadacitinib, and abrocitinib. Dupilumab, a monoclonal antibody targeting IL-4Rα, provides significant improvement in the molecular signature of barrier-related genes, inflammatory mediators, and cytokines.[72] This correlates with the clinical improvements in EASI, peak pruritus numerical rating score (NRS), and dermatology dife quality index (DLQI) observed in patients, with post hoc analysis showing similar efficacy across all racial subgroups.[73] Tralokinumab, a monoclonal antibody targeting IL-13, reduces investigator global assessment (IGA) scores and EASI-75, and provides patients with improvements in pruritus, sleep interference, and quality of life.[74] Upadacitinib and abrocitinib are both oral JAK1 inhibitors recently approved for the treatment of AD. Clinical trials of both biologics showed significant improvements in EASI-75 and vIGA in patients with moderate to severe AD.[75–78] Patient populations included White, Black, Asian, and Hispanic patients.

Cultural Considerations

Patients in African, Asian, and Hispanic cultures frequently employ complementary and alternative medicine techniques to treat skin conditions before seeking care from a dermatologist. For example, among Koreans, bath therapy and oriental medicine (use of herbs, acupuncture, and cupping) are commonly used to treat AD.[79] However, relapses, short-term alleviation, incomplete resolution, and post-inflammatory hyperpigmentation were all reasons for subsequently seeking medical treatment.

CLINICAL OUTCOMES

Clinical outcomes are difficult to measure in skin of color patients, as existing tools to assess AD are heavily reliant on erythema.[80] An alternative option is to use patient symptoms, including itch intensity, as markers of disease severity and treatment response in patients. Updates to diagnostic tools are needed to assist clinicians in early diagnosis and intervention of AD. We provide an adopted Hanifin and Rajka criteria for AD in skin of color populations (see **Fig. 11**), encompassing the various presentations of AD among a variety of races and ethnicities. This can assist clinicians in earlier diagnosis, thereby, creating opportunities to improve outcomes in skin of color patients.

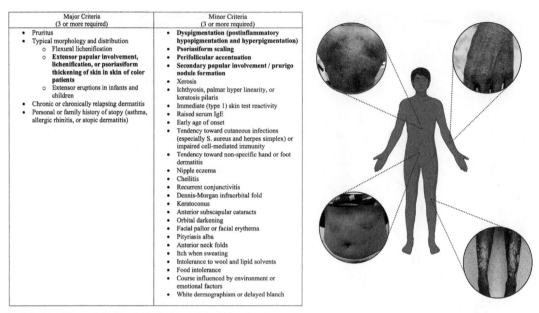

Major Criteria (3 or more required)	Minor Criteria (3 or more required)

• Pruritus
• Typical morphology and distribution
  o Flexural lichenification
  o **Extensor papular involvement, lichenification, or psoriasiform thickening of skin in skin of color patients**
  o Extensor eruptions in infants and children
• Chronic or chronically relapsing dermatitis
• Personal or family history of atopy (asthma, allergic rhinitis, or atopic dermatitis)
	• **Dyspigmentation (postinflammatory hypopigmentation and hyperpigmentation)**
	• **Psoriasiform scaling**
	• **Perifollicular accentuation**
	• **Secondary papular involvement / prurigo nodule formation**
	• Xerosis
	• Ichthyosis, palmar hyper linearity, or keratosis pilaris
	• Immediate (type 1) skin test reactivity
	• Raised serum IgE
	• Early age of onset
	• Tendency toward cutaneous infections (especially S. aureus and herpes simplex) or impaired cell-mediated immunity
	• Tendency toward non-specific hand or foot dermatitis
	• Nipple eczema
	• Cheilitis
	• Recurrent conjunctivitis
	• Dennis-Morgan infraorbital fold
	• Keratoconus
	• Anterior subscapular cataracts
	• Orbital darkening
	• Facial pallor or facial erythema
	• Pityriasis alba
	• Anterior neck folds
	• Itch when sweating
	• Intolerance to wool and lipid solvents
	• Food intolerance
	• Course influenced by environment or emotional factors
	• White dermographism or delayed blanch

Fig. 11. Hanifin and Rajka Criteria for AD in skin of color.

CLINICS CARE POINTS

- Skin of color patients are disproportionately affected by atopic dermatitis and suffer a greater disease burden, often presenting later in the disease process.

- Clinical manifestations of atopic dermatitis can vary in skin of color patients, often times with greater extensor and papular involvement in African Americans and psoriasiform scaling in Asian patients.

- Assessing itch intensity is a useful bedside tool to objectively assess disease severity in skin of color patients.

DICLOSURE

Dr Kwatra is an advisory board member/consultant for AbbVie, Aslan Pharmaceuticals, Arcutis Biotherapeutics, Castle Biosciences, Celldex Therapeutics, Galderma, Genzada Pharmaceuticals, Incyte Corporation, Johnson & Johnson, Leo Pharma, Novartis Pharmaceuticals Corporation, Pfizer, Regeneron Pharmaceuticals, and Sanofi, an Investigator for Galderma, Incyte, Pfizer, and Sanofi, as well as on the Board of Directors for the Skin of Color Society. Dr Kwatra is also supported by the National Institute of Arthritis and Musculoskeletal and Skin Diseases of the National Institutes of Health under Award Number K23AR077073. The content is solely the responsibility of the authors and does not necessarily represent the official views of the National Institutes of Health.

REFERENCES

1. Hadi HA, Tarmizi AI, Khalid KA, et al. The epidemiology and global burden of atopic dermatitis: a narrative review. Life 2021;11(9):936.
2. Shaw TE, Currie GP, Koudelka CW, et al. Eczema prevalence in the United States: data from the 2003 National Survey of Children's Health. J Invest Dermatol 2011;131(1):67–73.
3. Silverberg JI, Simpson EL. Associations of childhood eczema severity: a US population based study. Dermatitis 2014;25(3):107.
4. Chiesa Fuxench ZC, Block JK, Boguniewicz M, et al. Atopic dermatitis in america study: a cross-sectional study examining the prevalence and disease burden of atopic dermatitis in the US adult population. J Invest Dermatol 2019;139(3):583–90.
5. Hou A, Silverberg JI. Secular trends of atopic dermatitis and its comorbidities in United States children between 1997 and 2018. Arch Dermatol Res 2022;314(3):267–74.
6. Leasure A.C. and Cohen J.M., Prevalence of eczema among adults in the United States: a cross-sectional study in the All of Us research program, Arch Dermatol Res, 2022, 1–3. Epub ahead of print.
7. Silverberg JI, Gelfand JM, Margolis DJ, et al. Patient burden and quality of life in atopic dermatitis in US

adults: a population-based cross-sectional study. Ann Allergy Asthma Immunol 2018;121(3):340–7.

8. Roh YS, Huang AH, Sutaria N, et al. Real-world co-morbidities of atopic dermatitis in the US adult ambulatory population. J Am Acad Dermatol 2022; 86(4):835–45.

9. Drucker AM, Qureshi AA, Amand C, et al. Health care resource utilization and costs among adults with atopic dermatitis in the United States: a claims-based analysis. J Allergy Clin Immunol Pract 2018;6(4):1342–8.

10. Huang AH, Roh YS, Sutaria N, et al. Real-world co-morbidities of atopic dermatitis in the pediatric ambulatory population in the United States. J Am Acad Dermatol 2021;85(4):893–900.

11. Kwatra SG, Gruben D, Fung S, et al. Psychosocial comorbidities and health status among adults with moderate-to-severe atopic dermatitis: a 2017 us national health and wellness survey analysis. Adv Ther 2021;38(3):1627–37.

12. Chovatiya R., Begolka W.S., Thibau I.J., et al., Financial burden and impact of atopic dermatitis out-of-pocket healthcare expenses among black individuals in the United States, Arch Dermatol Res, 314 (8), 2022, 739–747.

13. Wongvibulsin S, Sutaria N, Kannan S, et al. Transcriptomic analysis of atopic dermatitis in African Americans is characterized by Th2/Th17-centered cutaneous immune activation. Sci Rep 2021;11(1): 11175.

14. Whang KA, Khanna R, Thomas J, et al. Racial and gender differences in the presentation of pruritus. Medicines 2019;6(4):98.

15. Kwatra SG, Misery L, Clibborn C, et al. Molecular and cellular mechanisms of itch and pain in atopic dermatitis and implications for novel therapeutics. Clin Transl Immunology 2022;11(5):e1390.

16. Kim BE, Leung DYM. Significance of skin barrier dysfunction in atopic dermatitis. Allergy Asthma Immunol Res 2018;10(3):207–15.

17. Sutaria N, Adawi W, Goldberg R, et al. Itch: pathogenesis and treatment. J Am Acad Dermatol 2021. https://doi.org/10.1016/J.JAAD.2021.07.078.

18. Persikov A v, Pillitteri RJ, Amin P, et al. Changes in the ceramide profile of atopic dermatitis patients. J Invest Dermatol 2010;130:2511–4.

19. Joo KM, Hwang JH, Bae S, et al. Relationship of ceramide–, and free fatty acid–cholesterol ratios in the stratum corneum with skin barrier function of normal, atopic dermatitis lesional and non-lesional skins. J Dermatol Sci 2015;77(1):71–4.

20. Muizzuddin N, Hellemans L, van Overloop L, et al. Structural and functional differences in barrier properties of African American, Caucasian and East Asian skin. J Dermatol Sci 2010;59(2):123–8.

21. Rodríguez E, Baurecht H, Herberich E, et al. Meta-analysis of filaggrin polymorphisms in eczema and asthma: robust risk factors in atopic disease. J Allergy Clin Immunol 2009;123(6):1361–70.e7.

22. Margolis DJ, Apter AJ, Gupta J, et al. The persistence of atopic dermatitis and filaggrin (FLG) mutations in a US longitudinal cohort. J Allergy Clin Immunol 2012;130(4):912–7.

23. Seykora J, Dentchev T, Margolis DJ. Filaggrin-2 barrier protein inversely varies with skin inflammation. Exp Dermatol 2015;24(9):720.

24. Margolis DJ, Gupta J, Apter AJ, et al. Filaggrin-2 variation is associated with more persistent atopic dermatitis in African American subjects. J Allergy Clin Immunol 2014;133(3):784–9.

25. Asad S, Winge MCG, Wahlgren C, et al. The tight junction gene Claudin-1 is associated with atopic dermatitis among Ethiopians. J Eur Acad Dermatol Venereol 2016;30(11):1939–41.

26. Homey B, Steinhoff M, Ruzicka T, et al. Cytokines and chemokines orchestrate atopic skin inflammation. J Allergy Clin Immunol 2006;118(1):178–89.

27. Sueki H, Whitaker-Menezes D, Kligman AM. Structural diversity of mast cell granules in black and white skin. Br J Dermatol 2001;144(1):85–93.

28. Sanyal RD, Pavel AB, Glickman J, et al. Atopic dermatitis in African American patients is TH2/TH22-skewed with TH1/TH17 attenuation. Ann Allergy Asthma Immunol 2019;122(1):99–110.e6.

29. Grundbacher FJ. Causes of variation in serum IgE levels in normal populations. J Allergy Clin Immunol 1975;56(2):104–11.

30. Hussein YM, Shalaby SM, Nassar A, et al. Association between genes encoding components of the IL-4/IL-4 receptor pathway and dermatitis in children. Gene 2014;545(2):276–81.

31. Guttman-Yassky E, Krueger JG. Atopic dermatitis and psoriasis: two different immune diseases or one spectrum? Curr Opin Immunol 2017;48: 68 73.

32. Lang CC v, Masenga J, Semango G, et al. Evidence for different immune signatures and sensitization patterns in sub-Saharan African vs. Central European atopic dermatitis patients. J Eur Acad Dermatol Venereol 2021;35(2):e140–2.

33. Ait-Khaled N, Odhiambo J, Pearce N, et al. Prevalence of symptoms of asthma, rhinitis and eczema in 13-to 14-year-old children in Africa: the international study of asthma and allergies in childhood phase III. Allergy 2007;62(3):247–58.

34. Callewaert C, Ravard Helffer K, Lebaron P. Skin Microbiome and its Interplay with the Environment. Am J Clin Dermatol 2020;21(1):4–11.

35. Croce EA, Levy ML, Adamson AS, et al. Reframing racial and ethnic disparities in atopic dermatitis in Black and Latinx populations. J Allergy Clin Immunol 2021;148(5):1104–11.

36. Tackett KJ, Jenkins F, Morrell DS, et al. Structural racism and its influence on the severity of atopic

dermatitis in African American children. Pediatr Dermatol 2020;37(1):142–6.

37. Biagini JM, Kroner JW, Baatyrbek kyzy A, et al. Longitudinal atopic dermatitis endotypes: an atopic march paradigm that includes Black children. J Allergy Clin Immunol 2022;149(5):1702–10.e4.

38. Williams HC, Jburney PG, Hay RJ, et al. The UK working party's diagnostic criteria for atopic dermatitis. I. Derivation of a minimum set of discriminators for atopic dermatitis. Br J Dermatol 1994;131(3): 383–96.

39. McLaurin CI. Pediatric dermatology in black patients. Dermatol Clin 1988;6(3):457–73.

40. Silverberg JI, Margolis DJ, Boguniewicz M, et al. Distribution of atopic dermatitis lesions in United States adults. J Eur Acad Dermatol Venereol 2019; 33(7):1341–8.

41. Nnoruka EN. Current epidemiology of atopic dermatitis in south-eastern Nigeria. Int J Dermatol 2004; 43(10):739–44.

42. Vachiramon V, Tey HL, Thompson AE, et al. Atopic dermatitis in African American children: addressing unmet needs of a common disease. Pediatr Dermatol 2012;29(4):395–402.

43. Allen HB, Jones NP, Bowen SE. Lichenoid and other clinical presentations of atopic dermatitis in an inner city practice. J Am Acad Dermatol 2008;58(3):503–4.

44. Ben-Gashir MA, Seed PT, Hay RJ. Reliance on erythema scores may mask severe atopic dermatitis in black children compared with their white counterparts. Br J Dermatol 2002;147(5):920–5.

45. Alexis AF, Sergay AB, Taylor SC. Common dermatologic disorders in skin of color: a comparative practice survey. Cutis 2007;80(5):387–94.

46. Kaufman BP, Guttman-Yassky E, Alexis AF. Atopic dermatitis in diverse racial and ethnic groups—Variations in epidemiology, genetics, clinical presentation and treatment. Exp Dermatol 2018;27(4): 340–57.

47. Zheng DX, Cwalina TB, Mulligan KM, et al. Delayed medical care due to transportation barriers among US children with atopic dermatitis. Pediatr Dermatol 2022;39(6):927–30.

48. Wan J, Oganisian A, Spieker AJ, et al. Racial/ethnic variation in use of ambulatory and emergency care for atopic dermatitis among US children. J Invest Dermatol 2019;139(9):1906–13.

49. Wan J, Margolis DJ, Mitra N, et al. Racial and ethnic differences in atopic dermatitis–related school absences among US children. JAMA Dermatol 2019; 155(8):973–5.

50. Hanifln JM, Rajka G. Diagnostic features of atopic dermatitis. Acta Derm Venereol 1980;92:44–7.

51. Huang AH, Kwatra SG, Khanna R, et al. Racial disparities in the clinical presentation and prognosis of patients with mycosis fungoides. J Natl Med Assoc 2019;111(6):633–9.

52. Kwon CD, Khanna R, Williams KA, et al. Diagnostic workup and evaluation of patients with prurigo nodularis. Medicines (Basel) 2019;6(4). https://doi.org/10.3390/medicines6040097.

53. Roh YS, Choi J, Sutaria N, et al. Itch: epidemiology, clinical presentation, and diagnostic workup. J Am Acad Dermatol 2022;86(1):1–14.

54. Huang AH, Williams KA, Kwatra SG. Prurigo nodularis: epidemiology and clinical features, 83. American Academy of Dermatology, Inc.; 2020. https://doi.org/10.1016/j.jaad.2020.04.183.

55. Wongvibulsin S, Sutaria N, Williams KA, et al. A nationwide study of prurigo nodularis: disease burden and healthcare utilization in the United States. J Invest Dermatol 2021. https://doi.org/10.1016/j.jid.2021.02.756.

56. Wongvibulsin S, Parthasarathy V, Pahalyants V, et al. Latent class analysis identification of prurigo nodularis comorbidity phenotypes. Br J Dermatol 2022; 186(5):903–5.

57. Bender AM, Tang O, Khanna R, et al. Racial differences in dermatologic conditions associated with HIV: a cross-sectional study of 4679 patients in an urban tertiary care center. J Am Acad Dermatol 2020;82(5):1117–23.

58. Sutaria N, Choi J, Roh YS, et al. Association of prurigo nodularis and infectious disease hospitalizations: a national cross-sectional study. Clin Exp Dermatol 2021. https://doi.org/10.1111/ced.14652.

59. Boozalis E, Tang O, Patel S, et al. Ethnic differences and comorbidities of 909 prurigo nodularis patients. J Am Acad Dermatol 2018;79(4):714–9.e3. https://doi.org/10.1016/j.jaad.2018.04.047.

60. Sutaria N, Alphonse MP, Marani M, et al. Cluster analysis of circulating plasma biomarkers in prurigo nodularis reveals a distinct systemic inflammatory signature in African Americans. J Invest Dermatol 2021. https://doi.org/10.1016/J.JID.2021.10.011.

61. Sutaria N, Adawi W, Brown I, et al. Racial disparities in mortality among patients with prurigo nodularis: a multi-center cohort study. J Am Acad Dermatol 2021. https://doi.org/10.1016/j.jaad.2021.09.028.

62. Sutaria N., Semenov Y.R. and Kwatra S.G., Understanding racial disparities in prurigo nodularis, J Am Acad Dermatol, 87 (3), E111-E112,2022.

63. Bell MA, Whang KA, Thomas J, et al. Racial and ethnic disparities in access to emerging and frontline therapies in common dermatological conditions: a cross-sectional study. J Natl Med Assoc 2020; 112(6):650–3.

64. Hirano SA, Murray SB, Harvey VM. Reporting, representation, and subgroup analysis of race and ethnicity in published clinical trials of atopic dermatitis in the United States between 2000 and 2009. Pediatr Dermatol 2012;29(6):749–55.

65. Eichenfield LF, Lucky AW, Langley RGB, et al. Use of pimecrolimus cream 1%(Elidel®) in the treatment of

atopic dermatitis in infants and children: the effects of ethnic origin and baseline disease severity on treatment outcome. Int J Dermatol 2005;44(1):70–5.

66. Callender VD, Alexis AF, Stein Gold LF, et al. Efficacy and safety of crisaborole ointment, 2%, for the treatment of mild-to-moderate atopic dermatitis across racial and ethnic groups. Am J Clin Dermatol 2019;20(5):711–23.

67. Eichenfield LF, Stein Gold LF, Chiesa Fuxench ZC, Venturanza ME, Brar KK. Safety and efficacy over 8 weeks and disease control over 52 weeks with ruxolitinib cream among Black or African American patients with atopic dermatitis: Pooled results from two phase 3 studies. Presented at: 2022 American Academy of Dermatology Annual Meeting. Abstract: 34794. American Academy of Dermatology Annual Meeting. Published online 2022.

68. Kim BS, Howell MD, Sun K, et al. Treatment of atopic dermatitis with ruxolitinib cream (JAK1/JAK2 inhibitor) or triamcinolone cream. J Allergy Clin Immunol 2020;145(2):572–82.

69. Nakagawa H, Nemoto O, Igarashi A, et al. Delgocitinib ointment, a topical Janus kinase inhibitor, in adult patients with moderate to severe atopic dermatitis: a phase 3, randomized, double-blind, vehicle-controlled study and an open-label, long-term extension study. J Am Acad Dermatol 2020; 82(4):823–31.

70. Vu YH, Hashimoto-Hachiya A, Takemura M, et al. IL-24 negatively regulates keratinocyte differentiation induced by Tapinarof, an aryl hydrocarbon receptor modulator: Implication in the treatment of atopic dermatitis. Int J Mol Sci 2020;21(24):9412.

71. Gooderham MJ, Kircik LH, Zirwas M, et al. The safety and efficacy of roflumilast cream 0.15% and 0.05% in atopic dermatitis: phase 2 proof-of-concept study. SKIN The Journal of Cutaneous Medicine 2020;4(6):s93.

72. Hamilton JD, Suárez-Farinas M, Dhingra N, et al. Dupilumab improves the molecular signature in skin of patients with moderate-to-severe atopic dermatitis. J Allergy Clin Immunol 2014;134(6):1293–300.

73. Alexis AF, Rendon M, Silverberg JI, et al. Efficacy of dupilumab in different racial subgroups of adults with moderate-to-severe atopic dermatitis in three randomized, placebo-controlled phase 3 trials. J Drugs Dermatol 2019;18(8):804–13.

74. Wollenberg A, Blauvelt A, Guttman-Yassky E, et al. Tralokinumab for moderate-to-severe atopic dermatitis: results from two 52-week, randomized, double-blind, multicentre, placebo-controlled phase III trials (ECZTRA 1 and ECZTRA 2). Br J Dermatol 2021; 184(3):437–49.

75. Guttman-Yassky E, Teixeira HD, Simpson EL, et al. Once-daily upadacitinib versus placebo in adolescents and adults with moderate-to-severe atopic dermatitis (Measure Up 1 and Measure Up 2): results from two replicate double-blind, randomised controlled phase 3 trials. Lancet 2021;397(10290): 2151–68.

76. Reich K, Teixeira HD, de Bruin-Weller M, et al. Safety and efficacy of upadacitinib in combination with topical corticosteroids in adolescents and adults with moderate-to-severe atopic dermatitis (AD Up): results from a randomised, double-blind, placebo-controlled, phase 3 trial. Lancet 2021;397(10290): 2169–81.

77. Reich K, Thyssen JP, Blauvelt A, et al. Efficacy and safety of abrocitinib versus dupilumab in adults with moderate-to-severe atopic dermatitis: a randomised, double-blind, multicentre phase 3 trial. Lancet 2022;400(10348):273–82.

78. Bieber T, Simpson EL, Silverberg JI, et al. Abrocitinib versus placebo or dupilumab for atopic dermatitis. N Engl J Med 2021;384(12):1101–12.

79. Kim G, Park J, Chin H, et al. Comparative analysis of the use of complementary and alternative medicine by Korean patients with androgenetic alopecia, atopic dermatitis and psoriasis. J Eur Acad Dermatol Venereol 2013;27(7).827–35.

80. Kaundinya T, Rakita U, Guraya A, et al. Differences in psychometric properties of clinician- and patient-reported outcome measures for atopic dermatitis by race and skin tone: a systematic review. J Invest Dermatol 2022;142(2):364–81.

Diagnosing Psoriasis in Skin of Color Patients

Rayva Khanna, MD[a], Ramona Khanna, BA[b], Seemal R. Desai, MD[c,d],*

KEYWORDS

• Psoriasis • Skin of color • Biologics • Vehicles • Lichen planus • Erythema • Dyspigmentation

KEY POINTS

- Psoriasis is often misdiagnosed in darker skin phenotypes due to lack of thick erythematous plaque with overlying scale in skin of color patients.
- To aid in the diagnosis, one should consider the anatomic locatio and clinical history.
- Psorasis should be on the differential diagnosis for skin of color patients with characteristics of hypertrophic lichen planus, sarcoidosis, cutaneous lupus, and tinea.

DIAGNOSING PSORIASIS IN SKIN OF COLOR

Introduction

Psoriasis is a chronic immune-mediated, genetic disease that presents primarily on the skin with systemic manifestations. However, there is a great deal of diversity in the presentation and manifestation in psoriasis. Diagnosis of patients with psoriasis can pose a challenge for dermatologists due to the lack of conspicuous "erythema" and overlap with features of other dermatological disorders. Delayed diagnosis or inadequate treatment of psoriasis can precipitate severe systemic involvement such as psoriatic arthritis and an increased risk for cardiac disease. Furthermore, undertreatment of psoriasis can lead to detrimental psychosocial consequences on cutaneous body image and quality of life.[1] Still, majority of data regarding biologic treatments and clinical data have been conducted on White patients.[2] Therefore, it is important to elucidate the unique presentation of patients with skin of color and summarize the therapeutic guidelines.

Clinical Presentation

Chronic plaque psoriasis presents as sharply demarcated plaques with significant erythema, thickening and overlying scale. However, there are notable differences in presentation of psoriasis in skin of color populations. Presentation of erythema and inflammation can present in a variety of ways depending on Fitzpatrick skin type. In active plaque psoriasis, darker skin (**Fig. 1**) tones may have less prominent erythema with light pink, violaceous or dark brown hues. Thus, psoriasis can be difficult to diagnose in these patients due to under recognition of erythema or misdiagnosis of violaceous or hyperpigmented lesions.

Dyspigmentation is a primary concern for patients diagnosed with psoriasis with higher Fitzpatrick skin types. It is theorized that the interleukin-17 (IL-17) tumor necrosis factor inhibits melanogenesis while simultaneously inducing melanocyte mitogens, leading to both hypo and hyperpigmented lesions in psoriasis patients. These macules and patches can persist from 3 months

The content in this article has not been published or submitted for publication elsewhere. All authors have contributed significantly and are in agreement with the content of the article.
IRB Status: Approval not required.
Patient Consent: Patient consent not required.
[a] Department of Internal Medicine, Medstar Washington Hospital Center, 110 Irving Street Northwest, Washington, DC 20010, USA; [b] Georgetown University School of Medicine, 3900 Reservoir Road Northwest, Washington, DC 20007, USA; [c] Innovative Dermatology, PA, 5655 West Spring Creek Parkway, Suite 105, Plano, TX 75024, USA; [d] Department of Dermatology, University of Texas Southwestern Medical Center, Dallas, TX, USA
* Corresponding author. Innovative Dermatology, PA, 5655 West Spring Creek Parkway, Suite 105, Plano, TX 75024.
E-mail address: seemald@yahoo.com

Dermatol Clin 41 (2023) 431–434
https://doi.org/10.1016/j.det.2023.02.002

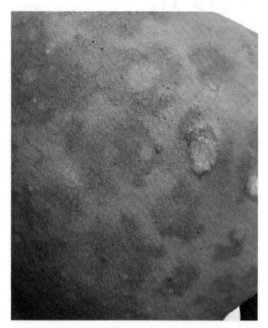

Fig. 1. Psoriasis in a darker skinned patient with markedly visible dysc.

until 1 year, increasing the burden of care for skin of color patients. In comparison to their White counterparts, Black patients noted a higher degree of dyspigmentation and less prominent erythema when diagnosed with psoriasis. Therefore, it is important to consider psoriasis on the differential diagnosis with clinical imitators such as tinea corporis, hypertrophic lichen planus, and cutaneous lupus.[3]

The presence of scaling is variable among different racial groups diagnosed with psoriasis. One survey of physicians stated that 55% of their Black patients with psoriasis presented with significantly increased scaling compared with their White patients. However, psoriasis in black patients can also present with minimal scale and skin thickening in contrast to White patients. Therefore, it is important to rule out diagnostic mimickers of psoriasis in this patient population—including tinea corporis. Additionally, Black patients traditionally have an increased body surface area (BSA) involvement with patients reporting 3% to 10% BSA of involvement compared with 1% to 2% BSA in White patients. However, it is important to note that disparities in access to care and delayed diagnosis may contribute to disease severity in these patients.

Furthermore, certain racial groups have a genetic predilection for subtypes of psoriasis. For instance, pustular psoriasis is more common in Asian and Hispanic populations.[3] There have also been reports of increased plaque psoriasis in the scalp of Black patients, thought to be due to less frequent hair washing practices. To accommodate to hair washing practices for a variety of hair types, formulations consistent with the patient's hair care should be prescribed (ie, foam, oils).

It is also important to note the differences in anatomical location of psoriatic lesions based on race or ethnicity. There is a lower rate of intertriginous psoriasis in East Asian and Black patients in comparison to White and Indian individuals.[4] Furthermore, there is less buttocks involvement of psoriasis Malay and Chinese individuals.

DIAGNOSIS

It is important to elaborate on and morphology, anatomical distribution, duration of lesions, and patient history when diagnosing psoriasis in skin of color. It is also important to consider psoriasis on the differential diagnosis in atypical appearing plaques on classic anatomical locations for psoriasis. To assess patients thoroughly, it is crucial to identify nail changes such as pitting, the presence of sharply demarcated plaques, and geographic distribution of classic psoriatic sites such as scalp, extensor surfaces, palms, soles, and intergluteal cleft. Furthermore, as noted above, hair washing practices vary based on hair type. Dermatologists should consider the patient's hair washing routine when diagnosing psoriasis and prescribing potential treatment formulations.

Differential Diagnosis

Due to the minimal skin thickening and scale, the differential diagnosis for psoriasis also includes tinea corporis, hypertrophic lichen planus, sarcoidosis, and cutaneous lupus.[2] The minimal scale accompanied by often annular borders and less prominent thickening in skin of color patients may raise concern for a fungal infection in patients who have plaque psoriasis. In such patients, conducting a minimally invasive fungal scraping can help rule out tinea infections. Furthermore, the often violaceous or purple hued nature of psoriatic plaques in skin of color patients can raise concern for lichen planus—specifically the hypertrophic subtype. Performing a thorough history, oral examination and assessing for anatomical distribution may help delineate lichen planus from psoriasis. Cutaneous lupus can often mimic plaque psoriasis as well. Particularly in patients of color, discoid lupus or sarcoidosis of the scalp can appear morphologically similar to psoriasis. Additionally, due to the pruritic nature, lack of characteristic silver scale, and sharped demarcated borders, plaque psoriasis may also be misdiagnosed as nummular eczema. Biopsy can serve as a useful tool in distinguishing psoriasis from clinical mimickers. It is essential to add psoriasis to the differential diagnosis when suspecting these conditions in skin of color patients.

Treatment/Long-Term Recommendations

Generally, the treatment guidelines for psoriasis are similar for patients across all skin phototypes.[5] However, it is important to consider cultural impacts of psoriasis treatment in different ethnic groups.[6] For example, side effects of certain therapies, such as phototherapy, may cause hyperpigmentation to sun-exposed areas, which may not be favorable in certain cultural groups that consider lighter skin complexions as desirable. This may lead to a reluctance to pursue UV treatment and/or influence compliance with therapy. Furthermore, overuse of topical steroids may create hypopigmentation, which is more prominent on skin of color patients. Such cultural implications must be considered to maximize patient compliance with treatment.

When managing scalp psoriasis in Black patients, topical hair regimens should consider hair texture and washing frequency.[2] Daily prescription shampoos may not be a suitable option for patients who refrain from doing so due to hair dryness and breakage. Instead, treatment should consider patient compliance and satisfaction to increase long-term outcomes. Thus, it is recommended to use a medicated shampoo once weekly and daily or bidaily topical corticosteroid in the vehicle of oils and emollient foams. For individuals who do not respond to topical or UV therapy, systemic medications such as self-injectable biologics such as infliximab, methotrexate, and apremilast are viable options.[7]

Clinical Outcomes/Long-Term Recommendations

Although testing for psoriasis biologics such as adalimumab, etanercept, and ustekinumab included a range of racial and ethnic groups, the proportions of these groups were not proportionally scaled to their representation in America.[2] In a Phase 4 study of biologic etanercept conducted by Shah and colleagues,[8] adverse event rates were measured and revealed no significant difference among different racial groups. When comparing different patient populations, the perception of treatment options differs among racial groups, which lead to differences in health outcomes. For example, despite the known efficacy of biologics in treating moderate-to-severe psoriasis, many patients with unfamiliarity of the therapies opted for less-efficient topical options.[6] Thus, differences in health literacy, income, and education differences may indicate an increased concern of adverse events in psoriasis treatment. For instance, due to high out-of-pocket costs, there is a decline of phototherapy use in the United States, regardless of its ability to act as an effective first-line treatment of moderate-to-severe psoriasis.[7] Therefore, when prescribing or recommending treatment in skin of color patients, dermatologist should be aware of cultural implications and long-term adherence to treatment before prescribing a vehicle.

SUMMARY

In conclusion, diagnosing psoriasis in patients of color can pose both diagnostic and treatment challenges. It is important to keep psoriasis on the differential diagnosis with conditions such as lichen planus, tinea corporis, and subcutaneous lupus for patients of color. Biopsy can help delineate the causes and guide treatment. Although there is no documented difference in efficacy of certain treatments for psoriasis based on racial group, cultural norms, hair washing practices, health literacy, and attitudes toward certain treatment options should be elicited in all patients.

CLINICS CARE POINTS

- Psoriasis is a multisystem autoimmune disease, which presents differently in skin of color populations.
- Psoriasis can present with less marked erythema and a variable amount of skin thickening and scale.
- Consider psoriasis on the differential diagnosis when suspecting lichen planus (particularly hypertrophic), tinea corporis, nummular eczema with a strange distribution, sarcoidosis, and cutaneous lupus (discoid).
- When treating scalp psoriasis in Black patients, prescribe an appropriate vehicle in conjunction with his/her hair-washing practices.
- When prescribing treatments for psoriasis, be aware to elicit cultural practices and attitudes toward treatment options to ensure compliance.
- There need to be more randomized control trials on efficacy of biologics to delineate differences in therapeutic benefit.

FUNDING SOURCES

This article has no funding source.

CONFLICT OF INTEREST

No conflicts of interest to declare.

REFERENCES

1. Hinkley SB, Holub SC, Menter A. The validity of cutaneous body image as a construct and as a mediator of the relationship between cutaneous disease and mental health. Dermatol Ther 2020;10(1):203–11.
2. Alexis AF, Blackcloud P. Psoriasis in skin of color: epidemiology, genetics, clinical presentation, and treatment nuances. J Clin Aesthet Dermatol 2014; 7(11):16–24.
3. Sangha AM. Special considerations in the diagnosis and treatment of psoriasis. J Clin Aesthet Dermatol 2021;14(12 Suppl 1):S24–5.
4. Gelfand JM, Stern RS, Nijsten T, et al. The prevalence of psoriasis in African Americans: results from a population-based study. J Am Acad Dermatol 2005; 52(1):23–6.
5. Kaufman BP, Alexis AF. Psoriasis in skin of color: insights into the epidemiology, clinical presentation, genetics, quality-of-life impact, and treatment of psoriasis in non-white racial/ethnic groups. Am J Clin Dermatol 2018;19(3):405–23.
6. Takeshita J, Eriksen WT, Raziano VT, et al. Racial differences in perceptions of psoriasis therapies: implications for racial disparities in psoriasis treatment. J Invest Dermatol 2019;139(8):1672–9.e1.
7. Takeshita J, Gelfand JM, Li P, et al. Psoriasis in the US medicare population: prevalence, treatment, and factors associated with biologic use. J Invest Dermatol 2015;135(12):2955–63.
8. Shah SK, Arthur A, Yang Y-C, et al. A retrospective study to investigate racial and ethnic variations in the treatment of psoriasis with etanercept. J Drugs Dermatol 2011;10(8):866–72.

Collagen Vascular Diseases
A Review of Cutaneous and Systemic Lupus Erythematosus, Dermatomyositis, and Distinguishing Features in Skin of Color

Victoria Lee, MD, PhD[a], Olayemi Sokumbi, MD[b], Oluwakemi Onajin, MD[a],*

KEYWORDS

- Collagen vascular diseases • Skin of color • Systemic lupus erythematosus
- Discoid lupus erythematosus • Subacute cutaneous lupus erythematosus • Dermatomyositis

KEY POINTS

- Differentiating the cutaneous manifestations of dermatomyositis (DM) from cutaneous lupus erythematosus (CLE) can be a diagnostic challenge for clinicians, as there are several clinical mimics.
- Histologic features of DM and CLE on skin biopsy can be indistinguishable, underscoring the importance of clinicopathologic correlation.
- DM and CLE in skin of color may seem more subtle and easily overlooked, and differ in color and pigmentation from classic descriptions in lighter skin tones.
- Patients with skin of color require unique management considerations due to their predisposition to dyspigmentation.

INTRODUCTION

Collagen vascular diseases such as lupus erythematosus (LE) and dermatomyositis (DM) occur 2 to 3 times more often among patients with skin of color, and symptoms develop at younger ages with more serious complications.[1] Patients with skin of color are disproportionally burdened by LE and often have higher disease activity at diagnosis, increased rates of end-organ damage, and poorer disease outcomes than white patients.[2–6] As African American ethnicity is a predictor of long-term organ damage and mortality,[5] it is essential that clinicians accurately recognize, diagnose, and promptly treat collagen vascular diseases in patients with skin of color.

Studies measuring clinicians' confidence assessing lupus-related rashes found significantly lower confidence in patients with skin of color than in patients with lighter skin tones.[7] Although curricular modules and educational tools involving skin of color during practitioners' early training are associated with higher physician confidence, studies show they insufficiently prepare clinicians for diagnosing and treating lupus-related rashes in long-term practice.[7] Moreover, systematic reviews of the literature have shown that darker skin tones are significantly underrepresented in cutaneous educational materials and published images of lupus and dermatomyositis, which further limits clinicians' ability to accurately diagnose and deliver appropriate care.[8,9] Interestingly, clinician confidence has been shown to correlate directly with the degree of continued clinical experience with patients with skin of color, more so than number of years in practice or clinical specialty.[7] Much less is known about clinician confidence in diagnosing dermatomyositis in patients with darker skin tones.

[a] Section of Dermatology, University of Chicago, 5841 South Maryland Ave, MC 5067, Chicago, IL 60637, USA;
[b] Department of Dermatology and Laboratory Medicine & Pathology, Mayo Clinic, 4500 San Pablo South, Jacksonville, FL 32224, USA
* Corresponding author.
E-mail address: oonajin@medicine.bsd.uchicago.edu

Dermatol Clin 41 (2023) 435–454
https://doi.org/10.1016/j.det.2023.02.009
0733-8635/23/© 2023 Elsevier Inc. All rights reserved.

In this article, the authors review DM and cutaneous lupus erythematosus (CLE), including acute cutaneous lupus erythematosus (ACLE), subacute cutaneous lupus erythematosus (SCLE), and discoid lupus erythematosus (DLE). The authors discuss the distinguishing features between these entities and highlight distinct presentations of these entities in skin of color to aid in prompt and correct diagnoses in this patient population.

CUTANEOUS LUPUS ERYTHEMATOSUS IN SKIN OF COLOR

CLE is a photosensitive cutaneous autoimmune disease that can be broadly classified into 3 subtypes based on morphology, histologic features, chronicity, and association with systemic lupus erythematosus (SLE): ACLE, SCLE, and chronic CLE (CCLE). Pigmentary changes are especially pronounced in skin of color. In CLE registries established at the University of Texas Southwestern, almost two-thirds of participants in the registry are those with skin of color, and the most common subtype of CLE represented is CCLE, specifically DLE.[10] Here, the authors review the distinguishing features between CLE subtypes, with a special focus on skin of color.

Differentiating Cutaneous Lupus Erythematosus Subtypes in Skin of Color

Although diagnostic criteria currently exist for SLE, there remains a need for systematic work to develop consensus definitions and diagnostic and classification criteria for CLE.[11,12] A formal process is currently underway, using the Delphi consensus method to develop such guidelines, with an initial focus on characterizing DLE.[13–16] To date, CLE lesions are diagnosed by subtype classification primarily based on morphology on clinical findings (Table 1), chronicity of lesions, histologic features in skin biopsy, and laboratory abnormalities.[17] A detailed skin examination is critical to the correct classification of CLE subtypes. Accurate diagnosis of CLE subtypes can be challenging. This challenge is further compounded in patients with skin of color, where clinical findings may be more subtle and representation of darker skin tones in published images remains sparse to date. Clinicians should note that erythema can often seem more violaceous, gray, or brown in darker skin tones, compared with the pink or red appearance in patients with lighter skin tones.

Clinical Presentation of Cutaneous Lupus Erythematosus Subtypes in Skin of Color

Acute cutaneous lupus erythematosus
ACLE is often the acute manifestation of SLE, and the clinical activity of these cutaneous lesions usually parallels the exacerbation of systemic organ disease.[18] These lesions are classically transient and sun-induced.[17] ACLE can be subdivided into localized ACLE or generalized ACLE. In the localized form, patients exhibit the hallmark "butterfly" malar rash, which is characterized by diffuse erythema over the bridge of the nose and cheeks (Fig. 1). These lesions may be accompanied by edema and scaling. Importantly, the erythema spares photo-protected areas such as the nasolabial folds, which is a feature that distinguishes it from dermatomyositis and other clinical mimics.[19] ACLE lesions are generally nonscarring, but dyspigmentation can occur.[17]

The generalized form of ACLE is characterized by widespread, symmetrically distributed erythematous macules and papules, which are occasionally edematous.[18] Often pruritic, this widespread eruption may be mistaken as a drug rash.[17] In addition, ACLE can rarely mimic toxic epidermal necrolysis (TEN), termed TEN-like ACLE (Fig. 2).[20] The skin lesions in TEN-like ACLE often presents initially on sun-exposed areas and involve one or more mucous membranes. Recognition of this rare form of ACLE is critical to the avoidance of misdiagnosis and the implementation of appropriate therapy.

Subtle erythematous rashes and photosensitivity may be challenging to detect in patients with darker skin. Occasionally, edema and scaling can be used to aid in the identification of CLE lesions. The presence of nonspecific cutaneous features such as Raynaud phenomenon or oral ulcers may also aid in the diagnosis of ACLE. Interestingly, studies have reported a high prevalence of diffuse blue-black melanonychia in patients with SLE of African descent, the mechanism of which is not entirely understood.[21] The differential diagnosis for ACLE includes dermatomyositis, rosacea, photosensitive eczema, contact dermatitis, seborrheic dermatitis, and polymorphous light eruption (Table 2).[19]

Subacute cutaneous lupus erythematosus
SCLE was originally recognized and described as a clinically and immunologically distinct subset of CLE by Sontheimer and Gilliam.[22,23] This disease entity is uncommon in patients of African, Korean, and Chinese descent.[24] SCLE lesions present with 1 of 2 morphologic patterns, annular/polycyclic or psoriasiform papulosquamous (Fig. 3 and Table 1). Photosensitivity is a major component of SCLE, and these lesions generally appear in a photoexposed distribution. It can be helpful to clinically define SCLE as a superficial inflammatory form of CLE, because this allows the differentiation

Table 1
Distinguishing cutaneous lupus erythematosus and dermatomyositis cutaneous involvement in skin of color

	ACLE	SCLE	CCLE (DLE)	DM[61,100]
Distinguishing clinical features	Localized: sun-induced, "butterfly" malar rash that spares nasolabial folds Generalized: photosensitive, pruritic eruption of symmetric macules and papules	Annular/polycyclic: erythematous plaques with raised borders in an annular or polycyclic configuration; may be vesicular, scaling, or crusted Papulosquamous/psoriasiform: erythematous hyperkeratotic plaques[18]	Well-circumscribed erythematous and indurated discoid patches or plaques, with adherent scale Chronic lesions develop peripheral hyperpigmentation and central hypopigmentation, atrophy, and telangiectasis	Pathognomonic: Gottron papules, Gottron sign, heliotrope erythema with edema Characteristic: periungual telangiectasia, shawl sign, holster sign, V-sign, atrophic erythematous scaly plaques of scalp Compatible: poikiloderma, periorbital edema, and facial swelling Less common: vesiculobullous/necrotic/ulcerative lesions, cutaneous vasculitis, calcinosis cutis Rare: mechanic's hands, flagellata erythema, follicular hyperkeratosis, panniculitis, mucinosis, erythroderma Recently described: digital pulp ulceration, Gottron papules/sign with ulceration, Hiker feet Nonspecific: photosensitivity, pruritus/burning, Raynaud phenomenon
Distribution	Localized: face Generalized: widespread	Upper thorax ("V" distribution), upper back, and other photoexposed areas	Localized (most common): classically head, scalp, and neck Disseminated (rare): generalized, often involving the hands	Variable

(continued on next page)

Table 1
(continued)

	ACLE	SCLE	CCLE (DLE)	DM[61,100]
Scarring or dyspigmentation	Nonscarring; can cause dyspigmentation	Nonscarring; vitiligo-like hypopigmentation	Scarring with dyspigmentation; scalp involvement may result in scarring alopecia	Dyspigmentation in poorly controlled DM inflammation[91] Hypopigmented and telangiectatic patches[96] Scarring, calcinosis, and/or lipoatrophy[63]
Duration of lesions	Transient, sun-induced, may persist days after photoexposure	More commonly drug-induced	More long-standing	Variable, chronic[72]

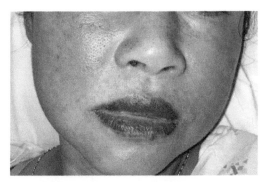

Fig. 1. Malar rash of ACLE sparing the nasolabial folds.

of SCLE from DLE via the lack of induration and scarring on physical examination.[25]

Around 50% of the patients with SCLE fulfill 4 or more of the American College of Rheumatology criteria for SLE.[26] However, these patients often have milder systemic disease activity, most commonly arthralgias and myalgias, and only 10% to 15% of patients will go on to develop renal involvement or severe systemic symptoms.[18,24,27] SCLE may be drug-induced in more than one-third of patients; thus a meticulous review of the patient's medication list is warranted on diagnosis.

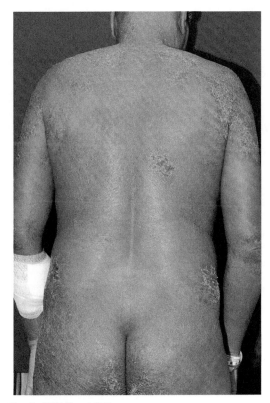

Fig. 2. TEN-like ACLE.

The most commonly implicated drugs include antifungals antihypertensives, diuretics, statins, and proton pump inhibitors.[28–33] Most cases of drug-induced SCLE spontaneously resolve on withdrawal of the offending drug.

Chronic cutaneous lupus erythematosus
CCLE is further categorized into DLE, hypertrophic discoid lupus erythematosus, lupus profundus (also known as lupus panniculitis), lupus erythematosus tumidus, and chilblain lupus erythematosus. Here, the authors focus their discussion specifically on DLE, the most common subtype of CCLE.

DLE is classically localized to the head, scalp, and neck areas (see **Table 1**).[34] Clinically, DLE is characterized by well-circumscribed erythematous keratotic patches or plaques, associated with peripheral hyperpigmentation and central hypopigmentation, atrophy, and telangiectasis (see **Table 1** and **Fig. 4**A–C).[19] In addition, DLE lesions show follicular dilatation with keratin plugging. Generalized DLE is a rarer form of DLE that presents in a disseminated fashion (see **Table 1**).[34] Patients with generalized DLE are more likely to progress to SLE.[35] DLE lesions are often scarring and dyspigmentation is common, especially in patients with darker skin tones (see **Table 1** and **Fig. 5**A–B).[36] A study of patients diagnosed with DLE at the University of Texas Southwestern found that Black patients with DLE had greater odds of having scalp and ear involvement (**Fig. 6**A), compared with non-Black patients with DLE,[36] although the mechanisms driving this phenomenon remains unclear. In addition, Black patients with DLE are more frequently affected by dyspigmentation and scarring alopecia (see **Fig. 6**B).[36]

DLE lesions can leave a long-lasting vitiligo-like hypopigmentation that is occasionally permanent.[37] These lesions are distinguished from vitiligo by the presence of telangiectasias within the hypopigmented areas (**Fig. 7**). The mechanisms of vitiligo-like dyspigmentation remain unknown but has been hypothesized to be a result of post-inflammatory hypopigmentation versus autoimmune destruction of melanocytes.

Distinguishing Histologic Features of Cutaneous Lupus Erythematosus Subtypes

Histologically, lesions of all CLE subtypes show extensive overlap in their histologic features, with interface dermatitis, degeneration of basal keratinocytes, dermal mucin, and superficial and/or deep perivascular and periadnexal lymphocytic infiltrate.[18] However, in ACLE lesions, these features are generally much less pronounced (**Fig. 8**A).[25] In contrast to DLE, ACLE lesions often

Table 2
Clinical mimics of cutaneous lupus erythematosus and dermatomyositis in skin of color

Diagnosis	Differential Diagnoses	Clinical Mimics
Acute cutaneous lupus erythematosus (ACLE)	Acne rosacea Steroid rosacea Photosensitive eczema Seborrheic dermatitis Contact dermatitis Polymorphous light eruption	Digital ulcers of MDA5 DM mimics digital ulcers of CLE and Raynaud phenomenon in SLE[61,87,88,100,110] Gottrons papules of DM can mimic ACLE on dorsal hands, which typically spares the MCP and PIP joints[113] Heliotrope erythema of DM occasionally involves the cheeks and nose, sparing the tip, which mimics the malar rash in ACLE[61]
Subacute cutaneous lupus erythematosus (SCLE)	Erythema multiforme Toxic epidermal necrolysis Eczema Psoriasis Pityriasis Vitiligo Dermatomyositis Cutaneous T-cell lymphoma Tinea corporis Erythema annulare centrifugum Erythema gyratum repens Photolichenoid drug eruption Granuloma annulare Pemphigus foliaceus Complement deficiency with lupus-like rash	Psoriasiform DM mimics psoriasiform subtype of SCLE[94–97] "V-sign" in DM mimics the photoexposed "V"-distribution of upper chest in SCLE[22,23,61]
Chronic cutaneous lupus erythematosus (CCLE)	DLE: Petaloid seborrheic dermatitis Acne vulgaris Psoriasis Lymphoma cutis Cutaneous T-cell lymphoma Granuloma faciale Polymorphous light eruption Sarcoidosis Vitiligo	Panniculitis in DM mimics LEP, both clinically and histologically[17,114]
Dermatomyositis (DM)	Systemic lupus erythematosus Hand dermatitis Psoriasis[75,77] Seborrheic dermatitis[75,77] Mycosis fungoides[61,72] Toxic irritant contact dermatitis[61,85,86] Pityriasis rubra pilaris[80–82] Rosacea Eczema Undifferentiated connective tissue disease (UCTD) Mixed connective tissue disease (MCTD)[62]	Severe edema of malar rash in ACLE mimics periorbital edema in DM[19] Generalized ACLE involving dorsal hands mimic Gottron papules[112]

Abbreviation: PIP, proximal interphalangeal.

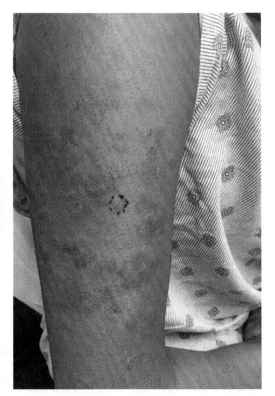

Fig. 3. SCLE presenting as papulosquamous eruption on outer arm.

in a speckled (particulate) pattern in epidermal nuclei.[40]

SCLE lesions show significant overlap in histologic features with those of DLE but can be described as more intermediate between the subtle findings of ACLE and those of DLE (see **Fig. 8**B).[25] Most of the SCLE lesions exhibit granular deposition of immunoreactants at the dermal-epidermal junction, similar to but with less intensity than that of DLE lesions.[22,41]

DLE lesions exhibit many of the classic histologic findings of CLE, and these features are often found to a greater degree than in those of other CLE subtypes.[25] The histologic hallmarks of DLE include hyperkeratosis, keratotic follicular plugging, dense superficial and deep perivascular and periadnexal lymphocytic infiltrate, basement membrane thickening, and dermal mucin deposition (see **Fig. 8**C). In addition, most of the DLE lesions will display a positive lupus band test in immunofluorescence studies, most commonly consisting of IgM and C3.[42]

Evaluation and Management of Cutaneous Lupus Erythematosus in Patients with Skin of Color

Studies investigating quality of life-specific measures in CLE indicate that CLE has profound effects on quality of life in patients with skin of color.[43] In addition, in a study of patients with CLE at the University of Pennsylvania, Black patients presented with greater initial measures of disease damage than white patients and showed higher measures of disease damage at follow-up.[44] These findings highlight the delay in care and importance of accurate diagnosis of CLE in patients with skin of color.

Because of the existing challenges in the accurate diagnosis of CLE subtypes, there is significant lag time in the prompt recognition of these entities in patients with skin of color.[6] As a result, skin of color patients with CLE often have worse disease outcomes when compared with white patients[5,6];

lack epidermal acanthosis, keratotic follicular plugging, or marked basement membrane thickening.[18,38] Direct immunofluorescence (DIF) studies show a positive lupus band test (a granular bandlike array of immunoglobulin and complement deposits at the dermal-epidermal junction of lesional skin) in more than 90% of patients with SLE and perivascular deposits in the upper dermis, most commonly immunoglobulin M (IgM).[17,18] A distinguishing feature of ACLE is that DIF studies will often show a positive lupus band test even in non–sun-exposed, clinically normal skin.[39] In addition, DIF also shows IgG deposition

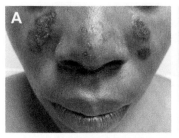
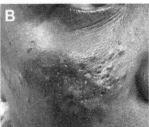
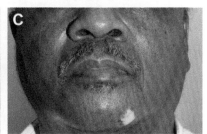

Fig. 4. (*A*) DLE. (*B*) Comedonal variant of DLE can mimic nodulocystic acne. (*C*) DLE presenting with atrophic pink and white patch with hyperpigmented borders.

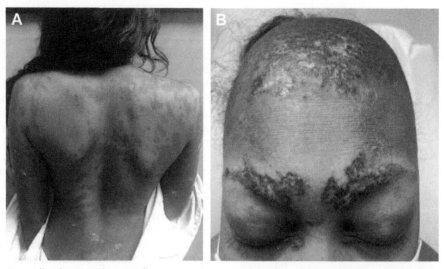

Fig. 5. (A) Generalized DLE with postinflammatory hyperpigmentation. (B) DLE resulting in scarring alopecia.

this underscores the need for a better representation of darker skin tones in published images and educational materials.

Clinicians should obtain a thorough medical history and document time of initial onset, possible triggers (such as sun exposure or new medications), associated symptoms, and family history of LE or autoimmunity. In addition, disease severity and damage may be documented with photographs to monitor disease progression longitudinally.[45] Skin biopsy should be performed initially to rule out mimics. As SCLE is frequently associated with the use of certain medications,

the patient's medication list should be reviewed and potential triggers should be stopped.[45] Clinicians should also assess whether the disease is active and document the degree of skin disease activity. Ongoing disease activity requires prompt and aggressive treatment to reduce the risk of scarring and dyspigmentation.

Skin of color patients with CLE require unique management considerations due to their predisposition to experiencing dyspigmentation on resolution of active disease.[19] Moreover, dyspigmentation is often more noticeable in patients with darker skin tones, as the contrast

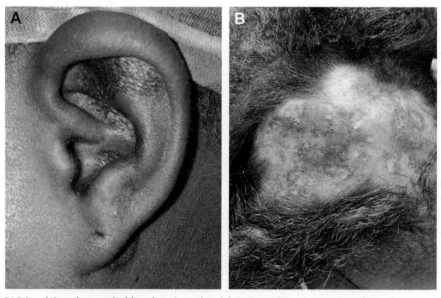

Fig. 6. (A) DLE involving the conchal bowl and scapha. (B) DLE resulting in scarring alopecia.

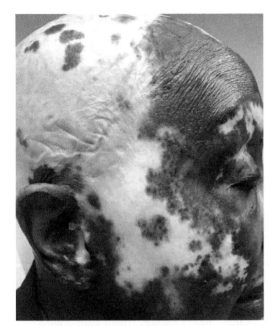

Fig. 7. Vitiligo-like dyspigmentation with telangiectasias and erythematous patches in a patient with DLE.

between affected and unaffected skin may be more pronounced. Patients with skin of color should receive counseling on the use of broad-spectrum mineral sunscreen and sun-protective clothing and should be encouraged to practice sun avoidance when possible.[46] Patients with skin of color should be educated on the importance of using formulations containing iron oxide, as studies have shown that these formulations mediated significant protections against visible light-induced pigmentation in individuals with Fitzpatrick skin phototypes IV and higher.[47] Furthermore, vitamin D insufficiency is a concern in all

dark-skinned individuals, and skin of color patients with CLE are especially predisposed to having lower vitamin D levels due to sun-protective practices.[48,49] As vitamin D has been shown to be immune-protective and antiinflammatory, skin of color patients with CLE should be counseled on the importance of vitamin D supplementation.[16,50]

As Black patients with DLE are more frequently affected by ear and scalp dyspigmentation and scarring alopecia, these patients should be counseled on gentle haircare practices and the use of sun-protective hats that cover the scalp to reduce further scalp damage.[36] Clinicians should familiarize themselves with common haircare practices among Black patients in order to facilitate a culturally competent approach to the evaluation and management of patients with DLE with scalp involvement.[51] Clinicians should be aware that once the scarring process has fully involved the hair follicles in DLE, hair loss is generally permanent.[52] It is important for clinicians to remember that in many patients with darker skin tones, the remnant of cutaneous disease damage and dyspigmentation may have a profound impact on the patient's quality of life.[43] Patients who wish to cover up dyspigmentation in areas of inactive lesions could consider using cosmetic skin care products such as foundation and tinted mineral sunscreen.[46]

Up to 20% of patients with CLE may progress to SLE.[10] In this regard, patients should be screened for internal organ involvement on initial diagnosis of CLE and at yearly intervals thereafter. Although all patients with CLE warrant a close follow-up, this is especially imperative in patients with skin of color, as they are disproportionally burdened by LE and often have worse disease outcomes than white patients.[5] In addition, patients with skin of color have a higher predisposition to renal

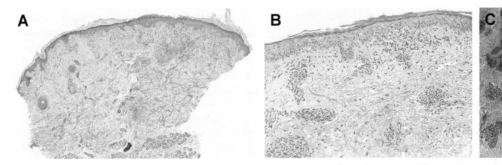

Fig. 8. (*A*) Biopsy of patient with ACLE demonstrating vacuolar interface alteration with prominent pigment incontinence, superficial perivascular lymphocytic inflammation, and dermal mucin (hematoxylin-eosin; original magnification: ×20). (*B*) SCLE lesion demonstrating vacuolar interface alteration with necrotic keratinocytes, perivascular inflammation, and dermal mucin (hematoxylin-eosin; original magnification: ×20). (*C*) Fairly dense superficial and deep perivascular, perifollicular, and perieccrine lymphocytic inflammation of DLE lesion (hematoxylin-eosin; original magnification: ×100).

involvement and progression to systemic disease than white patients[6] and should be properly counseled on reducing risk factors associated with systemic involvement or treatment resistance, such as smoking cessation.[53–58]

Clinic Care Points

- Subtle erythematous rashes of CLE and photosensitivity may be challenging to detect in patients with dark skin.
- Patients with CLE with skin of color require unique management considerations due to their predisposition to experiencing dyspigmentation.
- Patients with CLE with skin of color should receive counseling on the use of broad-spectrum sunscreen formulations containing iron oxide and vitamin D supplementation.
- Clinicians should recognize the importance of cultural competency when counseling patients with CLE with skin of color (eg, familiarity with common haircare practices and best sunscreens for darker skin).
- Patients with CLE should be properly counseled on reducing risk factors such as smoking cessation.

DERMATOMYOSITIS IN SKIN OF COLOR

DM is a systemic autoimmune disease included in the spectrum of immune-mediated disorders called idiopathic inflammatory myopathies, which can affect several organs other than skeletal muscle and skin.[59,60] DM is further classified into adult-onset and juvenile-onset DM, each comprising various subtypes.[61] Although DM classically involves myositis in addition to cutaneous findings, certain patients may present with amyopathic DM (ADM) or clinically amyopathic DM, which can further confound the diagnosis.[62,63]

The skin features in patients with DM are often quite variable and can be difficult to recognize, especially in patients with skin of color. Although African-Americans and Hispanics are disproportionally affected by inflammatory diseases such as DM, there is a significant underrepresentation of racial minorities and darker skin tones in the educational and medical literature depicting DM rashes.[9,64–67] This disparity contributes to the lack of proficiency in clinicians making a prompt diagnosis of DM in patients with skin of color. Accurate diagnosis of DM is paramount, as patients with DM have an increased risk for internal malignancy and interstitial lung disease, which can be present even among patients with purely cutaneous findings.[68–70] Thus, there is a need for clinicians to become familiar with the clinical and

histologic heterogeneity that can be seen in DM for patients with skin of color, in order to facilitate prompt diagnosis and management for this patient group.[45] Importantly, the clinical characteristics of DM can at times be difficult to discern from other connective tissue diseases such as CLE, and this challenge is compounded in skin of color, where clinician familiarity is often minimal. Here, the authors review the defining features of DM, with special remarks on skin of color. They then discuss how to differentiate DM from CLE in the subsequent section.

Clinical Presentation of Dermatomyositis in Skin of Color

A critical component in the diagnosis of DM involves the identification of cutaneous manifestations on physical examination; this is especially true because the histologic features of DM on skin biopsy can be subtle and is often indistinguishable from certain mimickers, such as CLE.[71] The pathognomonic skin findings of DM include Göttron sign, Göttron papules, and heliotrope erythema (see **Table 1**).[61,72] Gottron sign presents as erythematous macules along extensor tendons of the dorsal hands and fingers and often also on the knees and elbows.[61] Gottron papules are flat, violaceous papules and plaques found on the bony prominences of the dorsal metacarpophalangeal (MCP) and interphalangeal joints or along the nail contours.[72] In white patients, heliotrope erythema is classically characterized by violaceous erythema and edema, more often found on the upper eyelids. It can occasionally be found on the cheeks and nose and involves the nasolabial fold (**Fig. 9**), which should not be mistaken for the malar rash observed in patients with CLE that typically spares the nasolabial fold (see **Fig. 1** and **Table 2**).[61] However, heliotrope erythema and Gottron papules may be more subtle in darker skin types.[73] In skin of color patients, heliotrope erythema instead presents as deep brown or gray discoloration with or without edema over and around the eyes and eyelids (**Fig. 10**), whereas Gottron papules present as erythematous, hypopigmented or hyperpigmented papules along the extensor surfaces of the proximal interphalangeal joints (**Fig. 11A–B**).[74] Clinicians should recognize that pathognomonic findings of DM may present differently in patients with darker skin tones, which can make these features more subtle and more easily overlooked.

Other cutaneous findings in DM include periungal telangiectasia, dystrophic cuticles, and small hemorrhagic infarcts in the nailfold.[45] Patients may present with extensive macular purplish

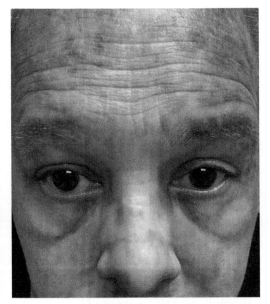

Fig. 9. DM presenting with violaceous patches and grayish brown macules on the face. Note involvement of nasolabial folds.

erythema or brown or gray patches that overlie the nape of the neck and posterior shoulders (shawl sign) (Fig. 12), extensor upper extremities (Fig. 13), dorsal hands, the lateral thighs or hips (holster sign), or the V-area of the upper chest (V-sign) (Fig. 14A–B) and forehead.[72,75,76] Patients may also present with intensely pruritic atrophic, erythematous, scaly plaques on the scalp, which can initially be misdiagnosed as psoriasis or seborrheic dermatitis (see Table 2).[75,77] Nonscarring generalized alopecia often accompanies the scalp eruptions.[72] Photosensitive poikiloderma, hypo- or hyperpigmentation, telangiectasia, and atrophy can involve the upper chest (Fig. 15), buttocks,

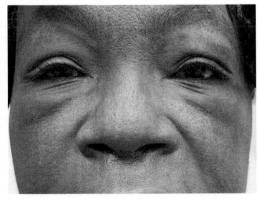

Fig. 10. Periorbital edema with thin violaceous and greyish brown plaques on the face.

thighs, or hips.[61,72] Other compatible skin findings include periorbital and facial edema with or without erythema.[77–79]

Some patients with DM may present with follicular hyperkeratosis, which is a rare variant of DM termed "Wong-type DM" that may mimic many dermatoses including pityriasis rubra pilaris or CLE (see Table 2).[80–82] This rare entity was recently described in an African-American female patient as skin-colored hyperkeratotic follicular papules with subtle erythema and dyspigmentation in areas of resolved erythema.[83] Flagellate erythema is occasionally reported in association with DM and presents as linear, zebralike patterns of erythematous streaks on an edematous background that can be itching or painful.[61] In patients with skin of color, flagellate dermatoses may be characterized as dull, erythematous-to-hyperpigmented linear streaks (Fig. 16).[84] Other rare skin findings are listed in Table 2.[61,85,86] Another finding involves digital pulp ulcerations, which have been associated with the anti-MDA5 subset of patients with DM and with underlying vasculopathy and interstitial lung disease (Fig. 17A–C).[87–90]

Importantly, physicians should also be aware that significant postinflammatory pigmentary alterations may confound the diagnoses of DM in patients with skin of color. For example, poorly controlled inflammation in DM may create prominent dyspigmentation that may mimic vitiligo or systemic sclerosis (Fig. 18), and postinflammatory hyperpigmentation in DM can mimic lichen planus pigmentosus (Fig. 19).[91] Lastly, lesions in DM can occasionally present as scaly plaques resembling psoriasis or psoriasiform SCLE.[92–97]

Notably, a significant proportion of patients may present with cutaneous lesions of classic DM but lack clinical or laboratory evidence of muscle involvement. In this case, patients are classified as having ADM. Although diagnostic criteria currently exist for ADM, its validation and continued improvement is a subject of ongoing debate.[62,63,98,99] The lack of myositis in patients with ADM often confounds the clinical picture, leading to misdiagnoses (see Table 2).[62]

Distinguishing Histologic Features of Dermatomyositis

Although DM can present with a spectrum of histologic changes, skin biopsies play an important role in ruling out mimickers of DM. Histologic findings of DM are characterized by hyperkeratosis, epidermal atrophy, basement membrane thickening, vacuolar interface dermatitis, increased dermal edema and mucin deposits, mild-to-moderate mononuclear

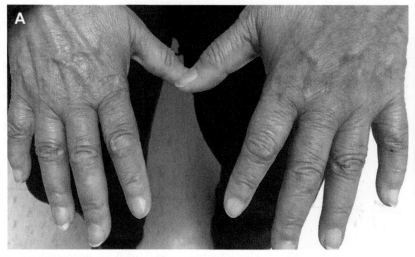
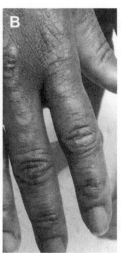

Fig. 11. (*A–B*) Gottron papules in DM.

cell inflammatory infiltrates, and perivascular infiltrates of CD4+ lymphocytes (**Fig. 20**).[71,100] However, the absence of interface dermatitis on skin biopsy does not rule out DM.[45]

It is important to note that the histopathology of cutaneous DM lesions can often be indistinguishable from that of acute cutaneous lesions of SLE. In a blinded study of DM versus SLE skin biopsies, the histologic grading of SLE skin biopsies was found to be nearly identical to that of DM skin biopsies.[71] These findings underscore the importance of clinicopathologic correlation in reaching accurate diagnosis of DM versus SLE and further highlight the need for increased clinician familiarity with cutaneous and clinical presentations of DM versus SLE in patients with skin of color.

Evaluation and Management of Dermatomyositis in Patients with Skin of Color

The heterogeneous and variable presentations of DM can pose a diagnostic challenge for clinicians, and the difficulty in recognizing DM rashes in patients with skin of color is further exacerbated by the scarce depictions of DM lesions on darker skin tones in the medical literature.[9] Studies have shown that quality of life was worse for patients with DM than for patients with other skin diseases.[101] It is important that clinicians routinely assess how DM skin disease is affecting the patient's quality of life and avoid undertreating the cutaneous components of this disease. Photosensitivity, pruritus, and mental health effects all contributed to poor quality of life observed in patients with DM.[14,102,103] In the United States, African-Americans and Hispanics are disproportionally affected by inflammatory

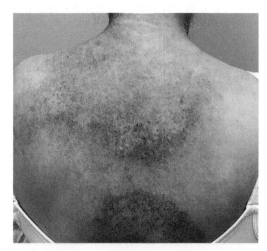

Fig. 12. Shawl sign in DM.

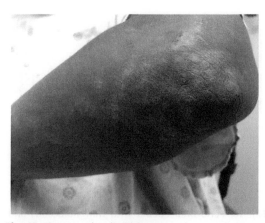

Fig. 13. Gottron sign in DM.

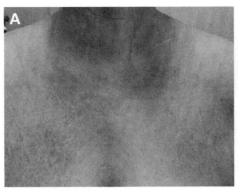
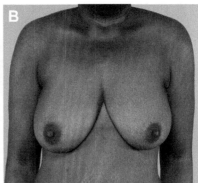

Fig. 14. (A–B) "V" sign in DM.

diseases such as DM and SLE.[64–66] The disparity in access to specialty care, along with lack of physician familiarity with skin findings on darker skin tones, lends to worst disease outcomes in this patient group.[64–66] In addition, morbidity and mortality risks are significantly elevated in patients with DM who are undiagnosed or misdiagnosed due to its association with malignancy and systemic involvement.[104] Thus, clinicians should become comfortable in the proper evaluation and management of DM for patients with skin of color in order to facilitate prompt diagnosis, appropriate screening and treatment initiation for these patients.[45]

Skin biopsies play an important role in ruling out mimickers of DM, although it is important to note that DM can present with a spectrum of histologic changes and the presence of interface dermatitis is not required for diagnosis of DM.[71] In addition, dermoscopy should be used routinely to detect periungual telangiectasias, which is a sensitive marker for DM.[45] In patients with skin of color, dyspigmentation can be a particular concern due to the prominent contrast between affected and unaffected areas. Recently, a case of significant depigmentation was described in a darker-skinned individual with TIF1-associated classic DM.[91] Patients with DM with skin of color should be counseled on photoprotective measures and the use of broad-spectrum mineral sunscreens containing iron oxide. Often, topical therapies alone are insufficient to successfully treat skin disease, and skin-directed systemic therapies may be required.[45,91,105]

Clinic Care Points

- Diagnosis of DM relies heavily on clinical and cutaneous findings, which can be widely heterogeneous in this disease entity.
- Pathognomonic findings of DM may present differently in patients with darker skin tones, which can make these features more subtle and more easily overlooked (eg, heliotrope erythema presents as deep brown or gray discoloration with or without edema, Gottron papules present as hyperpigmented papules).
- Postinflammatory dyspigmentation in patients with DM with skin of color may mimic vitiligo or systemic sclerosis.

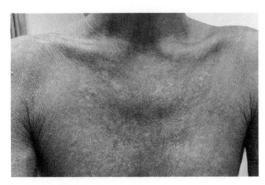

Fig. 15. Poikiloderma in DM.

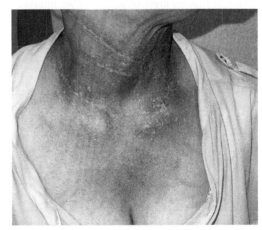

Fig. 16. Poikiloderma and flagellate erythema in DM.

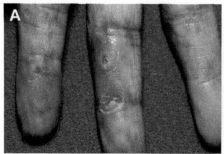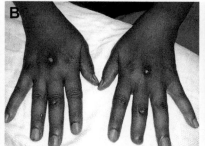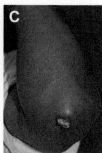

Fig. 17. (A–C) MDA5 dermatomyositis presenting with cutaneous ulcerations.

- Lack of muscle involvement in patients with ADM often leads to misdiagnoses, with CLE being the most common.
- Myositis-specific autoantibodies (MSA) profiles should be routinely utilized to guide diagnosis, prognosis, treatment recommendations and follow-up guidelines for DM.
- All patients with DM should be evaluated for malignancy, interstitial lung disease, and extracutaneous systemic involvement at the time of initial DM diagnosis.

DIFFERENTIATING CUTANEOUS LUPUS ERYTHEMATOSUS FROM DERMATOMYOSITIS

Distinguishing between cutaneous lesions of DM versus CLE can pose a diagnostic challenge for clinicians, as both can present with variable and similar clinical characteristics. In a recent study, 37% of patients with DM were initially misdiagnosed as having CLE, with a median delay of 15.5 months before the proper diagnosis of DM was reached[106]; this is especially true in the case of ADM, in which the purely cutaneous findings of ADM may be initially mistaken as CLE due to the lack of muscle involvement.[62,106] As interface dermatitis is a common histopathologic feature of both diseases, clinicopathologic correlation and clinician familiarity with the variable mimicking features of DM versus CLE is critical in making the correct diagnosis.[71,106,107] Importantly, the cutaneous lesions in patients with darker skin tones may be more subtle or easily overlooked and may appear differently in color and pigmentation from the classic presentations described in patients with lighter skin tones.[74] The consequences of misdiagnosis can be severe with DM, as patients with DM have an increased risk for internal malignancy and interstitial lung disease, and will require thorough workup and screening for these disease sequelae at the time of DM diagnosis.[68–70] In the following section, the authors discuss the

Fig. 18. Prominent dyspigmentation in DM mimicking systemic sclerosis.

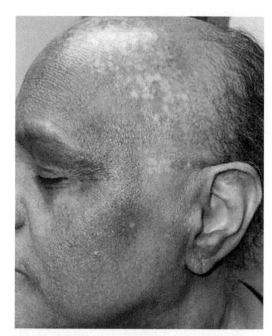

Fig. 19. Greyish brown patches and violaceous erythema involving the face, scalp, and ears.

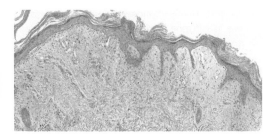

Fig. 20. Biopsy of Gottron papule with hyperkeratosis, interface dermatitis, pigment incontinence, dermal edema, and superficial perivascular inflammation (hematoxylin-eosin; original magnification: ×40).

cutaneous features of CLE that can be mistaken for features observed in DM and vice versa (see **Table 2**).

CLINICAL MIMICS OF CUTANEOUS LUPUS ERYTHEMATOSUS VERSUS DERMATOMYOSITIS

Although most of the patients with DM exhibit digital involvement, it is also a frequent feature in SLE or CLE.[106,108,109] Consequently, the differential diagnosis is often complicated when digital involvement occurs. For instance, digital pulp ulcerations, a finding commonly associated with anti-MDA5 DM, mimics the digital ulcerations seen in CLE (see **Fig. 17**A–C).[87,88,110] In addition, ulcerations may occur with Raynaud phenomenon, which is a nonspecific finding seen in both DM and SLE.[61,100] Although periungual telangiectasias is a sensitive marker for DM, it is also a feature that can be observed in CLE.[45] Studies attempting to distinguish nailfold capillaroscopy (NFC) findings between DM and CLE failed to differentiate between the 2 diseases when digital lesions were present, and the most frequent NFC finding in DM was that of a scleroderma pattern.[110]

When patients exhibit purely cutaneous manifestations of DM, the EULAR/ACR diagnostic criteria for ADM is often used, which focuses on the pathognomonic findings of heliotrope rash, Gottron sign, and Gottron papules.[62,111] However, these clinical characteristics can at times be confused for those of CLE. For instance, heliotrope erythema can occasionally involve the cheeks and nose, which mimics the malar rash observed in ACLE, although the nasolabial fold is notably spared in ACLE (see **Figs. 1** and **10**).[61] In contrast, edema of the malar rash seen in ACLE can sometimes be severe and may resemble the periorbital edema found in DM.[19] When lesions in generalized ACLE involve the dorsum of the hands, these lesions may resemble the Gottron

papules of DM. However, the distinction lies in the fact that DM primarily affects the bony prominences of the dorsal distal interphalangeal, proximal interphalangeal, and MCP joints, whereas these areas are often spared in ACLE (see **Table 2**).[112,113]

Another point of confusion may be when differentiating the "V-sign" observed in DM from the photoexposed "V"-distribution of lesions seen on the upper chest in SCLE.[22,23,61] In this scenario, clinicians should make note of the morphology of lesions, which may seem annular and polycyclic in SCLE but not in DM.[22,23,72,75,76] However, this would be difficult in the case of psoriasiform or papulosquamous SCLE, as psoriasiform plaques can also be observed in DM.[92–97]

Lastly, panniculitis is a rare feature of DM that can seem identical to lupus erythematosus panniculitis (LEP), both clinically and histologically.[17,114] In this case, other clinical features should be elicited to distinguish between the 2 entities, such as muscle involvement or other pathognomonic findings of DM. It should be noted that photosensitivity is a nonspecific feature of both DM and CLE.[100] Patients with DM often complain of treatment-refractory pruritus that can be intense enough to disturb sleep, a phenomenon that rarely affects patients with CLE.[61,115–118] In summary, clinicians should take care to distinguish between the various mimickers of CLE and DM and should consider the broader clinical picture when making the diagnosis.

CLINICS CARE POINTS

- Histologic features of DM on skin biopsy can be indistinguishable from mimics such as CLE, underscoring the importance of clinicopathologic correlation.

- Periungual telangiectasia, a sensitive feature of DM, cannot reliably distinguish DM from CLE.

- Digital pulp ulcerations of anti-MDA5 DM mimic digital ulcerations seen in CLE.

- Heliotrope erythema in DM occasionally involves the cheeks and nose, sparing the tip, which mimics malar rash in ACLE.

- Psoriasiform plaques in DM mimic the psoriasiform subtype of SCLE.

- Panniculitis in DM can seem identical to LEP, both clinically and histologically.

- Patients with DM often complain of treatment-refractory pruritus, which rarely affects patients with CLE.

SUMMARY

The histopathology of cutaneous DM is subtle and can often be indistinguishable from ACLE, underscoring the importance of clinicopathologic correlation. Differentiating the cutaneous manifestations of DM from CLE can be a diagnostic challenge for clinicians, as there are several clinical mimics, and the differential diagnosis is often complicated when digital involvement occurs. In addition, the pathognomonic findings of DM and CLE may present with differences in color and pigmentation in patients with darker skin tones, which can make these features more subtle and more easily overlooked. There is a need for increased representation of darker skin tones in depictions of DM and CLE in order to improve physician recognition of these disease entities in skin of color.

DISCLOSURE

The authors have no conflicts of interest to disclose.

REFERENCES

1. Somers EC, Marder W, Cagnoli P, et al. Population-Based Incidence and Prevalence of Systemic Lupus Erythematosus The Michigan Lupus Epidemiology and Surveillance Program. Arthritis Rheumatol 2014;66:369–78.
2. Mccarty DJ, Manzi S, Medsger TA, et al. Incidence of systemic lupus erythematosus. Race and gender differences. Arthritis Rheum 1995;38:1260–70.
3. Chiu YM, Lai CH. Nationwide population-based epidemiologic study of systemic lupus erythematosus in Taiwan. Lupus 2010;19:1250–5.
4. Mok CC, To CH, Ho LY, et al. Incidence and Mortality of Systemic Lupus Erythematosus in a Southern Chinese Population, 2000–2006. J Rheumatol 2008;35.
5. Babaoglu H, Li J, Goldman D, et al. Predictors of predominant Lupus Low Disease Activity State (LLDAS-50). Lupus 2019;28:1648–55.
6. Lewandowski LB, Schanberg LE, Thielman N, et al. Severe disease presentation and poor outcomes among pediatric systemic lupus erythematosus patients in South Africa. Lupus 2017;26:186–94.
7. Kannuthurai V, Murray J, Chen L, et al. Health care practitioners' confidence assessing lupus-related rashes in patients of color. Lupus 2021;30:1998–2002.
8. Rana A, Witt A, Jones H, et al. Representation of Skin Colors in Images of Patients With Lupus Erythematosus. Arthritis Care Res 2021. https://doi.org/10.1002/ACR.24712.
9. Babool S, Bhai SF, Sanderson C, et al. Racial disparities in skin tone representation of dermatomyositis rashes: a systematic review. Rheumatology 2022;61:2255–61.
10. O'Brien JC, Chong BF. Not Just Skin Deep: Systemic Disease Involvement in Patients With Cutaneous Lupus. J Invest Dermatol Symp Proc 2017;18:S69–74.
11. Aringer M., Costenbader K., Daikh D., et al., European League Against Rheumatism/American College of Rheumatology classification criteria for systemic lupus erythematosus, Ann Rheum Dis, 78, 2019, 1151–1159.
12. Petri M, Orbai AM, Alarcón GS, et al. Derivation and validation of the Systemic Lupus International Collaborating Clinics classification criteria for systemic lupus erythematosus. Arthritis Rheum 2012;64:2677–86.
13. Elman S.A., Joyce C., Braudis K., et al., Creation and Validation of Classification Criteria for Discoid Lupus Erythematosus, JAMA Dermatol, 156, 2020, 901–906.
14. Schultz H.Y., Dutz J.P., Furukawa F., et al., From Pathogenesis, Epidemiology, and Genetics to Definitions, Diagnosis, and Treatments of Cutaneous Lupus Erythematosus and Dermatomyositis: A Report from the 3rd International Conference on Cutaneous Lupus Erythematosus (ICCLE) 2013, J Invest Dermatol, 2015, 135 7-13512, Nature Publishing Group.
15. Merola JF, Nyberg F, Furukawa F, et al. Redefining cutaneous lupus erythematosus: a proposed international consensus approach and results of a preliminary questionnaire. Lupus Sci Med 2015;2.
16. Hejazi EZ, Werth VP. Cutaneous Lupus Erythematosus: An Update on Pathogenesis, Diagnosis and Treatment. Am J Clin Dermatol 2016;17:135–46.
17. Okon LG, Werth VP. Cutaneous lupus erythematosus: diagnosis and treatment. Best Pract Res Clin Rheumatol 2013;27:391–404.
18. Li Q., Wu H., Liao W., et al., A comprehensive review of immune-mediated dermatopathology in systemic lupus erythematosus, J Autoimmun, 93, 2018, 1–15.
19. Watson R. Cutaneous lesions in systemic lupus erythematosus. Med Clin North Am 1989;73:1091–111.
20. Romero LS, Bari O, Smith CJF, et al. Toxic epidermal necrolysis-like acute cutaneous lupus erythematosus: report of a case and review of the literature. Dermatol Online J 2018;24.
21. Koch K, Tikly M. Spectrum of cutaneous lupus erythematosus in South Africans with systemic lupus erythematosus. Lupus 2019;28:1021–6.
22. Sontheimer RD, Thomas JR, Gilliam JN. Subacute Cutaneous Lupus Erythematosus: A Cutaneous

Marker for a Distinct Lupus Erythematosus Subset. Arch Dermatol 1979;115:1409–15.

23. Sontheimer RD. Subacute Cutaneous lupus Erythematosus: A Decade's Perspective. Med Clin 1989;73.

24. Sontheimer RD. Subacute cutaneous lupus erythematosus: 25-year evolution of a prototypic subset (subphenotype) of lupus erythematosus defined by characteristic cutaneous, pathological, immunological, and genetic findings. Autoimmun Rev 2005;4:253–63.

25. Sepehr A, Wenson S, Tahan SR. Histopathologic manifestations of systemic diseases: the example of cutaneous lupus erythematosus. J Cutan Pathol 2010;37(Suppl 1):112–24.

26. Cohen MR, Crosby D. Systemic disease in subacute cutaneous lupus erythematosus: a controlled comparison with systemic lupus erythematosus. J Rheumatol 1994;21:1665–9.

27. Ribero S, Sciascia S, Borradori L, et al. The Cutaneous Spectrum of Lupus Erythematosus. Clin Rev Allergy Immunol 2017;53:291–305.

28. Grönhagen CM, Fored CM, Linder M, et al. Subacute cutaneous lupus erythematosus and its association with drugs: a population-based matched case-control study of 234 patients in Sweden. Br J Dermatol 2012;167:296–305.

29. Lowe G, Henderson CL, Grau RH, et al. A systematic review of drug-induced subacute cutaneous lupus erythematosus. Br J Dermatol 2011;164:465–72.

30. Dalle Vedove C, Simon J, Girolomoni G. Medikamenteninduzierter Lupus erythematodes unter besonderer Berucksichtigung von Hautmanifestationen und Anti-TNFα-Therapeutika. J Ger Soc Dermatol 2012;10:889–97.

31. Stavropoulos PG, Goules Av, Avgerinou G, et al. Pathogenesis of subacute cutaneous lupus erythematosus. J Eur Acad Dermatol Venereol 2008;22:1281–9.

32. Wiznia LE, Subtil A, Choi JN. Subacute cutaneous lupus erythematosus induced by chemotherapy: Gemcitabine as a causative agent. JAMA Dermatol 2013;149:1071–5.

33. Michaelis TC, Sontheimer RD, Lowe GC. An update in drug-induced subacute cutaneous lupus erythematosus. Dermatol Online J 2016;23. https://doi.org/10.5070/d3233034281. Preprint at.

34. Lenormand C, Lipsker D. Lupus erythematosus: Significance of dermatologic findings. Ann Dermatol Venereol 2021;148:6–15.

35. Hochberg M.C., Boyd R.E., Ahearn J.M., et al., Systemic lupus erythematosus: a review of clinico-laboratory features and immunogenetic markers in 150 patients with emphasis on demographic subsets, *Medicine (Baltim)*, 64, 1985, 285–295.

36. Joseph AK, Windsor B, Hynan LS, et al. Discoid lupus erythematosus skin lesion distribution and characteristics in Black patients: a retrospective cohort study. Lupus Sci Med 2021;8.

37. Kuhn A, Sticherling M, Bonsmann G. Clinical manifestations of cutaneous lupus erythematosus. J Dtsch Dermatol Ges 2007;5:1124–37.

38. Monthgomery H, Prunieras M. Histopathology of cutaneous lesions in systemic lupus erythematosus. AMA Arch Derm 1956;74:177–90.

39. Harrist TJ, Mihm MC. The specificity and clinical usefulness of the lupus band test. Arthritis Rheum 1980;23:479–90.

40. Prystowsky SD, Tuffanelli DL. Speckled (Particulate) Epidermal Nuclear IgG Deposition in Normal Skin: Correlation of Clinical Features and Laboratory Findings in 46 Patients With a Subset of Connective Tissue Disease Characterized by Antibody to Extractable Nuclear Antigen. Arch Dermatol 1978;114:705–10.

41. David-Bajar KM, Bennion SD, Despain JD, et al. histologic, and immunofluorescent distinctions between subacute cutaneous lupus erythematosus and discoid lupus erythematosus. J Invest Dermatol 1992;99:251–7.

42. Patel P, Werth V. Cutaneous lupus erythematosus: a review. Dermatol Clin 2002;20:373–85.

43. Vasquez R, Wang D, Tran QP, et al. A multicentre, cross-sectional study on quality of life in patients with cutaneous lupus erythematosus. Br J Dermatol 2013;168:145–53.

44. Verma SM, Okawa J, Propert KJ, et al. The impact of skin damage due to cutaneous lupus on quality of life. Br J Dermatol 2014;170:315–21.

45. Fett NM, Fiorentino D, Werth VP. Practice and Educational Gaps in Lupus, Dermatomyositis, and Morphea. Dermatol Clin 2016;34:243–50.

46. Song H, Beckles A, Salian P, et al. Sunscreen recommendations for patients with skin of color in the popular press and in the dermatology clinic. Int J Womens Dermatol 2020;7:165–70.

47. Dumbuya H, Grimes PE, Lynch S, et al. Impact of Iron-Oxide Containing Formulations Against Visible Light-Induced Skin Pigmentation in Skin of Color Individuals. J Drugs Dermatol 2020;19:712–7.

48. Word AP, Perese F, Tseng LC, et al. 25-Hydroxyvitamin D levels in African-American and Caucasian/Hispanic subjects with cutaneous lupus erythematosus. Br J Dermatol 2012;166:372–9.

49. Heine G, Lahl A, Müller C, et al. Vitamin D deficiency in patients with cutaneous lupus erythematosus is prevalent throughout the year. Br J Dermatol 2010;163:863–5.

50. Kamen D, Aranow C. Vitamin D in systemic lupus erythematosus. Curr Opin Rheumatol 2008;20:532–7.

51. Haskin A, Aguh C. All hairstyles are not created equal: What the dermatologist needs to know about black hairstyling practices and the risk of

traction alopecia (TA). J Am Acad Dermatol 2016;
75:606–11.

52. Udompanich S, Chanprapaph K, Suchonwanit P. Hair and Scalp Changes in Cutaneous and Systemic Lupus Erythematosus. Am J Clin Dermatol 2018;19:679–94. https://doi.org/10.1007/s40257-018-0363-8. Preprint at.

53. Kuhn A, Sigges J, Biazar C, et al. Influence of smoking on disease severity and antimalarial therapy in cutaneous lupus erythematosus: analysis of 1002 patients from the EUSCLE database. Br J Dermatol 2014;171:571–9.

54. Gallego H, Crutchfield CE 3rd, Lewis EJ, et al. Report of an association between discoid lupus erythematosus and smoking. Cutis 1999;63:231–4.

55. Miot HA, Miot LDB, Haddad GR. Association between discoid lupus erythematosus and cigarette smoking. Dermatology 2005;211:118–22.

56. Wahie S, Daly AK, Cordell HJ, et al. Clinical and pharmacogenetic influences on response to hydroxychloroquine in discoid lupus erythematosus: a retrospective cohort study. J Invest Dermatol 2011;131:1981–6.

57. Piette EW, Foering KP, Chang AY, et al. Impact of smoking in cutaneous lupus erythematosus. Arch Dermatol 2012;148:317–22.

58. Chasset F, Francès C, Barete S, et al. Influence of smoking on the efficacy of antimalarials in cutaneous lupus: a meta-analysis of the literature. J Am Acad Dermatol 2015;72:634–9.

59. Lundberg IE, Miller FW, Tjärnlund A, et al. Diagnosis and classification of idiopathic inflammatory myopathies. J Intern Med 2016;280:39–51.

60. Lundberg IE, de Visser M, Werth VP. Classification of myositis. Nat Rev Rheumatol 2018;14:269–78.

61. Mainetti C, Terziroli Beretta-Piccoli B, Selmi C. Cutaneous Manifestations of Dermatomyositis: a Comprehensive Review. Clin Rev Allergy Immunol 2017;53:337–56.

62. Concha JSS, Tarazi M, Kushner CJ, et al. The diagnosis and classification of amyopathic dermatomyositis: a historical review and assessment of existing criteria. Br J Dermatol 2019;180:1001–8.

63. Fernandez AP. Connective Tissue Disease: Current Concepts. Dermatol Clin 2019;37:37–48.

64. Goonesekera S, Bansal A, Tadwalkar S, et al. The Prevalence of Systemic Sclerosis, Dermatomyositis/Polymyositis, and Giant Cell Arteritis in the United States by Race and Ethnicity: An Analysis Using Electronic Health Records [abstract]. Arthritis Rheumatol 2020;72.

65. Feldman CH, Hiraki LT, Liu J, et al. Epidemiology and sociodemographics of systemic lupus erythematosus and lupus nephritis among US adults with Medicaid coverage, 2000-2004. Arthritis Rheum 2013;65:753–63.

66. Buster KJ, Stevens EI, Elmets CA. Dermatologic health disparities. Dermatol Clin 2012;30:53–9.

67. Smoyer-Tomic KE, Amato AA, Fernandes AW. Incidence and prevalence of idiopathic inflammatory myopathies among commercially insured, Medicare supplemental insured, and Medicaid enrolled populations: an administrative claims analysis. BMC Musculoskelet Disord 2012;13.

68. El-Azhary RA, Pakzad SY. Amyopathic dermatomyositis: retrospective review of 37 cases. J Am Acad Dermatol 2002;46:560–5.

69. Gerami P, Schope JM, McDonald L, et al. A systematic review of adult-onset clinically amyopathic dermatomyositis (dermatomyositis siné myositis): a missing link within the spectrum of the idiopathic inflammatory myopathies. J Am Acad Dermatol 2006;54:597–613.

70. Ghazi E, Sontheimer RD, Werth VP. The importance of including amyopathic dermatomyositis in the idiopathic inflammatory myositis spectrum. Clin Exp Rheumatol 2013;31:128–34.

71. Smith ES, Hallman JR, DeLuca AM, et al. Dermatomyositis: a clinicopathological study of 40 patients. Am J Dermatopathol 2009;31:61–7.

72. Bogdanov I, Kazandjieva J, Darlenski R, et al. Dermatomyositis: Current concepts. Clin Dermatol 2018;36:450–8.

73. Auriemma M, Capo A, Meogrossi G, et al. Cutaneous signs of classical dermatomyositis. G Ital Dermatol Venereol 2014;149:505–17.

74. Bridges BF. The rashes of dermatomyositis in a black patient. Am J Med 1991;91:661–2.

75. Sontheimer RD. Dermatomyositis: an overview of recent progress with emphasis on dermatologic aspects. Dermatol Clin 2002;20:387–408.

76. Gordon P., Cooper R., Chinoy H., et al., AB0629 Design of A Randomized, Double-Blind, Placebo-Controlled Phase 2 Clinical Trial of The Toll-like Receptor Antagonist IMO-8400 in Patients with Dermatomyositis, Ann Rheum Dis, 75, 2016, 1119.

77. Santmyire-Rosenberger B, Dugan EM. Skin involvement in dermatomyositis. Curr Opin Rheumatol 2003;15:714–22.

78. Rafailidis PI, Kapaskelis A, Falagas ME. Periorbital and facial swelling due to dermatomyositis. CMAJ (Can Med Assoc J) 2007;176:1580–1.

79. Hall VC, Keeling JH, Davis MDP. Periorbital edema as the presenting sign of dermatomyositis. Int J Dermatol 2003;42:466–7.

80. Lupton JR, Figueroa P, Berberian BJ, et al. An unusual presentation of dermatomyositis: the type Wong variant revisited. J Am Acad Dermatol 2000;43:908–12.

81. Mutasim DF, Egesi A, Spicknall KE. Wong-type dermatomyositis: a mimic of many dermatoses. J Cutan Pathol 2016;43:781–6.

82. Wong KO. Dermatomyositis: a clinical investigation of twenty-three cases in Hong Kong. Br J Dermatol 1969;81:544–7.

83. Bax CE, Chakka S, Concha JSS, et al. The effects of immunostimulatory herbal supplements on autoimmune skin diseases. J Am Acad Dermatol 2021;84:1051–8.

84. Pangti R, Gupta S. Flagellate Dermatitis Associated With Dermatomyositis in Skin of Color. J Cutan Med Surg 2022;26:313.

85. Stahl NI, Klippel JH, Decker JL. A cutaneous lesion associated with myositis. Ann Intern Med 1979;91:577–9.

86. Sohara E, Saraya T, Sato S, et al. Mechanic's hands revisited: is this sign still useful for diagnosis in patients with lung involvement of collagen vascular diseases? BMC Res Notes 2014;7.

87. Ward I, Hiles P, Arroyo R, et al. Digital Pulp Ulcerations and Inverse Gottron Papules in Melanoma Differentiation-Associated Gene 5-Related Dermatomyositis. J Clin Rheumatol 2016;22:274–5.

88. Narang NS, Casciola-Rosen L, Li S, et al. Cutaneous ulceration in dermatomyositis: association with anti-melanoma differentiation-associated gene 5 antibodies and interstitial lung disease. Arthritis Care Res 2015;67:667–72.

89. Kurtzman DJB, Vleugels RA. Anti-melanoma differentiation-associated gene 5 (MDA5) dermatomyositis: A concise review with an emphasis on distinctive clinical features. J Am Acad Dermatol 2018;78:776–85.

90. Cao H, Pan M, Kang Y, et al. Clinical manifestations of dermatomyositis and clinically amyopathic dermatomyositis patients with positive expression of anti-melanoma differentiation-associated gene 5 antibody. Arthritis Care Res 2012;64:1602–10.

91. Gutierrez D, Svigos K, Femia A, et al. Prominent dyspigmentation in a patient with dermatomyositis and TIF1-γ autoantibodies. JAAD Case Rep 2022;22:107–9.

92. Sarin KY, Chung L, Kim J, et al. Molecular profiling to diagnose a case of atypical dermatomyositis. J Invest Dermatol 2013;133:2796–9.

93. Rathore U, Haldule S, Gupta L. Psoriasiform rashes as the first manifestation of anti-MDA5 associated myositis. Rheumatology 2021;60:3483.

94. Wolstencroft PW, Fiorentino DF. Dermatomyositis Clinical and Pathological Phenotypes Associated with Myositis-Specific Autoantibodies. Curr Rheumatol Rep 2018;20.

95. Bernet LL, Lewis MA, Rieger KE, et al. Ovoid Palatal Patch in Dermatomyositis: A Novel Finding Associated With Anti-TIF1γ (p155) Antibodies. JAMA Dermatol 2016;152:1049–51.

96. Fiorentino DF, Kuo K, Chung L, et al. Distinctive cutaneous and systemic features associated with antitranscriptional intermediary factor-1γ antibodies in adults with dermatomyositis. J Am Acad Dermatol 2015;72:449–55.

97. Casal-Dominguez M, Pinal-Fernandez I, Mego M, et al. High-resolution manometry in patients with idiopathic inflammatory myopathy: Elevated prevalence of esophageal involvement and differences according to autoantibody status and clinical subset. Muscle Nerve 2017;56:386–92.

98. Concha JSS, Pena S, Gaffney RG, et al. Developing classification criteria for skin-predominant dermatomyositis: the Delphi process. Br J Dermatol 2020;182:410–7.

99. Euwer RL, Sontheimer RD. Amyopathic dermatomyositis (dermatomyositis siné myositis). Presentation of six new cases and review of the literature. J Am Acad Dermatol 1991;24:959–66.

100. DeWane ME, Waldman R, Lu J. Dermatomyositis: Clinical features and pathogenesis. J Am Acad Dermatol 2020;82:267–81.

101. Goreshi R, Chock M, Foering K, et al. Quality of life in dermatomyositis. J Am Acad Dermatol 2011;65:1107–16.

102. Bailey EE, Fiorentino DF. Amyopathic dermatomyositis: definitions, diagnosis, and management. Curr Rheumatol Rep 2014;16.

103. Robinson ES, Feng R, Okawa J, et al. Improvement in the cutaneous disease activity of patients with dermatomyositis is associated with a better quality of life. Br J Dermatol 2015;172:169–74.

104. Bronner IM, van der Meulen MF, de Visser M, et al. Long-term outcome in polymyositis and dermatomyositis. Ann Rheum Dis 2006;65:1456–61.

105. Anyanwu CO, Chansky PB, Feng R, et al. The systemic management of cutaneous dermatomyositis: Results of a stepwise strategy. Int J Womens Dermatol 2017;3:189–94.

106. da Silva DM, Patel B, Werth VP. Dermatomyositis: A diagnostic dilemma. J Am Acad Dermatol 2018;79:371–3.

107. Magro CM, Segal JP, Crowson AN, et al. The phenotypic profile of dermatomyositis and lupus erythematosus: a comparative analysis. J Cutan Pathol 2010;37:659–71.

108. Patel B, Khan N, Werth VP. Applicability of EULAR/ACR classification criteria for dermatomyositis to amyopathic disease. J Am Acad Dermatol 2018;79:77–83.e1.

109. Bouaziz J.D., Barete S., Le Pelletier F., et al., Cutaneous lesions of the digits in systemic lupus erythematosus: 50 cases, *Lupus*, 16, 2007, 163–167.

110. Monfort JB, Chasset F, Barbaud A, et al. Nailfold capillaroscopy findings in cutaneous lupus erythematosus patients with or without digital lesions and

comparison with dermatomyositis patients: A prospective study. Lupus 2021;30:1207–13.

111. Lundberg IE, Tjärnlund A, Bottai M, et al. European League Against Rheumatism/American College of Rheumatology Classification Criteria for Adult and Juvenile Idiopathic Inflammatory Myopathies and Their Major Subgroups. Arthritis Rheumatol 2017; 69:2271–82.

112. Rothfield N, Sontheimer RD, Bernstein M. Lupus erythematosus: systemic and cutaneous manifestations. Clin Dermatol 2006;24:348–62.

113. Jain S, Sharma A. Lupus versus dermatomyositis: the hands say it all. Rheumatology 2020;59:2647.

114. Ginter DC, Ramien ML, Brundler MA, et al. A rare case of suspected lupus erythematous panniculitis as the presenting skin feature of juvenile dermatomyositis: A case report. SAGE Open Med Case Rep 2022;10.

115. Callen JP. Cutaneous manifestations of dermatomyositis and their management. Curr Rheumatol Rep 2010;12:192–7.

116. Muro Y, Sugiura K, Akiyama M. Cutaneous Manifestations in Dermatomyositis: Key Clinical and Serological Features-a Comprehensive Review. Clin Rev Allergy Immunol 2016;51:293–302.

117. Vleugels RA, Callen JP. Dermatomyositis. In: Dermatological signs of systemic disease. Elsevier; 2017.

118. Vleugels RA, Callen JP. Dermatomyositis. In: treatment of skin disease. Comprehensive therapeutic strategies. Elsevier Saunders; 2014.

Cutaneous Sarcoidosis

Nnenna Ezeh, MD[a,1], Avrom Caplan, MD[b], Misha Rosenbach, MD[c,2], Sotonye Imadojemu, MD, MBE[d,*]

KEYWORDS

- Sarcoidosis • Cutaneous sarcoidosis • Lupus pernio • Sarcoidosis disparities
- Sarcoidosis in skin of color

KEY POINTS

- Sarcoidosis is a chronic, multiorgan, inflammatory disorder that commonly presents on the skin, thus there are significant implications on diagnosis and management in patients with darkly pigmented skin.
- There are significant racial disparities in prevalence, severity, and outcomes; however, there is a dearth of studies investigating the impact of structural racism.
- Clinicians should adopt a comprehensive systemic approach to working up potential patients with sarcoidosis with treatment targeting the most impacted organ systems with topical therapies, immunomodulators, and systemic immunosuppressants.

INTRODUCTION

Sarcoidosis is a chronic inflammatory disorder, which is characterized by noncaseating granulomas impairing organ function. It is a multisystem condition that can affect any organ in the body, causing significant morbidity and mortality through organ damage, chronic dysfunction, and scarring. Understanding and recognizing cutaneous sarcoidosis is paramount. Skin is the second most common organ affected in sarcoidosis, affected in approximately 25% to 40% of cases reported and, in some studies, was the initial presenting symptom in up to 88% of cases.[1–10] This article will review updates on epidemiology and pathogenesis, clinical presentation with focus on presentation in darker pigmented skin in patients of color, diagnosis, and management of cutaneous sarcoidosis to better aid dermatologists in caring for patients of color with sarcoidosis.[11–13]

EPIDEMIOLOGY

Systemic sarcoidosis occurs worldwide, affecting people of all age, sex, ethnicity, and race. Large generalizable epidemiologic assessments of sarcoidosis have been hindered by inconsistency in case definition, poor diagnostic sensitivity with varied methods, multiple subphenotypes, and varying levels of access to care.[14] This influences the accuracy of estimates of the burden of sarcoidosis as well as highlights disparities in disease manifestations, phenotype, and mortality related to age, sex, geographic location, genetic background, race and ethnicity, or environmental triggers.[15]

The best available evidence suggests that the prevalence of sarcoidosis ranges from 1 to 5 per 100,000 in countries including South Korea, Taiwan, Japan, Spain to 140 to 160 per 100,000 in Sweden and Canada.[15] In the United States,

[a] Harvard Combined Dermatology Residency, Massachusetts General Hospital, Boston, MA, USA; [b] Ronald O. Perelman Department of Dermatology, NYU School of Medicine, 222 East 41st Street, 16th Floor, New York, NY 10016, USA; [c] Department of Dermatology, University of Pennsylvania, Philadelphia, PA, USA; [d] Department of Dermatology, Brigham and Women's Hospital, Harvard Medical School, 221 Longwood Avenue, Boston, MA 02115, USA
[1] Present address: 221 Longwood Avenue, Boston, MA 02115, USA.
[2] Present address: 2506 Pine Street, Philadelphia PA 19103, USA.
* Corresponding author.
E-mail address: Simadojemu@bwh.Harvard.edu

Dermatol Clin 41 (2023) 455–470
https://doi.org/10.1016/j.det.2023.02.012

the estimated prevalence is on average 60 per 100,000, varying greatly based on race from 19 in Asian Americans to 140 in Black American.[16] A bimodal distribution in incidence has been demonstrated with peaks in the third and fourth decades followed by the sixth decade.[17] Women have a higher incidence of sarcoidosis compared with men and generally were older than men when diagnosed, 30 to 50 years in men versus 50 to 60 years in women.[18] In late-onset sarcoidosis, recent studies in France showed asthenia, uveitis, and specific skin lesions were more common with less pulmonary and lymphatic involvement.[19,20] Studies have detected seasonal variability in incidence, with the highest incidence rates reported during the winter and the lowest reported in autumn.[21]

Race has been noted as an important source of variation in sarcoidosis epidemiology. However, race, a social construct, has often been used in research studies as a proxy for unmeasured genetic factors, leading to generalizations regarding biologic risk. This obfuscates the role of systemic racism have as legitimate and clinically relevant cause of poor health and outcomes.[22,23] For example, racist housing practices could potentially manifest in racial minorities having increased exposure to environmental triggers leading to increased prevalence of sarcoidosis. Similarly, neighborhood disadvantage and segregated communities has been shown to increase the risk of asthma and atopic dermatitis in marginalized racial groups.[24–28] Future research should include large, matched epidemiologic studies conducted in racially diverse populations through large population data sets and registries. In addition, studies directly measuring the impact of discrimination, structural racism, and access to quality care on patients diagnosed with sarcoidosis will help clarify any impact of these factors on sarcoidosis pathogenesis and quality of life.[29,30]

Studies have consistently demonstrated a high incidence of sarcoidosis among Black women and identified this population as being at an elevated risk for systemic complications of sarcoidosis as well as severe and fatal outcomes.[31–34] In a multicenter, multiethnic European cohort, 5 clinical phenotypes were isolated with non-White patients having phenotypes with more severe internal disease and lupus pernio.[35] In the United States, the annual incidence of sarcoidosis is consistently higher among non-Hispanic Black Americans estimated at 35.5 per 100,000 compared with 10.9 per 100,000 in white Americans and 3 to 4 per 100,000 in Asian Americans.[16,17,36–38] However, in French Guadeloupe and West Africa, in which inhabitants share genetic ancestry with Black Americans, the incidence of sarcoidosis seems to be much lower.[39] This conveys that ancestry and genetics is not the full explanation for this racial disparity. In a prospective, multicenter study of sarcoidosis, Black patients were more likely to have a family income of less than US$20,000 and public insurance suggesting, that Black patients were more likely to have financial barriers, delaying timely access to care.[40]

Black patients, overall, are more likely to have cutaneous sarcoidosis. Additionally, Black patients tend to present with cutaneous sarcoidosis at a younger age, a trend, which was also observed in patients who were evaluated for ocular disease.[31,41] Additionally, the clinical subphenotype of Lofgren syndrome characterized by fever, arthritis, erythema nodosum, and bilateral hilar lymphadenopathy is associated with favorable prognosis in White patients of northern European ancestry with specific human leukocyte antigen (HLA) subtypes but is uncommon in Black and Asian populations that lack those HLA subtypes.[42,43] If extracutaneous disease was noted, Black patients had more organ systems affected, including cardiac disease and pulmonary disease, specifically pulmonary hypertension.[31] These disparities are notable as cardiac sarcoidosis and pulmonary hypertension can be fatal and serve as possible explanations of the higher mortality rate seen in this group.[44–46] In longitudinal studies, Black patients had a higher likelihood of more severe disease, new organ involvement and more frequently required systemic medication compared with White patients.[34,47–49] Furthermore, Black patients have higher rates of hospitalization up to 9 times higher compared with White patients.[41] In another retrospective study, there was a near doubling of hospitalization in Black, female and older patients in a retrospective study.[42] Moreover, the age-adjusted sarcoidosis-specific mortality rate is higher for Black Americans compared with White Americans in 2008 to 2016, up to 9 times as high in Black women compared with White women with Black patients dying at an earlier age.[50–52] This study also investigated the role of geographic location and urbanization in sarcoidosis incidence among Black Americans. They found the lowest rates of sarcoidosis in southern states and the highest rates in small rather than large metropolitan areas.[50] The extent to which institutional and structural racism contribute to these disparities warrants a dedicated study to better understand the epidemiologic complexities and to ultimately provide the most optimal care for patients with sarcoidosis.

PATHOGENESIS

The development of sarcoidosis is thought to be secondary to a genetic predisposition combined with an environmental insult causing the histologic hallmark of granulomatous inflammation.

Genetic Factors

A genetic predisposition is supported by cases showing familial clustering, a high concordance rate in monozygotic twins, and by genetic variation studies.[53–56] In Black patients with at least one first-degree relative with sarcoidosis, the risk of sarcoidosis is 2.5 to 2.9 times higher compared with White individuals, with the risk increasing with multiple affected relatives.[53,54,56] Genetic variants may increase susceptibility to environmental triggers. For example, a case-control study of first responders in the 2001 World Trade Center attacks identified specific genetic variations in firefighters who developed sarcoidosis that were not present in those who did not develop the disease.[57] Additionally, there were similarities between variants seen in cases of sarcoidosis without known environmental exposure and World Trade Center-related sarcoidosis.[57]

Sarcoidosis is considered a polygenic disease with several gene variants associated with a large array of phenotypes, prognoses, and therapeutic responses. However, most of the genetic background of sarcoidosis remains unknown.[58] The HLA-DRB1 gene locus has been extensively identified for its importance in predicting disease progression and risks versus protection from sarcoidosis.[43,58,59] In Black Americans, HLA-DQB1 alleles resulted in both increased susceptibility to sarcoidosis and progression of disease in a family-based genetic association analysis.[60] Further stratification of Black families by genetically determined ancestry revealed linkage differences by subpopulation, with previously reported linkage signals on chromosome 5 at 1p22, 3p21-14, 11p15, and 17q21 specific to ancestral heritage.[61] For example, in a study involving 301 patients with Löfgren syndrome, complete resolution within 2 years occurred in DRB1*03-positive patients. On the contrary, HLA-DRB1*15 (DR15) and DRB1*14 (DR14) have been associated with chronic nonresolving disease, diffuse endobronchial involvement, and severe multiorgan involvement.[62] Other implicated genes have included ANXA11, BTNL2, XAF1, NOTCH4, IL-23R, ACE, TLR9, NOD2, tumor necrosis factor (TNF)-α, and TGF-ß1 but have yet to be associated with specific clinical phenotypes.[63–69]

In a recent whole-genome study of family with high rates of sarcoidosis, Janus kinase 2, among others, was isolated as a potential gene of interest.[70] The JAK phosphorylates signal transducer and activates STAT, a transcription factor with broad effects on cell differentiation and the immune system.[71] The JAK/STAT signal transduction pathway connected to a number of cytokines including interleukin (IL)-12 and IL-23, which mediate T helper 1 (Th1) and Th17 cell response, respectively, as well as interferon (IFN-)γ, type I interferons, IL-2, IL-4, IL-6, IL-10, IL-13, and granulocyte-macrophage colony-stimulating factor. Many of these factors and cytokines have been implicated in granuloma formation in sarcoidosis.[43,72–75] There is an increasing evidence base supporting the association of the JAK/STAT pathway in sarcoidosis pathogenesis including a study, which revealed activation of JAK-STAT signaling at the microRNA level in peripheral blood.[76] Additionally, many case series and translational investigations describe resolution of sarcoidosis and decreased JAK-STAT activity in patients treated with JAK inhibitors.[72,77–79]

Environmental Triggers

Various infectious and noninfectious antigens such as a misfolded self-antigen, or organic or inorganic environmental molecules, have been implicated as potential triggers in the immune-inflammatory events that lead to granuloma formation.[58] A dysregulated immune response against one or more disease-promoting antigens results in an inflammatory process to eliminate the offending antigen leading to granuloma formation.[43] Both environmental and occupational triggers have been hypothesized given the wide variation in incidence based on geographic location even within countries.

Infectious antigens range from stronger associations with mycobacteria and Propionibacterium acnes to possible links with rubella virus to more inconclusive links to Borrelia, Rickettsia, and human herpesvirus-8 that may trigger inflammation as opposed to viable infections.[43,80–87] Noninfectious exposures such as inorganic aerosolized metals or combustible materials such as wood and toner ink have been described to trigger sarcoidosis or sarcoidosis-like granulomatous diseases.[12,88–93] Additionally, sarcoidosis has been diagnosed at higher rates in firefighters, first responders, health-care workers, and agricultural employees.[92,94,95] The role of vitamin D mechanisms has yet to be conclusively explained but is being studied. Autoimmunity also has been implicated with vimentin, a cytoskeletal protein, as potential target given humoral responses to the protein have been shown to be associated to patients with HLA-DRB1*03-positive sarcoidosis.[96,97]

As aforementioned, objective measurements of racism and the sequelae of structural racism as environmental triggers have been understudied as a risk factor for sarcoidosis. Racial discrimination can manifest in various avenues of society including employment, housing, education, health care, and can directly influence socioeconomic standings.[98–101] This can create chronic stress that results in maladaptive coping mechanisms including tobacco smoking, which has been linked to ocular sarcoidosis and possibly cutaneous granulomas in retrospective studies.[102,103] A retrospective study from Sweden showed that a high neighborhood deprivation (a composite of income, education, unemployment, social welfare assistance) was associated with a 20% increased odds of having sarcoidosis.[104] Additionally, racial discrimination can trigger a "weathering" or accelerated physiologic deterioration in Black Americans and has been associated with chronically high levels of proinflammatory cytokines, increasing the risk for inflammatory and chronic conditions such as cardiovascular disease.[105–113] In a disease that similarly disproportionately affects Black Americans, observational studies of Black female patients with systemic lupus erythematosus (SLE) showed increased frequencies of self-reported racial discrimination or vicarious racism stress were associated with an increased SLE activity and irreversible organ damage.[114–116]

Granuloma Formation

Once both genetic and environment insults occur, a predominantly Th1 immune response, helped by the innate immune system and Th17 response is initiated to drive granuloma formation followed by either persistent or resolving disease. Subclinical inflammation with each exposure begins with the activation of membrane-bound pattern recognition receptors (eg, toll-like receptors). When stimulated, macrophages and other innate immune cells promote transcription factors, resulting in the production of cytokines and chemokines such as CD4+ and CD8+ cells.[14] IL-13, a potentially significant cytokine to target, promotes the differentiation of alveolar macrophage 2 and monocytes into antigen-presenting cells. The mammalian target of rapamycin complex (mTORC1) of the mTOR pathway, a potent repressor of autophagy, is activated, which promotes and sustains further granuloma formation.[117,118] Ongoing hypotheses propose that dysregulation of autophagy may lead to aberrant degradation of cellular byproducts and affect antigenic presentation.[119] Many cytokines are involved in this process including IL-1, IL-2, IL-12, IL-17, IL-18, IL-23 with IFN-γ, and

TNF-α playing key roles including activating the previously discussed JAK-STAT pathway.[74] If the antigen can be eliminated, the response will shut down. Conversely, if the antigen persists, granuloma formation occurs through the persistent activation of IFN-γ and TNF-α triggering a complex fibrotic process stimulated by the release of TGF-β and IL-10.[120] Circulating fibrocytes can differentiate into fibroblasts and release collagen and other profibrotic substances.[121] FoxP3-expressing regulatory T (Treg) cells have the ability to aid in granuloma resolution but often are dysfunctional.[58]

Clinical Presentations

Cutaneous disease is often the first sign of systemic sarcoidosis, and commonly, many patients have initially skin-limited disease. Cutaneous manifestations can be divided into 2 major categories: lesions specific to sarcoidosis, with characteristic sarcoidal granulomas, and nonspecific lesions resulting from the systemic immunologic response. Specifically, when evaluating patients with darker pigmented skin, lesions can appear pink, red-brown, yellow-brown, purple-brown, or even gray. Erythema can be more subtle and can seem brown or purple. The various specific sarcoidosis findings are detailed in **Table 1** (selected examples in **Figs. 1–3**). Patients of color are more likely to present with specific manifestations compared with nonspecific lesions. Lupus pernio,[122,123] papule/plaque,[124,125] hypopigmented, verrucous, ulcers, psoriasiform, and scalp sarcoidosis occur more frequently in Black patients than in White patients.[2,122–124,126–133] Certain variants of cutaneous sarcoidosis carry potential prognostic implications and are discussed further below.

Lupus Pernio

The clinical variant, lupus pernio, consisting of violaceous, firm papules, and nodules that may develop scale. It is most often seen on the central

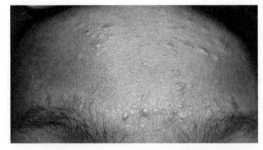

Fig. 1. Papular sarcoidosis: flesh colored papular lesions are shown on the forehead here. Papular sarcoidosis is a very common morphologic subtype.

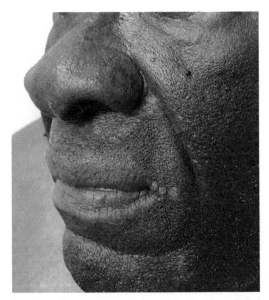

Fig. 2. Erythematous papules and plaques: slightly pink lesions with a vaguely annular architecture are seen in the perinasal area, with additional papules on the lip.

face, especially the distal nose, ears, lips, face, and less seen on hands and feet. It is characterized by a later age of onset and is disproportionately seen in Black and female patients.[123,126] It can present with a few small nodules on the nose, spread insidiously with progressive infiltration and induration into bone and cartilage. Lesions wrapping inward from the alar rim to obliterate the nasal mucosa can be seen on clinical examination and suggest the possibility of additional upper airway involvement. In addition to the standard workup for extracutaneous disease, the evaluation of a patient with lupus pernio should prompt otorhinolaryngology evaluation because sinus disease can be severe in patients with lupus pernio. It can be disfiguring and is associated with a more chronic or refractory course.[134] It can present as an isolated skin lesion but more often is an early systemic manifestation. Lupus pernio is associated with an increased risk of extracutaneous, especially upper respiratory and pulmonary, involvement as well as bone involvement. Lupus pernio warrants a thorough workup and often requires aggressive systemic therapy, specifically including the use of TNF-inhibitors.[122,123,135–137]

Scar Sarcoidosis

Cutaneous sarcoidosis may occur in scar tissue, at traumatized sites, and around imbedded foreign material, such as tattoos.[138,139] This can include scars from surgical incisions, venipuncture, acne,

herpes zoster virus, and other forms of skin trauma. They can become raised and erythematous to violaceous. Lesions developing in old, chronic scars may be confused with hypertrophic scars or keloids.[140] Tattoo involvement can be mistaken for granulomatous hypersensitivity reactions to tattoo pigment or infections such as syphilis or atypical mycobacterial infections. The appearance of disease in previously inactive scars is thought to herald increased disease activity.[139]

Subcutaneous Sarcoidosis

Subcutaneous sarcoidosis presents as asymptomatic smooth cutaneous nodules located in the deep dermis and subcutis.[140] It is sometimes referred to as Darier-Roussy sarcoidosis.[128,141] They typically present on the trunk and extremities, mainly arms.[142] They can be distributed in a

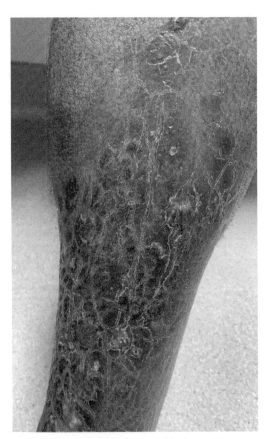

Fig. 3. Ichthyosiform sarcoidosis: this rare morphology is clinically challenging to distinguish from other forms of acquired ichthyosis however, a biopsy would typically show sarcoidal granulomatous inflammation. This patient has also had ulcerative sarcoidosis within the ichthyosiform lesions and has healing ulcers and scars at sites of earlier severe inflammation.

Table 1
Specific cutaneous sarcoidosis manifestations

Common	Papules and nodules	• Red-brown to purple-brown micropapules, papules, and nodules usually located on extensor surfaces or face, particularly the nasolabial folds, periorbital, perioral regions. Can originate within scars
	Plaques	• Red-brown to purple-brown well-demarcated, round to oval infiltrated plaques on the trunk and extremities predominantly but also the scalp and face. Can be annular with peripheral elevation or with white-gray scale • More likely to have chronic or scarring disease compared with papular lesions
	Lupus pernio	• Red-brown to purple-brown smooth indurated papules and nodules present symmetrically on the central face, also ears. Can present with beaded appearance with notching along the nasal rim • Often disfiguring and chronic
Uncommon or rare	Atrophic and ulcerative	• Easily ulcerative depressed plaques with roller borders • May have surrounding yellow-brown plaques with telangiectasias • Favors head and neck • Can originate de novo or in preestablished specific lesions
	Angiolupoid	• Pink to purple-brown papules and plaques with pronounced overlying telangiectasias on face • Commonly diagnosed as lupus pernio but usually more discrete and less extensive
	Erythrodermic	• Indurated red-yellow brown or purple-brown confluent plaques with overlying fine scale or desquamation
	Hypopigmented	• Skin colored to yellow-brown macules on extremities. Can be more noticeable or prominent in darkly pigmented skin • Present in isolation or papules and plaques • Better diagnostic value if biopsy of indurated hypopigmented lesions or associated papule
	Ichthyosiform	• Brown or white-gray polygonal with scale more adherent in center than edge, appearing pasted on • Present on lower legs • High rates of progression to systemic sarcoidosis
	Mucosal	• Can vary from papules, plaques, nodules with localized edema or infiltrative thickening. Located on buccal mucosa, gingiva, hard palate, tongue, posterior pharynx, and salivary glands
	Nail	• Thinning, brittle nails, thickened nails, pitting, ridging, trachyonychia, hyperpigmentation, clubbing or pseudo-clubbing, onycholysis, or destruction of the nail plate and scarring (ie, pterygium)
	Psoriasiform	• Red to pink-brown plaques with overlying scale resembling psoriasis primarily on the legs • Unlike psoriasis, heals with scarring and hyperpigmentation
	Scalp	• Scarring or nonscarring alopecia, localized or diffuse • Range in lesions resembling alopecia areata-like macules, seborrheic dermatitis-like scaly plaques to infiltrated plaques and nodules
	Subcutaneous nodules	• Firm, mobile, painless, oval, flesh-colored to purple-brown subcutaneous nodules on the trunk or extremities
	Verrucous	• Hyperkeratotic pink to red-brown wart-like papules and plaques possibly with overlying white-gray scale

Data from Caplan A, Rosenbach M, Imadojemu S. Cutaneous Sarcoidosis. Semin Respir Crit Care Med. 2020;41(5):689-699, Rosenbach, Misha A., et al. "Non-Infectious Granulomas." *Dermatology*, Fourth Edition, 2018, pp. 1644–63 and Heath CR, David J, Taylor SC. Sarcoidosis: Are there differences in your skin of color patients? *J Am Acad Dermatol*. 2012;66(1):121.e1-14.

linear fashion in a lymphangitic or sporotrichoid pattern. It presents more commonly in White patients.[143] Some argue that subcutaneous sarcoidosis is associated with benign systemic disease but this assertion is debated.[128,142]

Erythema Nodosum

Erythema nodosum is the most common nonspecific sarcoidosis lesion, developing in up to 25% of patients.[140] It is a reactive panniculitis that seems as erythematous to violaceous to brown, tender, warm subcutaneous nodules, predominantly located on the pretibial leg. It presents usually with arthralgias, lower extremity edema, and fever. Erythema nodosum has been associated with a favorable prognosis, a pattern most commonly seen in White patients of Scandinavian European descent.[144,145] Of note, a variant called erythema nodosum-like sarcoid has been described in a Japanese cohort, which, by contrast, is a specific cutaneous sarcoidosis manifestation.[146] It resembles erythema nodosum solely in appearance as sarcoid granulomas are seen histologically.

Löfgren syndrome consists of the tetrad of erythema nodosum, bilateral hilar lymphadenopathy, migratory polyarthralgia, and fever.[140] Löfgren syndrome is associated with a good prognosis with spontaneous resolution within 2 years, although it can be very symptomatic.[147,148] It is typically managed with nonsteroidal anti-inflammatory drugs but can demand systemic corticosteroids.

Other nonspecific cutaneous findings of sarcoidosis include calcinosis cutis, clubbing, and prurigo.[140]

DIAGNOSTICS AND EVALUATION
Clinicopathologic Diagnosis

The diagnosis of sarcoidosis is clinicopathologic, ruling out other causes of granulomatous disease in conjunction with a systemic evaluation given the high prevalence of concomitant systemic sarcoidosis. Cutaneous histopathology of sarcoid-specific lesions can present a high-yield source of diagnostic information. Punch or incisional biopsy is preferred over superficial shave biopsy, as granulomatous involvement can be superficial, deep within the dermis, or in subcutaneous tissue.[12,149,150]

Typical biopsies of sarcoid-specific lesions demonstrate "naked granulomas"—noncaseating aggregates of epithelioid histiocytes without inflammatory cells. Multinucleated giant cells—typically of the Langerhans or foreign-body type—are often present. These giant cells at times show asteroid bodies (eosinophilic starburst inclusions) within their cytoplasm or Schaumann bodies

(laminated, cytoplasmic calcifications) but neither Schaumann bodies nor asteroid bodies are specific to sarcoidosis.[151] Although naked granulomas are typical, sparse infiltrates of lymphocytes and plasma cells and focal necrosis have been reported. These findings should not preclude a diagnosis of sarcoidosis in the right clinical and pathologic setting.[12,150,151]

The clinical differential diagnosis is broad given the numerous presentations but includes granuloma annulare, leprosy, tuberculosis, lichen planus, SLE, secondary or tertiary syphilis, leukemia cutis, necrobiosis lipoidica, and leishmaniasis. The differential diagnosis of naked granulomas includes cutaneous Crohn disease, orofacial granulomatosis (Melkersson-Rosenthal syndrome), granulomatous rosacea, silica, beryllium, zirconium granulomas, and tuberculoid leprosy. Perineural infiltration of granulomas has rarely been reported in sarcoidosis and cannot definitely differentiate tuberculoid leprosy from sarcoidosis.[151] Foreign body reactions, infections (including deep fungal infections), immunodeficiency disorders, drug eruptions, and other entities may also show granulomas on biopsy.[12,151,152] Therefore, all slides with granulomas should be stained for infections, and tissue culture should be considered based on clinical suspicion. Additionally, all slides should be polarized for foreign material. Notably, up to 25% of sarcoidal granulomas can contain foreign body material, which should not exclude a diagnosis of sarcoidosis.[12,150–153] Clinical correlation and additional workup is required when foreign body material is evident on biopsy.

Uncommonly, patients present with sarcoid-like skin lesions and sarcoidal granulomas on biopsy without other diagnoses to explain these findings and without another organ involvement. These patients can be diagnosed with "sarcoid-like granulomatous disease of unknown significance," although many refer to them as having "isolated cutaneous sarcoidosis."[12] It is controversial whether patients with isolated skin findings can be diagnosed with sarcoidosis because strict definitions require involvement of at least 2 organ systems.[12,154]

Workup and Evaluation

Skin involvement can be objectively and systematically evaluated. Clinical assessment tools such as the Cutaneous Sarcoidosis Activity and Morphology Instrument and the Sarcoidosis Activity and Severity Index can be used to measure clinical response to treatment.[155,156] Evaluating a patient with suspected sarcoidosis combines clinical, pathologic, and radiographic analysis to both establish a diagnosis and evaluate for systemic disease.[12,157] A thorough history must be taken to screen for extracutaneous sarcoidosis and to help eliminate other diagnoses (occupational history, exposures, travel, and family history).[12,158] Collaboration with specialists in pulmonology, cardiology, ophthalmology, otolaryngology, neurology, and endocrinology among others may be necessary to investigate and further manage extracutaneous involvement.[159] Extracutaneous manifestations can include pulmonary (interstitial lung disease, pulmonary hypertension), cardiovascular (palpitations, conduction disease, sudden cardiac death), ocular (uveitis, conjunctivitis), neurologic (nerve palsies, neuropsychiatric symptoms or seizures), among others. Nonspecific or parasarcoid symptoms such as fatigue, exercise intolerance, cognitive impairment, and small fiber neuropathy can greatly affect quality of life and wellness.[29,160–164] Workup includes a chest X-ray, pulmonary function testing to evaluate for interstitial lung disease, ophthalmologic examination, and an electrocardiogram (ECG). Some experts advocate a baseline echocardiogram and 24-hour Holter monitor in all patients with sarcoidosis, and those tests should be considered in patients with any history of palpitations because an ECG

may miss cardiac sarcoidosis.[12,31,165] One study found that cardiac sarcoidosis is more likely to occur in Black patients with sarcoidosis as compared with other groups.[31] Although controversy exists, cardiac sarcoidosis may be better imaged with either PET scanning or dedicated cardiac MRI.[14] Laboratory analysis should include a complete blood count, comprehensive metabolic panel, urinalysis (if a history of nephrolithiasis), vitamin D (both 25-hydroxyvitamin-D and 1,25-dihydroxyvitamin D3), and thyroid testing.[12,158] Biomarkers may be more useful as evidence of active inflammation as opposed to pathognomonic tests.[166] For example, the serum angiotensin-converting enzyme is elevated in only 50% to 60% of patients with sarcoidosis, lacking diagnostic specificity with limited use for therapeutic response.[166–168] Other proposed biomarkers, including soluble IL-2 receptor, C-reactive protein, serum amyloid A (SAA), and chitotriosidase, may aid in assessing the disease activity but are either expensive, not available, or lack broad studies demonstrating reliability. FDG PET-computed tomography may be more effective for detecting tissue-specific inflammatory activity and identifying site for diagnostic biopsies[14] and may be an option to track disease activity and response in some patients.

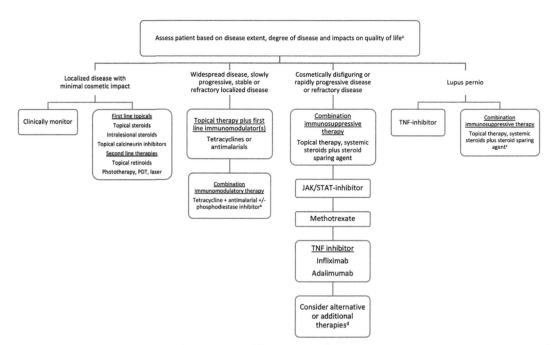

Fig. 4. Cutaneous sarcoidosis treatment algorithm.[140] [a]Give 3 mo of therapy before assessing treatment efficacy. [b]Second-line immunomodulation: pentoxifylline and isotretinoin. [c]Second-line immunosuppressives: leflunomide, thalidomide, lenalidomide, mycophenolate mofetil, and azathioprine. [d]Additional/alternative therapies include IL-6 inhibitors, rituximab. (*Adapted from* Imadojemu S, Wanat KA, Noe M, English JC, Rosenbach M. Cutaneous sarcoidosis. In: Baughman RP, Valeyre D, eds. *Sarcoidosis, a clinician's guide*. Vol 2019; 127–144.)

MANAGEMENT

Management of sarcoidosis poses significant challenges due to its clinical diversity. For most patients, there is spontaneous resolution without the need for systemic therapies. Because there are no Food and Drug Administration–approved cutaneous sarcoidosis therapies, retrospective case series and expert opinion offer treatment guidance from a range of local therapies, immunomodulatory systemic therapies, and immunosuppressive therapies.

In general, treatment can include topical therapy, systemic immunomodulatory therapy, and systemic immunosuppressive therapy. **Fig. 4** describes a proposed treatment algorithm. First-line therapy for mild local cutaneous sarcoidosis includes a combination topical and intralesional corticosteroids, topical calcineurin inhibitors, along with antimalarials,[6,140,169,170] and doxycycline (minimal risk for hyperpigmentation and autoimmune sequelae).[11,140] Small case series and case reports with post hoc analysis have shown limited benefit in phosphodiesterase (PDE4) inhibitors having a steroid-sparing effect in pulmonary sarcoid but cutaneous effects have yet to be fully studied.[171,172]

For moderate-to-severe disease, refractory, disfiguring, or destructive lesions, systemic corticosteroids and methotrexate are first line[140,173–176] except in patients with thick plaque sarcoidosis or lupus pernio. Those patients should be immediately considered for TNF-inhibitor therapy, which has demonstrated efficacy in multiple studies and case series.[177–184]

Emerging therapies with an increasing evidence base as a beneficial treatment of sarcoidosis include topical and systemic JAK inhibitors,[77,78,185–192] with open-label clinical trials showing improvement in pulmonary and cutaneous sarcoidosis.[190,193] A monoclonal antibody to IL-6 currently in a clinical trial as inhibition has been linked to reduction in SAA and granulomatous formation (ClinicalTrials.gov identifier: NCT04008069). Unfortunately, IL-12/-23 inhibitors have been studied in a randomized control trial and failed to show efficacy and were shown to exacerbate or induce disease in case reports.[194–196] IL-17 inhibitors have been reported to paradoxically induce granulomatous inflammation in early reports.[197]

Box 1
Workup recommendations in patients with cutaneous sarcoidosis

History including full review of systems, occupational/environmental exposures

Physical examination including ophthalmologic examination

Complete blood count

Comprehensive metabolic panel including creatinine, liver function tests, and calcium

Urinalysis if history of nephrolithiasis

Vitamin D_{25} and Vitamin D1, 25

Thyroid function tests

Chest X-ray

Pulmonary function tests including diffusion capacity for carbon monoxide

Electrocardiogram; if palpitations noted, cardiology referral for further testing (transthoracic echocardiogram, Holter monitor/event monitor/EP evaluation, cardiac MRI, cardiac PET)[a]

Can consider:

- Biomarkers such as angiotensin converting enzyme or others[b] for disease activity
- FDG PET-CT for identifying potential biopsy sites or disease activity

[a]Some cardiac experts prefer cardiac MRI or PET to evaluate for cardiac sarcoidosis. [b]Soluble interleukin-2 receptor, C-reactive protein, serum amyloid A (SAA) and chitotriosidase can aid in disease activity assessments but can be expensive or inconsistently available.

SUMMARY

Sarcoidosis is a multiorgan disease with high levels of cutaneous involvement. Although the exact cause is still unclear, it is thought that genetic predisposition combined with an environmental insult triggers granuloma formation. Black Americans are disproportionately affected by this condition with more severe and disfiguring disease as well higher rates of increased morbidity and mortality. This is likely due to ethnic and familial variations in pathogenic genes coupled with environmental triggers that likely include structural and institutional racism. Future studies should specifically look at the role of racism in the development of sarcoidosis. Evaluation of patients with cutaneous sarcoidosis should include workup (**Box 1**) for systemic involvement. Treatment should be focused on severely impacted organs and symptoms negatively affecting quality of life with the use of topical, immunomodulatory, and/or immunosuppressive medications.

DISCLOSURES

M. Rosenbach receives research support from Processa Pharmaceuticals. He has consulted for Processa, AbbVie, Janssen, Merck, Novartis, and Xentria. He is a member of the Foundation for Sarcoidosis Research Scientific Advisory Board. A. Caplan, N. Ezeh and S. Imadojemu have no disclosures.

REFERENCES

1. Baughman RP, Teirstein AS, Judson MA, et al. Clinical characteristics of patients in a case control study of sarcoidosis. Am J Respir Crit Care Med 2001;164(10 Pt 1):1885–9.

2. Mañá J, Marcoval J. Skin manifestations of sarcoidosis. Presse Med 2012;41(6, Part 2):e355–74.

3. Löfgren S. Diagnosis and incidence of sarcoidosis. Br J Tubercul Dis Chest 1957;51(1):8–13.

4. Longcope WT, Freiman DG. A study of sarcoidosis; based on a combined investigation of 160 cases including 30 autopsies from The Johns Hopkins Hospital and Massachusetts General Hospital. Medicine (Baltim) 1952;31(1):1–132.

5. Mayock RL, Bertrand P, Morrison CE, et al. Manifestations of sarcoidosis: analysis of 145 patients, with a review of nine series selected from the literature. Am J Med 1963;35(1):67–89.

6. Siltzbach LE, James DG, Neville E, et al. Course and prognosis of sarcoidosis around the world. Am J Med 1974;57(6):847–52.

7. Yanardağ H, Pamuk ÖN, Karayel T. Cutaneous involvement in sarcoidosis: analysis of the features in 170 patients. Respir Med 2003;97(8):978–82.

8. Ishak R, Kurban M, Kibbi AG, et al. Cutaneous sarcoidosis: clinicopathologic study of 76 patients from Lebanon. Int J Dermatol 2015;54(1):33–41.

9. Abed Dickson M, Hernández BA, Marciano S, et al. Prevalence and characteristics of cutaneous sarcoidosis in Argentina. Int J Womens Dermatol 2021;7(3):280–4.

10. Marcoval J, Mañá J, Rubio M. Specific cutaneous lesions in patients with systemic sarcoidosis: relationship to severity and chronicity of disease. Clin Exp Dermatol 2011;36(7):739–44.

11. Caplan A, Rosenbach M, Imadojemu S. Cutaneous sarcoidosis. Semin Respir Crit Care Med 2020; 41(5):689–99.

12. Wanat KA, Rosenbach M. A practical approach to cutaneous sarcoidosis. Am J Clin Dermatol 2014; 15(4):283–97.

13. Wu JH, Imadojemu S, Caplan AS. The evolving landscape of cutaneous sarcoidosis: pathogenic insight, clinical challenges, and new frontiers in therapy. Am J Clin Dermatol 2022. https://doi.org/ 10.1007/s40257-022-00693-0.

14. Drent M, Crouser ED, Grunewald J. Challenges of sarcoidosis and its management. N Engl J Med 2021;385(11):1018–32.

15. Arkema EV, Cozier YC. Sarcoidosis epidemiology: recent estimates of incidence, prevalence and risk factors. Curr Opin Pulm Med 2020;26(5):527–34.

16. Baughman RP, Field S, Costabel U, et al. Sarcoidosis in america. analysis based on health care use. Ann Am Thorac Soc 2016;13(8):1244–52.

17. Brito-Zerón P, Sellarés J, Bosch X, et al. Epidemiologic patterns of disease expression in sarcoidosis: age, gender and ethnicity-related differences. Clin Exp Rheumatol 2016;34(3):380–8.

18. Zhou Y, Gerke AK, Lower EE, et al. The impact of demographic disparities in the presentation of sarcoidosis: A multicenter prospective study. Respir Med 2021;187:106564.

19. Bert A, Gilbert T, Cottin V, et al. Sarcoidosis diagnosed in the elderly: a case-control study. QJM 2021;114(4):238–45.

20. Varron L, Cottin V, Schott AM, et al. Late-onset sarcoidosis: a comparative study. Medicine (Baltim) 2012;91(3):137–43.

21. Ungprasert P, Crowson CS, Matteson EL. Seasonal variation in incidence of sarcoidosis: a population-based study, 1976-2013. Thorax 2016;71(12):1164–6.

22. On racism: a new standard for publishing on racial health inequities | Health affairs forefront. Available at: https://www.healthaffairs.org/do/10.1377/ forefront.20200630.939347/full/. Accessed June 15, 2022.

23. Ford CL, Airhihenbuwa CO. Critical race theory, race equity, and public health: toward antiracism praxis. Am J Public Health 2010;100(Suppl 1): S30–5.

24. Tackett KJ, Jenkins F, Morrell DS, et al. Structural racism and its influence on the severity of atopic dermatitis in African American children. Pediatr Dermatol 2020;37(1):142–6.

25. Hughes HK, Matsui EC, Tschudy MM, et al. Pediatric asthma health disparities: race, hardship, housing, and asthma in a national survey. Acad Pediatr 2017;17(2):127–34.

26. Rosenbaum E. Racial/ethnic differences in asthma prevalence: the role of housing and neighborhood environments. J Health Soc Behav 2008;49(2): 131–45.

27. Brewer M, Kimbro RT, Denney JT, et al. Does neighborhood social and environmental context impact race/ethnic disparities in childhood asthma? Health Place 2017;44:86–93.

28. Martinez A, de la Rosa R, Mujahid M, et al. Structural racism and its pathways to asthma and atopic dermatitis. J Allergy Clin Immunol 2021;148(5): 1112–20.

29. Saketkoo LA, Russell AM, Jensen K, et al. Health-related quality of life (HRQoL) in sarcoidosis:

diagnosis, management, and health outcomes. Diagnostics 2021;11(6):1089.

30. Hena KM. Sarcoidosis epidemiology: race matters. Front Immunol 2020;11:537382.

31. Kassamali B, Villa-Ruiz C, Kus KJB, et al. Increased risk of systemic and cardiac sarcoidosis in Black patients with cutaneous sarcoidosis. J Am Acad Dermatol 2022;86(5):1178–80.

32. Tukey MH, Berman JS, Boggs DA, et al. Mortality among African American women with sarcoidosis: data from the Black Women's Health Study. Sarcoidosis Vasc Diffuse Lung Dis 2013;30(2):128–33.

33. Cozier YC, Berman JS, Palmer JR, et al. Sarcoidosis in black women in the United States: data from the Black Women's Health Study. Chest 2011;139(1):144–50.

34. Judson MA, Boan AD, Lackland DT. The clinical course of sarcoidosis: presentation, diagnosis, and treatment in a large white and black cohort in the United States. Sarcoidosis Vasc Diffuse Lung Dis 2012;29(2):119–27.

35. Lhote R, Annesi-Maesano I, Nunes H, et al. Clinical phenotypes of extrapulmonary sarcoidosis: an analysis of a French, multi-ethnic, multicentre cohort. Eur Respir J 2021;57(4):2001160.

36. Birnbaum AD, Rifkin LM. Sarcoidosis: sex-dependent variations in presentation and management. J Ophthalmol 2014;2014:236905.

37. Rybicki BA, Maliarik MJ, Major M, et al. Epidemiology, demographics, and genetics of sarcoidosis. Semin Respir Infect 1998;13(3):166–73.

38. Rybicki BA, Iannuzzi MC. Epidemiology of sarcoidosis: recent advances and future prospects. Semin Respir Crit Care Med 2007;28(1):22–35.

39. Coquart N, Cadelis G, Tressières B, et al. Epidemiology of sarcoidosis in Afro-Caribbean people: a 7-year retrospective study in Guadeloupe. Int J Dermatol 2015;54(2):188–92.

40. Rabin DL, Thompson B, Brown KM, et al. Sarcoidosis: social predictors of severity at presentation. Eur Respir J 2004;24(4):601–8.

41. Evans M, Sharma O, LaBree L, et al. Differences in clinical findings between Caucasians and African Americans with biopsy-proven sarcoidosis. Ophthalmology 2007;114(2):325–33.

42. Ungprasert P, Wetter DA, Crowson CS, et al. Epidemiology of cutaneous sarcoidosis, 1976-2013: a population-based study from Olmsted County, Minnesota. J Eur Acad Dermatol Venereol 2016;30(10):1799–804.

43. Grunewald J, Grutters JC, Arkema EV, et al. Sarcoidosis. Nat Rev Dis Primers 2019;5(1):45.

44. Gideon NM, Mannino DM. Sarcoidosis mortality in the United States 1979-1991: an analysis of multiple-cause mortality data. Am J Med 1996;100(4):423–7.

45. Iwai K, Sekiguti M, Hosoda Y, et al. Racial difference in cardiac sarcoidosis incidence observed at autopsy. Sarcoidosis 1994;11(1):26–31.

46. Mirsaeidi M, Machado RF, Schraufnagel D, et al. Racial difference in sarcoidosis mortality in the United States. Chest 2015;147(2):438–49.

47. Judson MA, Baughman RP, Thompson BW, et al. Two year prognosis of sarcoidosis: the ACCESS experience. Sarcoidosis Vasc Diffuse Lung Dis 2003;20(3):204–11.

48. Foreman MG, Mannino DM, Kamugisha L, et al. Hospitalization for patients with sarcoidosis: 1979-2000. Sarcoidosis Vasc Diffuse Lung Dis 2006;23(2):124–9.

49. Gerke AK, Yang M, Tang F, et al. Increased hospitalizations among sarcoidosis patients from 1998 to 2008: a population-based cohort study. BMC Pulm Med 2012;12:19.

50. Ogundipe F, Mehari A, Gillum R. Disparities in sarcoidosis mortality by region, urbanization, and race in the united states: a multiple cause of death analysis. Am J Med 2019;132(9):1062–8.e3.

51. Kearney GD, Obi ON, Maddipati V, et al. Sarcoidosis deaths in the United States: 1999-2016. Respir Med 2019;149:30–5.

52. Wills AB, Adjemian J, Fontana JR, et al. Sarcoidosis-associated hospitalizations in the United States, 2002 to 2012. Ann Am Thorac Soc 2018;15(12):1490–3.

53. Rybicki BA, Kirkey KL, Major M, et al. Familial risk ratio of sarcoidosis in African-American sibs and parents. Am J Epidemiol 2001;153(2):188–93.

54. Rybicki BA, Iannuzzi MC, Frederick MM, et al. Familial aggregation of sarcoidosis. A case-control etiologic study of sarcoidosis (ACCESS). Am J Respir Crit Care Med 2001;164(11):2085–91.

55. Sverrild A, Backer V, Kyvik KO, et al. Heredity in sarcoidosis: a registry-based twin study. Thorax 2008;63(10):894–6.

56. Rossides M, Grunewald J, Eklund A, et al. Familial aggregation and heritability of sarcoidosis: a Swedish nested case-control study. Eur Respir J 2018;52(2):1800385.

57. Cleven KL, Ye K, Zeig-Owens R, et al. Genetic variants associated with FDNY WTC-related sarcoidosis. Int J Environ Res Public Health 2019;16(10):E1830.

58. Bennett D, Bargagli E, Refini RM, et al. New concepts in the pathogenesis of sarcoidosis. Expet Rev Respir Med 2019;13(10):981–91.

59. Levin AM, Adrianto I, Datta I, et al. Association of HLA-DRB1 with sarcoidosis susceptibility and progression in African Americans. Am J Respir Cell Mol Biol 2015;53(2):206–16.

60. Rybicki BA, Maliarik MJ, Poisson LM, et al. The major histocompatibility complex gene region and sarcoidosis susceptibility in African Americans. Am J Respir Crit Care Med 2003;167(3):444–9.

61. Thompson CL, Rybicki BA, Iannuzzi MC, et al. Reduction of sample heterogeneity through use of population substructure: an example from a population of African American families with sarcoidosis. Am J Hum Genet 2006;79(4):606–13.

62. Yanardag H, Tetikkurt C, Bilir M, et al. Association of HLA antigens with the clinical course of sarcoidosis and familial disease. Monaldi Arch Chest Dis 2017;87(3):835.

63. Morais A, Lima B, Alves H, et al. Associations between sarcoidosis clinical course and ANXA11 rs1049550 C/T, BTNL2 rs2076530 G/A, and HLA class I and II alleles. Clin Respir J 2018;12(2): 532–7.

64. Calender A, Weichhart T, Valeyre D, et al. Current insights in genetics of sarcoidosis: functional and clinical impacts. J Clin Monit 2020;9(8):2633.

65. Schnerch J, Prasse A, Vlachakis D, et al. Functional toll-like receptor 9 expression and CXCR3 ligand release in pulmonary sarcoidosis. Am J Respir Cell Mol Biol 2016;55(5):749–57.

66. Bello GA, Adrianto I, Dumancas GG, et al. Role of NOD2 pathway genes in sarcoidosis cases with clinical characteristics of blau syndrome. Am J Respir Crit Care Med 2015;192(9):1133–5.

67. Wolin A, Lahtela EL, Anttila V, et al. SNP variants in major histocompatibility complex are associated with sarcoidosis susceptibility-a joint analysis in four european populations. Front Immunol 2017;8: 422.

68. Zhou H, Diao M, Zhang M. The association between ANXA11 gene polymorphisms and sarcoidosis: a meta-analysis and systematic review. Sarcoidosis Vasc Diffuse Lung Dis 2016;33(2): 102–11.

69. Rivera NV, Patasova K, Kullberg S, et al. A gene-environment interaction between smoking and gene polymorphisms provides a high risk of two subgroups of sarcoidosis. Sci Rep 2019;9(1): 18633.

70. Fritz D, Ferwerda B, Brouwer MC, et al. Whole genome sequencing identifies variants associated with sarcoidosis in a family with a high prevalence of sarcoidosis. Clin Rheumatol 2021;40(9): 3735–43.

71. Villarino AV, Kanno Y, O'Shea JJ. Mechanisms and consequences of Jak-STAT signaling in the immune system. Nat Immunol 2017;18(4):374–84.

72. Wang A, Singh K, Ibrahim W, et al. The promise of JAK inhibitors for treatment of sarcoidosis and other inflammatory disorders with macrophage activation: a review of the literature. Yale J Biol Med 2020;93(1):187–95.

73. Morris R, Kershaw NJ, Babon JJ. The molecular details of cytokine signaling via the JAK/STAT pathway. Protein Sci 2018;27(12):1984–2009.

74. Sakthivel P, Bruder D. Mechanism of granuloma formation in sarcoidosis. Curr Opin Hematol 2017; 24(1):59–65.

75. Floss DM, Moll JM, Scheller J. IL-12 and IL-23-close relatives with structural homologies but distinct immunological functions. Cells 2020; 9(10):2184.

76. Zhou T, Casanova N, Pouladi N, et al. Identification of Jak-STAT signaling involvement in sarcoidosis severity via a novel microRNA-regulated peripheral blood mononuclear cell gene signature. Sci Rep 2017;7(1):4237.

77. Damsky W, Young BD, Sloan B, et al. Treatment of multiorgan sarcoidosis with tofacitinib. ACR Open Rheumatol 2020;2(2):106–9.

78. Damsky W, Thakral D, McGeary MK, et al. Janus kinase inhibition induces disease remission in cutaneous sarcoidosis and granuloma annulare. J Am Acad Dermatol 2020;82(3):612–21.

79. Talty R, Damsky W, King B. Treatment of cutaneous sarcoidosis with tofacitinib: a case report and review of evidence for Janus kinase inhibition in sarcoidosis. JAAD Case Rep 2021;16:62–4.

80. Zhou Y, Hu Y, Li H. Role of propionibacterium acnes in sarcoidosis: a meta-analysis. Sarcoidosis Vasc Diffuse Lung Dis 2013;30(4):262–7.

81. Shields BE, Perelygina L, Samimi S, et al. Granulomatous dermatitis associated with rubella virus infection in an adult with immunodeficiency. JAMA Dermatol 2021;157(7):842–7.

82. Knoell KA, Jr JDH, Stoler MH, et al. Absence of human herpesvirus 8 in sarcoidosis and crohn disease granulomas. Arch Dermatol 2005;141(7): 909–10.

83. Esteves T, Aparicio G, Garcia-Patos V. Is there any association between sarcoidosis and infectious agents?: A systematic review and meta-analysis. BMC Pulm Med 2016;16(1):165.

84. Derler AM, Eisendle K, Baltaci M, et al. High prevalence of "Borrelia-like" organisms in skin biopsies of sarcoidosis patients from Western Austria. J Cutan Pathol 2009;36(12):1262–8.

85. Song Z, Marzilli L, Greenlee BM, et al. Mycobacterial catalase-peroxidase is a tissue antigen and target of the adaptive immune response in systemic sarcoidosis. J Exp Med 2005;201(5):755–67.

86. Drake WP, Culver DA, Baughman RP, et al. Phase II investigation of the efficacy of antimycobacterial therapy in chronic pulmonary sarcoidosis. Chest 2021;159(5):1902–12.

87. Chen ES, Wahlstrom J, Song Z, et al. T cell responses to mycobacterial catalase-peroxidase profile a pathogenic antigen in systemic sarcoidosis. J Immunol 2008;181(12):8784–96.

88. Bindoli S, Dagan A, Torres-Ruiz JJ, et al. Sarcoidosis and autoimmunity: from genetic background

to environmental factors. Isr Med Assoc J 2016; 18(3–4):197–202.

89. Oliver LC, Zarnke AM. Sarcoidosis: an occupational disease? Chest 2021;160(4):1360–7.

90. Armbruster C, Dekan G, Hovorka A. Granulomatous pneumonitis and mediastinal lymphadenopathy due to photocopier toner dust. Lancet 1996; 348(9028):690–690.

91. Newman KL, Newman LS. Occupational causes of sarcoidosis. Curr Opin Allergy Clin Immunol 2012; 12(2):145–50.

92. Newman LS, Rose CS, Bresnitz EA, et al. A case control etiologic study of sarcoidosis: environmental and occupational risk factors. Am J Respir Crit Care Med 2004;170(12):1324–30.

93. Kim YC, Triffet MK, Gibson LE. Foreign bodies in sarcoidosis. Am J Dermatopathol 2000;22(5): 408–12.

94. Hena KM, Yip J, Jaber N, et al. Clinical course of sarcoidosis in world trade center-exposed firefighters. Chest 2018;153(1):114–23.

95. Izbicki G, Chavko R, Banauch GI, et al. World Trade Center "sarcoid-like" granulomatous pulmonary disease in New York City Fire Department rescue workers. Chest 2007;131(5):1414–23.

96. Musaelyan A, Lapin S, Nazarov V, et al. Vimentin as antigenic target in autoimmunity: a comprehensive review. Autoimmun Rev 2018;17(9):926–34.

97. Kinloch AJ, Kaiser Y, Wolfgeher D, et al. In situ humoral immunity to vimentin in HLA-DRB1*03(+) patients with pulmonary sarcoidosis. Front Immunol 2018;9:1516-1516.

98. Williams DR, Mohammed SA. Racism and health I: pathways and scientific evidence. Am Behav Sci 2013;57(8).

99. Pager D, Shepherd H. The sociology of discrimination: racial discrimination in employment, housing, credit, and consumer markets. Annu Rev Sociol 2008;34:181–209,

100. Bailey ZD, Krieger N, Agénor M, et al. Structural racism and health inequities in the USA: evidence and interventions. Lancet 2017;389(10077):1453–63.

101. Chae DH, Nuru-Jeter AM, Lincoln KD, et al. Conceptualizing racial disparities in health: advancement of a socio-psychobiological approach. Du Bois Rev 2011;8(1):63–77.

102. Ronsmans S, De Ridder J, Vandebroek E, et al. Associations between occupational and environmental exposures and organ involvement in sarcoidosis: a retrospective case-case analysis. Respir Res 2021;22(1):224.

103. Janot AC, Huscher D, Walker M, et al. Cigarette smoking and male sex are independent and age concomitant risk factors for the development of ocular sarcoidosis in a New Orleans sarcoidosis population. Sarcoidosis Vasc Diffuse Lung Dis 2015;32(2):138–43.

104. Li X, Sundquist J, Hamano T, et al. Neighborhood deprivation and risks of autoimmune disorders: a national cohort study in Sweden. Int J Environ Res Public Health 2019;16(20):E3798.

105. Chae DH, Walters KL. Racial discrimination and racial identity attitudes in relation to self-rated health and physical pain and impairment among two-spirit American Indians/Alaska Natives. Am J Public Health 2009;99(Suppl 1):S144–51.

106. Chae DH, Nuru-Jeter AM, Adler NE, et al. Discrimination, racial bias, and telomere length in African-American men. Am J Prev Med 2014;46(2):103–11.

107. Chae DH, Nuru-Jeter AM, Lincoln KD, et al. Racial discrimination, mood disorders, and cardiovascular disease among black americans. Ann Epidemiol 2012;22(2):104–11.

108. Brody GH, Yu T, Miller GE, et al. Discrimination, racial identity, and cytokine levels among African-American adolescents. J Adolesc Health 2015; 56(5):496–501.

109. Stepanikova I, Bateman LB, Oates GR. Systemic inflammation in midlife: race, socioeconomic status, and perceived discrimination. Am J Prev Med 2017;52(1S1):S63–76.

110. Beatty DL, Matthews KA, Bromberger JT, et al. Everyday discrimination prospectively predicts inflammation across 7-years in racially diverse midlife women: study of women's health across the nation. J Soc Issues 2014;70(2):298–314.

111. Lewis TT, Aiello AE, Leurgans S, et al. Self-reported experiences of everyday discrimination are associated with elevated C-reactive protein levels in older African-American adults. Brain Behav Immun 2010; 24(3):438–43.

112. Geronimus AT, Hicken M, Keene D, et al. Weathering" and age patterns of allostatic load scores among blacks and whites in the United States. Am J Public Health 2006;96(5):826–33.

113. McEwen BS. Stress, adaptation, and disease. Allostasis and allostatic load. Ann N Y Acad Sci 1998; 840:33–44.

114. Martz CD, Allen AM, Fuller-Rowell TE, et al. Vicarious racism stress and disease activity: the black women's experiences living with lupus (BeWELL) study. J Racial Ethn Health Disparities 2019;6(5):1044–51.

115. Chae DH, Martz CD, Fuller-Rowell TE, et al. Racial discrimination, disease activity, and organ damage: the black women's experiences living with lupus (BeWELL) study. Am J Epidemiol 2019; 188(8):1434–43.

116. Chae DH, Drenkard CM, Lewis TT, et al. Discrimination and cumulative disease damage among african american women with systemic lupus erythematosus. Am J Public Health 2015;105(10):2099–107.

117. Pacheco Y, Lim CX, Weichhart T, et al. Sarcoidosis and the mTOR, Rac1, and Autophagy Triad. Trends Immunol 2020;41(4):286–99.

118. Miyara M, Amoura Z, Parizot C, et al. The immune paradox of sarcoidosis and regulatory T cells. J Exp Med 2006;203(2):359–70.

119. Dikic I, Elazar Z. Mechanism and medical implications of mammalian autophagy. Nat Rev Mol Cell Biol 2018;19(6):349–64.

120. Celada LJ, Drake WP. Targeting CD4(+) T cells for the treatment of sarcoidosis: a promising strategy? Immunotherapy 2015;7(1):57–66.

121. Elżbieta R, Iwona K, Joanna B, et al. Role of fibrocytes and endothelial progenitor cells among low-differentiated CD34+ cells in the progression of lung sarcoidosis. BMC Pulm Med 2020;20(1):306.

122. Redissi A., Penmetsa G.K. and Litaiem N., Lupus Pernio. In: StatPearls. StatPearls Publishing, Available at: http://www.ncbi.nlm.nih.gov/books/NBK536968/. Accessed June 16, 2022.

123. Spiteri MA, Matthey F, Gordon T, et al. Lupus pernio: a clinico-radiological study of thirty-five cases. Br J Dermatol 1985;112(3):315–22.

124. Minus HR, Grimes PE. Cutaneous manifestations of sarcoidosis in blacks. Cutis 1983;32(4):361–3, 372.

125. Elgart ML. Cutaneous sarcoidosis: definitions and types of lesions. Clin Dermatol 1986;4(4):35–45.

126. Marchell RM, Judson MA. Cutaneous sarcoidosis. Semin Respir Crit Care Med 2010;31(4):442–51.

127. Albertini JG, Tyler W, Miller OF. Ulcerative sarcoidosis. Case report and review of the literature. Arch Dermatol 1997;133(2):215–9.

128. Ando M, Miyazaki E, Hatano Y. Subcutaneous sarcoidosis: a clinical analysis of nine patients. Clin Rheumatol 2016;35(9):2277–81.

129. Olive KE, Kataria YP. Cutaneous manifestations of sarcoidosis. Relationships to other organ system involvement, abnormal laboratory measurements, and disease course. Arch Intern Med 1985;145(10):1811–4.

130. Burgoyne JS, Wood MG. Psoriasiform sarcoidosis. Arch Dermatol 1972;106(6):896–8.

131. Mitsuishi T, Nogita T, Kawashima M. Psoriasiform sarcoidosis with ulceration. Int J Dermatol 1992;31(5):339–40.

132. Katta R, Nelson B, Chen D, et al. Sarcoidosis of the scalp: a case series and review of the literature. J Am Acad Dermatol 2000;42(4):690–2.

133. Jacyk WK. Cutaneous sarcoidosis in black South Africans. Int J Dermatol 1999;38(11):841–5.

134. Mana J, Marcoval J, Graells J, et al. Cutaneous involvement in sarcoidosis. Relationship to systemic disease. Arch Dermatol 1997;133(7):882–8.

135. Nagai Y, Igarashi N, Ishikawa O. Lupus pernio with multiple bone cysts in the fingers. J Dermatol 2010;37(9):812–4.

136. Efthimiou P, Kukar M. Lupus pernio: sarcoid-specific cutaneous manifestation associated with chronic sarcoid arthropathy. J Clin Rheumatol 2011;17(6):343–343.

137. Stagaki E, Mountford WK, Lackland DT, et al. The treatment of lupus pernio: results of 116 treatment courses in 54 patients. Chest 2009;135(2):468–76.

138. Atci T, Baykal C, Kaya Bingöl Z, et al. Scar sarcoidosis: 11 patients with variable clinical features and invariable pulmonary involvement. Clin Exp Dermatol 2019;826:44.

139. Martires K, Shvartsbeyn M, Brinster N, et al. Sarcoidosis. Dermatol Online J 2015;21(12):53306–3308.

140. Imadojemu S, Wanat KA, Noe M, et al. Cutaneous sarcoidosis. In: Baughman RP, Valeyre D, editors. Sarcoidosis, a clinician's guide. 1st edition. St. Louis (MO: Elsevier; 2019. p. 127–44.

141. Adamson HG. Tuberculide of the type called "sarcoid" of Darier- Roussy. Proc R Soc Med 1912;5(Dermatol Sect):132–3.

142. O'Neill JL, Moustafa F, Teague D, et al. Subcutaneous sarcoidosis without systemic involvement. Dermatol Online J 2014;20(8).

143. Heath CR, David J, Taylor SC. Sarcoidosis: Are there differences in your skin of color patients? J Am Acad Dermatol 2012;66(1). 121.e1-14.

144. Neville E, Walker AN, James DG. Prognostic factors predicting the outcome of sarcoidosis: an analysis of 818 patients. Q J Med 1983;52(208):525–33.

145. Milman N, Selroos O. Pulmonary sarcoidosis in the Nordic countries 1950-1982. II Course and prognosis. Sarcoidosis 1990;7(2):113–8.

146. Ishikawa M, Yamamoto T. Erythema nodosum-like sarcoid lesion: a specific skin manifestation occasionally seen in Japanese sarcoidosis patients. Sarcoidosis Vasc Diffuse Lung Dis 2022;39(1):e2022013.

147. Wanat KA, Rosenbach M. Cutaneous sarcoidosis. Clin Chest Med 2015;36(4):685–702.

148. James DG, Thomson AD, Willcox A. Erythema nodosum as a manifestation of sarcoidosis. Lancet 1956;271(6936):218–21.

149. Rabinowitz LO, Zaim MT. A clinicopathologic approach to gran- ulomatous dermatoses. J Am Acad Dermatol 1996;35(4):588–600.

150. Cardoso JC, Cravo M, Reis JP, et al. Cutaneous sarcoidosis: a histopathological study. J Eur Acad Dermatol Venereol 2009;678:23.

151. Ball NJ, Kho GT, Martinka M. The histologic spectrum of cutane- ous sarcoidosis: a study of twenty-eight cases. J Cutan Pathol 2004;31(2):160–8.

152. Callen JP. The presence of foreign bodies does not exclude the diagnosis of sarcoidosis. Arch Dermatol 2001;137(4):485–6.

153. Marcoval J, Mañá J, Moreno A, et al. Foreign bodies in granulomatous cutaneous lesions of

patients with systemic sarcoidosis. Arch Dermatol 2001;137(4):427–30.

154. Judson MA, Baughman RP. How many organs need to be involved to diagnose sarcoidosis?: An unanswered question that, hopefully, will become irrelevant. *Sarcoidosis Vasc Diffuse Lung. Dis* 2014;31(1):6–7.

155. Rosenbach M, Yeung H, Chu EY. Reliability and convergent validity of the cutaneous sarcoidosis activity and morphology instrument for assessing cutaneous sarcoidosis. JAMA Dermatol 2013; 149(5):550–6.

156. Yeung H, Farber S, Birnbaum BK. Reliability and validity of cutaneous sarcoidosis outcome instruments among dermatolo- gists, pulmonologists, and rheumatologists. JAMA Dermatol 2015;151(12):1317–22.

157. Judson MA. The diagnosis of sarcoidosis. Curr Opin Pulm Med 2019;25(5):484–96.

158. Costabel U, Guzman J, Baughman RP. Systemic evaluation of a potential cutaneous sarcoidosis patient. Clin Dermatol 2007;303AD:25.

159. Imadojemu S, Rosenbach M. Advances in inflammatory granu- lomatous skin diseases. Dermatol Clin 2019;37(1):49–64.

160. Hoitsma E, Marziniak M, Faber CG, et al. Small fibre neuropathy in sarcoidosis. Lancet 2002; 359(9323):2085–6.

161. Drent M, Costabel U, Crouser ED, et al. Misconceptions regarding symptoms of sarcoidosis. Lancet Respir Med 2021;9(8):816–8.

162. Hendriks C, Drent M, De Kleijn W, et al. Everyday cognitive failure and depressive symptoms predict fatigue in sarcoidosis: a prospective follow-up study. Respir Med 2018;138S:S24–30.

163. Voortman M, Fritz D, Vogels OJM, et al. Small fiber neuropathy: a disabling and underrecognized syndrome. Curr Opin Pulm Med 2017;23(5): 447–57.

164. Tavee J, Culver D. Nonorgan manifestations of sarcoidosis. Curr Opin Pulm Med 2019;25(5):533–8.

165. Villa-Ruiz C, Lo K, Desai S, et al. Practice gaps in the evaluation of systemic involvement in patients with cutaneous sarcoidosis presenting to a dermatologist: a retrospective review of 48 patients. J Am Acad Dermatol 2021;85(3):794–6.

166. Kraaijvanger R, Janssen Bonás M, Vorselaars ADM, et al. Biomarkers in the diagnosis and prognosis of sarcoidosis: current use and future prospects. Front Immunol 2020;11:1443.

167. Eurelings LEM, Miedema JR, Dalm VASH, et al. Sensitivity and specificity of serum soluble interleukin-2 receptor for diagnosing sarcoidosis in a population of patients suspected of sarcoidosis. PLoS One 2019;14(10):e0223897.

168. Paolino A, Galloway J, Birring S, et al. Clinical phenotypes and therapeutic responses in cutaneous-predominant sarcoidosis: 6-year experience in a tertiary referral service. Clin Exp Dermatol 2021; 46(6):1038–45.

169. Morse SI, Cohn ZA, Hirsch JG, et al. The treatment of sarcoidosis with chloroquine. Am J Med 1961; 30:779–84.

170. Jones E, Callen JP. Hydroxychloroquine is effective therapy for control of cutaneous sarcoidal granulomas. J Am Acad Dermatol 1990;23(3, Pt 1): 487–9.

171. Baughman RP, Judson MA, Ingledue R, et al. Efficacy and safety of apremilast in chronic cutaneous sarcoidosis. Arch Dermatol 2012;148(2):262–4.

172. Park MK, Fontana B Jr, Babaali H, et al. Steroid-sparing effects of pentoxifylline in pulmonary sarcoidosis. Sarcoidosis Vasc Diffuse Lung Dis 2009;26(2):121–31.

173. Veien NK, Brodthagen H. Cutaneous sarcoidosis treated with methotrexate. Br J Dermatol 1977; 97(2):213–6.

174. Lower EE, Baughman RP. The use of low dose methotrexate in refractory sarcoidosis. Am J Med Sci 1990;299(3):153–7.

175. Lower EE, Baughman RP. Prolonged use of methotrexate for sarcoidosis. Arch Intern Med 1995; 155(8):846–51.

176. Hrin ML, Williams JA, Bowers NL, et al. Methotrexate for cutaneous sarcoidosis: a dermatology-based case series of 23 patients. J Cutan Med Surg 2022. https://doi.org/10.1177/120347542211 01361. 12034754221101360.

177. Stagaki E, Mountford WK, Lackland DT, Judson MA. The treatment of lupus pernio: results of 116 treatment courses in 54 patients. Chest 2009;135(2):468–76.

178. Thielen AM, Barde C, Saurat JH, et al. Refractory chronic cutaneous sarcoidosis responsive to dose escalation of TNF- alpha antagonists. Dermatology 2009;219(1):59–62.

179. Tu J, Chan J. Cutaneous sarcoidosis and infliximab: evidence for efficacy in refractory disease. Australas J Dermatol 2014;55(4):279–81.

180. Tuchinda P, Bremmer M, Gaspari AA. A case series of refractory cutaneous sarcoidosis successfully treated with infliximab. Dermatol Ther (Heidelb) 2012;2(1):11.

181. Wanat KA, Rosenbach M. Case series demonstrating improvement in chronic cutaneous sarcoidosis following treatment with TNF inhibitors. Arch Dermatol 2012;148(9):1097–100.

182. Judson MA. Successful treatment of lupus pernio with adalimumab. Arch Dermatol 2011;147(11): 1332–3.

183. Heffernan MP, Smith DI. Adalimumab for treatment of cutaneous sarcoidosis. Arch Dermatol 2006; 142(1):17–9.

184. Baughman RP, Judson MA, Lower EE. Sarcoidosis Investi- gators. Infliximab for chronic cutaneous

sarcoidosis: a subset analysis from a double-blind randomized clinical trial. Sarcoidosis Vasc Diffuse Lung Dis 2016;32(4):289–95.

185. Wei JJ, Kallenbach LR, Kreider M, et al. Resolution of cutaneous sarcoidosis after Janus kinase inhibitor therapy for concomitant polycythemia vera. JAAD Case Rep 2019;5(4):360–1.

186. Rotenberg C, Besnard V, Brillet PY, et al. Dramatic response of refractory sarcoidosis under ruxolitinib in a patient with associated JAK2-mutated polycythemia. Eur Respir J 2018;20;52(6):1801482.

187. Rosenbach M. Janus kinase inhibitors offer promise for a new era of targeted treatment for granulomatous disorders. J Am Acad Dermatol 2020; 82(3):e91–2.

188. Scheinberg M, Maluf F, Wagner J. Steroid-resistant sarcoidosis treated with baricitinib. Ann Rheum Dis 2020;79(9):1259–60.

189. Levraut M, Martis N, Viau P, et al. Refractory sarcoidosis-like systemic granulomatosis responding to ruxolitinib. Ann Rheum Dis 2019;78(11): 1606–7.

190. Friedman MA, Le B, Stevens J, et al. Tofacitinib as a steroid-sparing therapy in pulmonary sarcoidosis, an open-label prospective proof-of-concept study. Lung 2021;199(2):147–53.

191. Alam M, Fang V, Rosenbach M. Treatment of cutaneous sarcoidosis with tofacitinib 2% ointment and extra virgin olive oil. JAAD Case Rep 2021;9:1–3.

192. Singh K, Wang A, Heald P, et al. Treatment of angiolupoid sarcoidosis with tofacitinib ointment 2% and pulsed dye laser therapy. JAAD Case Rep 2021;7:122–4.

193. Damsky W, Wang A, Kim DJ, et al. Inhibition of type 1 immunity with tofacitinib is associated with marked improvement in longstanding sarcoidosis. Nat Commun 2022;13(1):3140.

194. Gad MM, Bazarbashi N, Kaur M, et al. Sarcoid-like phenomenon—ustekinumab induced granulomatous reaction mimicking diffuse metastatic disease: a case report and review of the literature. J Med Case Rep 2019;13(1):257.

195. Powell JB, Matthews P, Rattehalli R, et al. Acute systemic sarcoidosis complicating ustekinumab therapy for chronic plaque psoriasis. Br J Dermatol 2015;172(3):834–6.

196. Thomas AS, Rosenbaum JT. Poor control of sarcoidosis-related panuveitis with an antibody to IL-23. Ocul Immunol Inflamm 2020;28(3):491–3.

197. Hornick N, Wang A, Lim Y. Development or worsening of sarcoidosis associated with IL-17 blockade for psoriasis. J Eur Acad Dermatol Venereol 2020. https://doi.org/10.1111/jdv.16451.

Hidradenitis Suppurativa

Toni Jenkins, MS[a], Jahdonna Isaac, MS, MD[b], Alicia Edwards, MS[a],
Ginette A. Okoye, MD[b],*

KEYWORDS

- Skin of color • Diagnosis • Health disparities • Hidradenitis suppurativa • Boils • Sinus tracts
- Acne inversa

KEY POINTS

- Hidradenitis suppurativa (HS) is diagnosed clinically, and it is characterized by recurrent nodules and abscesses, and chronic sinus tracts and scarring in intertriginous locations.
- Its highest prevalence in the United States is among women, especially of African American or biracial descent.
- In addition to the cutaneous manifestation, HS is associated with comorbidities such as obesity, cardiovascular disease, chronic pain, and other inflammatory diseases such as inflammatory bowel disease and pyoderma gangrenosum.
- Treatment approach is multimodal and aims to address underlying follicular occlusion, inflammation, bacterial overgrowth, hormonal and metabolic dysregulation and lifestyle modifications.

INTRODUCTION

Hidradenitis suppurativa (HS) is a chronic inflammatory disorder of the hair follicles in the apocrine gland-rich and intertriginous areas of the body. The disease is characterized by postpubertal onset of recurrent painful nodules and enduring sinus tracts, as well as long-term sequelae such as scarring, lymphedema, contractures, and squamous cell carcinoma (SCC).[1,2] The pathogenesis of HS is likely multifactorial, involving genetic susceptibility in some patients,[3] hair follicle occlusion,[4] hormonal dysregulation,[5] microbiome dysregulation,[6,7] and immune dysregulation.[7] External factors such as smoking, diet, and friction shearing forces on the skin may also play a role in some patients.[8,9]

HS is a debilitating disease that significantly affects patients' quality of life. Patients with HS have more absenteeism from school and work due to disease flares and medical appointments.[10] It affects productivity in the workforce and negatively influences opportunities for advancement, resulting in slower income growth, lower annual incomes, and a higher risk of leaving the workforce.[10,11] HS can also significantly affect patients' sexual health given the locations affected, malodorous drainage, scarring, and pain.[12,13] The latter is a significant, and often undertreated issue in HS. Moreover, patients living with HS are more likely to suffer from anxiety and depression,[14] substance use disorders, and are at an increased risk for completed suicide.[15,16]

EPIDEMIOLOGY

In the United States, the prevalence of HS is approximately 0.10%, with the highest occurrences noted among women, biracial groups and African Americans.[17] The latter group has an estimated prevalence of 296 per 100 000 (95% CI, 291–300 per 100 000, P < .001); more than 3 times that of White patients (95 per 100 000; CI, 94–96 per 100 000, P < .001).[17] Incidence rates vary but in one study, the incidence of HS globally was estimated to be between 0.00033% and 4.1%.[1] Epidemiologically, HS has been associated with cigarette smoking, obesity,[8] and a low

a Howard University College of Medicine, 520 West Street NW, Washington, DC 20059, USA; b Department of Dermatology, Howard University, 2041 Georgia Avenue NW, Towers Suite 4300, Washington, DC 20060, USA
* Corresponding author.
E-mail address: ginette.okoye@Howard.edu

Dermatol Clin 41 (2023) 471–479
https://doi.org/10.1016/j.det.2023.02.001
0733-8635/23/© 2023 Elsevier Inc. All rights reserved.

socioeconomic status.[18] There seems to be geographic clusters of HS prevalence in the United States with significant overlap with the map of obesity rates.[19,20]

HS usually presents after puberty and in some, but not all, patients abates after menopause.[21] The peak age of presentation is in patients aged between 30 and 39 years,[17] disrupting the crucial work-related, social, and family activities that tend to ensue in this age group.

The prevalence of HS in the pediatric and adolescent populations seems to be increasing[22] with an average age of onset of 12.5 years.[23] Similar to adults, HS in pediatric patients is associated with obesity and is more common in female patients.[23]

HS has also been associated with significant health-care utilization and higher-cost care, including Emergency Department visit, outpatient care, inpatient care, and high-cost medications.[24–26] This burden is unequally distributed with African American patients with HS more likely to be hospitalized.[25] Additionally, African American and Hispanic patients with HS have increased health-care utilization compared with their White counterparts.[25]

CLINICAL FINDINGS

HS is classically described as occurring in the intertriginous areas of the skin such as the axillae, inframammary area, inguinal folds, gluteal cleft, and perianal area. However, lesions can occur anywhere there is skin-on-skin contact including the posterior neck, intermammary cleft, abdominal and flank folds, and medial thighs. Acute lesions are characterized by painful deep-seated nodules (**Fig. 1**) that often rupture and drain purulent malodorous or sanguineous material. The resulting ulcers are often slow to heal. Other acute lesions of HS include pustules and perifollicular inflammatory papules. Because the disease progresses, adjacent nodules connect via sinus tracts (**Fig. 2**), which are deep dermal tunnels with an epithelialized lining and associated inflammation.[27] These sinus tracts are chronic persistent lesions that do not usually resolve without surgical intervention. Other chronic changes associated with HS include "double-comedones"[28–30] (**Fig. 3**), postinflammatory hyperpigmentation (PIH), atrophic, hypertrophic, and keloidal scarring, and contractures in severe cases.

The pain and contractures of HS can lead to gait abnormalities and decreased range of motion of the extremities. Additionally, systemic symptoms sometimes accompany flares of cutaneous lesions, such as fever, chills, myalgias, arthralgias,

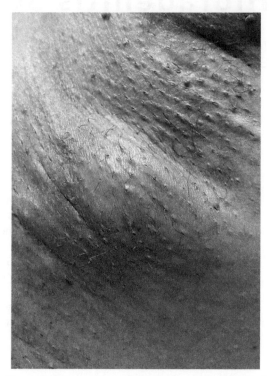

Fig. 1. Inflammatory nodule seen in early stages of HS.

and fatigue. In rare cases, the chronic inflammation of HS leads to the development of SCC. Unfortunately, SCCs can be clinically and histologically difficult to distinguish from HS lesions, leading to delays in diagnosis and poorer outcomes.[2,31]

DIAGNOSIS

Currently, there is no definitive histologic or serologic diagnostic test for HS. HS is diagnosed clinically, using 3 diagnostic criteria (**Box 1**). Diagnostic delays are common; ranging between 7.2 and 10.2 years in adult populations and nearly 2 years in pediatric patients.[23,32,33] Some of the factors contributing to this delay include the clinical overlap with other diagnoses (eg, folliculitis and epidermal inclusion cysts), phenotypic variation seen among patients, and unequal access to dermatologic care in the populations commonly affected by HS.[18] Furthermore, many patients with HS first present to nondermatologists at the onset of their disease.[33] The lack of familiarity with HS among nondermatology providers such as emergency room, primary care, surgical, and gynecologic providers may also contribute to these delays.[33]

When diagnosing HS, the patient should have classic HS lesions (eg, inflammatory nodules, abscesses, and/or sinus tracts) in the typical locations

Fig. 2. Sinus tracts are epithelialized tunnels in the deep dermis. Deroofing surgery (also called marsupialization) can be an effective management strategy for these chronic lesions.

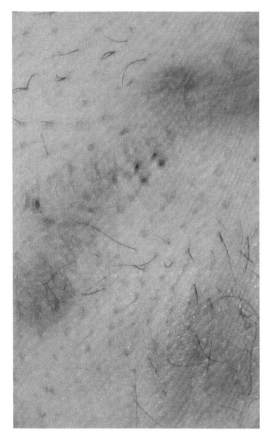

Fig. 3. Double-comedones, also called "double-ended pseudocomedones" are sequelae of the inflammation and fibrosis of HS.[29,30,53]

and evidence of other disorders of follicular occlusion (eg, severe acne, dissecting cellulitis of the scalp, or pilonidal disease). To elicit a more accurate history from patients, it is important to use the lay terms for HS such as "boils," "bumps," or "scars," and the lay terms for surgical procedures such as "lancing," "draining," or "sweat gland surgery." Once the diagnosis is established, various grading systems have been used in both clinical

such as intertriginous areas or other areas of friction. The third criterion is arguably the most important factor: chronicity and recurrence. There must be 2 or more recurrences during a 6-month period, or evidence of chronicity such as PIH or scarring (Fig. 4) from previous lesions[1] (see Box 1).

Other aspects of the patient's history and physical examination that suggest a diagnosis of HS include a positive family history, surgical scars in the axillae or groin from earlier incision and drainage procedures or larger excisions (Fig. 5),

---

Box 1
Diagnostic criteria for hidradenitis suppurativa[1]

- Classical HS lesions (eg, inflammatory nodules, cysts, abscesses, and/or sinus tracts)
- Classical locations of intertriginous areas or areas of increased skin friction/shearing forces
- Chronicity and recurrence: 2 or more recurrences within a 6-mo period and/or clinical evidence of chronicity such as PIH and scarring

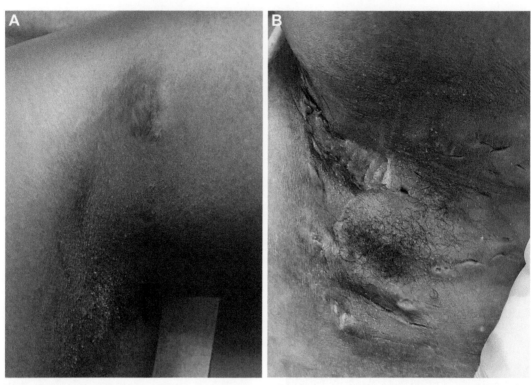

Fig. 4. (*A*) Atrophic scars in an anatomic area commonly affected by HS can be a clue to the diagnosis. (*B*) Ulceration and PIH seen in chronic advanced HS plaques.

practice and clinical trials to assess the severity of disease. Although there are significant limitations to its use, the Hurley Staging System is still the most commonly used grading system in clinical practice because it is quick, easy to use, and easy to explain to patients. Hurley stage I disease is defined as one or more lesions (eg, nodules) without sinus tracts; stage II is defined as one or more widely separated lesions with sinus tract formation and scarring; and stage III as multiple lesions connected via sinus tracts and extensive

scarring involving an entire anatomic area (eg, the entire axillary vault)[34] (**Fig. 6**). The Sartorius grading system is more complex and rarely used in clinical practice. It incorporates anatomical locations, number, and types of lesions as well as distance between active lesions and presence or absence of normal skin between lesions to determine the severity of disease.[35,36]

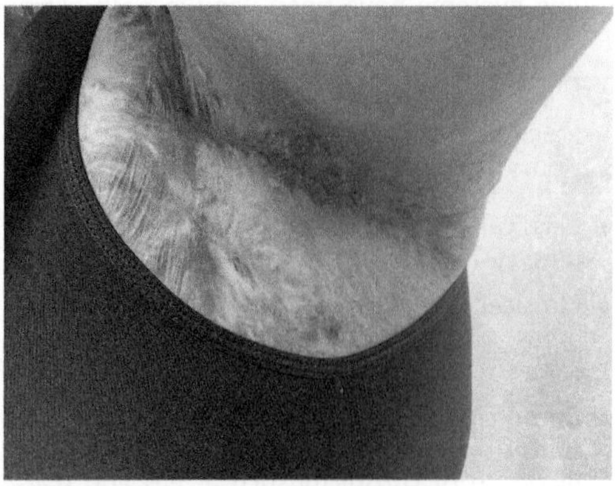

COMORBIDITIES

HS is associated with various psychiatric, metabolic, and inflammatory comorbidities.[37] Many studies show that HS significantly affects the quality of life. This likely explains the higher prevalence of depression, anxiety, and completed suicide among this group.[14–16] The chronic pain experienced by patients with HS may also contribute to the increased rates of substance use disorder.[15] Additionally, there is an increased prevalence of obesity, metabolic syndrome, and dyslipidemia. The relationship between obesity and HS is complex and has not yet been fully elucidated. Obesity results in increased body folds/intertriginous areas and is considered to be a proinflammatory state. These factors may play a role in the development and/or exacerbation of HS[38] but there are many nonobese patients with HS and many patients

Fig. 5. Patient with large postsurgical scar secondary to axillary HS excision.

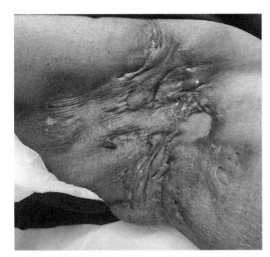

Fig. 6. HS Hurley stage III. Multiple HS lesions connected via sinus tracts and forming ulcers involving the entire axillary vault.

who do not experience improvement in their HS despite significant weight loss. Due to elevated levels of interleukin (IL)-6, IL-32, and tumor necrosis factor alpha (TNF-α), HS has been associated with chronic inflammation, thrombosis, and endothelial dysfunction.[11,39] This supports the known association between HS and other cardiovascular risk factors.[11,40] Both inflammatory bowel diseases (IBDs) and spondyloarthritis have been linked to HS. For instance, Crohn disease shows a 3-fold increased risk in patients with HS.[39] These inflammatory disorders share a similar cytokine profile, which could explain their mutual features of chronic inflammation and/or recurrent granulomatous and suppurative lesions associated with underlying sinus tracts. Other rare autoinflammatory syndromes are also associated with HS such as PASH (pyoderma gangrenosum, acne, and suppurative hidradenitis) or PAPASH (pyogenic arthritis, pyoderma gangrenosum, acne, and suppurative hidradenitis). These syndromic forms of HS appear driven by IL-1 dysregulation leading to neutrophilic overactivation, another important mediator in the pathogenesis of HS.[41]

DIFFERENTIAL DIAGNOSIS

The differential diagnosis of HS (Table 1) is varied and may range from infectious, granulomatous, autoinflammatory, and malignant processes. One approach is to divide this differential based on clinical morphology and chronicity of lesions. Acute lesions may be similar to epidermal inclusion cysts, staphylococcal infections including boils, carbuncles, and folliculitis, or acne fulminans. As lesions progress, they may form ulcers akin to

pyoderma gangrenosum, Crohn disease, cutaneous tuberculosis, mycetoma, lymphogranuloma venereum (LGV), and herpes simplex infection. Chronic lesions can have a more atrophic, scarred, and indurated appearance due to recurrent tissue inflammation and remodeling. SCC, chronic lymphedema, acne keloidalis nuchae, and dissecting cellulitis of the scalp should thus be considered in the differential diagnosis of chronic lesions.

TREATMENT

A multimodal approach is fundamental when treating patients with HS. One may establish a therapeutic ladder based on the severity of disease while targeting 5 different components of the disease[42,43] (Fig. 7). The first addresses the dysregulation in follicular occlusion and includes various treatments such a topical or systemic retinoids,[44] topical resorcinol,[42] and laser hair reduction.[45] The second involves the reduction of systemic inflammation associated with HS. Different emerging modalities have been used such as biologics (eg, TNF-α inhibitors), other immunoregulators (eg, Janus kinase inhibitors, phosphodiesterase 4 inhibitors), systemic and intralesional steroids as well as other oral anti-inflammatory agents such as colchicine and dapsone.[44] Hormonal regulations through medications such as metformin, combined oral contraceptive pills, spironolactone, and finasteride may be helpful in patients with hormonally driven flares.[44] Antimicrobials are a mainstay of therapy and considered first line to help reduce the bacterial and inflammatory burden of HS. Typical regimens include antimicrobial soaps such as benzoyl peroxide, chlorhexidine gluconate wash, and bleach baths. Antibiotics such as doxycycline, clindamycin in combination with rifampin and ertapenem are often used to control flares.[44,46] The last category involves lifestyle modifications and limiting exacerbating factors such as friction, heat, moisture, and smoking while promoting healthy weight management and dietary modifications.[8] Nevertheless, there are limitations to medical management, and severe and refractory disease often requires surgical intervention to achieve symptomatic control.[45]

Emerging therapies for HS include biologics and small molecules with the aim of utilizing more personalized and targeted treatment regimens.[42] TNF-α inhibitors, IL-1, IL-17, IL-12/IL-23, IL-36 antagonists, anti-C5a agents, JAK inhibitors are among various treatment being tested in clinical trials.[42] Despite the increased prevalence of HS in populations of color, these patients are often underrepresented in clinical trials. Improved

Table 1
Differential diagnosis of hidradenitis suppurativa

	Acute HS	Ulcerative HS	Chronic HS
DDx	• Epidermal inclusion cyst • Carbuncle/Furuncle • Folliculitis • Steatocystoma • Acne fulminans	• LGV • Pyoderma gangrenosum • Crohn disease • Acne fulminans • Herpes simplex • Mycetoma • Cutaneous tuberculosis	• SCC • Lymphedema • Acne keloidalis nuchae • Dissecting cellulitis of the scalp

representation is important to confirm that the treatment outcomes observed in these studies are applicable to diverse patient populations.[47,48]

CLINICAL OUTCOMES/LONG-TERM RECOMMENDATIONS

HS can be a chronic lifelong condition. Treatments alleviate symptoms and improve quality of life but the condition tends to be cyclical and require sustained maintenance therapy to prevent recurrence. Clinical outcomes are closely linked to early disease detection and management.[49] As such,

the aim of therapy is to address flares and prevent further disease progression. Many lifestyle factors can contribute to disease severity. Smoking and obesity may be associated with poorer outcomes in HS and contribute to the cardiovascular comorbidities associated with the disease. Therefore, even in the absence of definitive evidence of the link between diet and obesity and HS, patients should be encouraged to avoid smoking and maintain a healthy diet as part of their long-term treatment plan.[50] Exercise and bariatric surgery have also shown to correlate with improved HS symptoms.[51] However, these recommendations

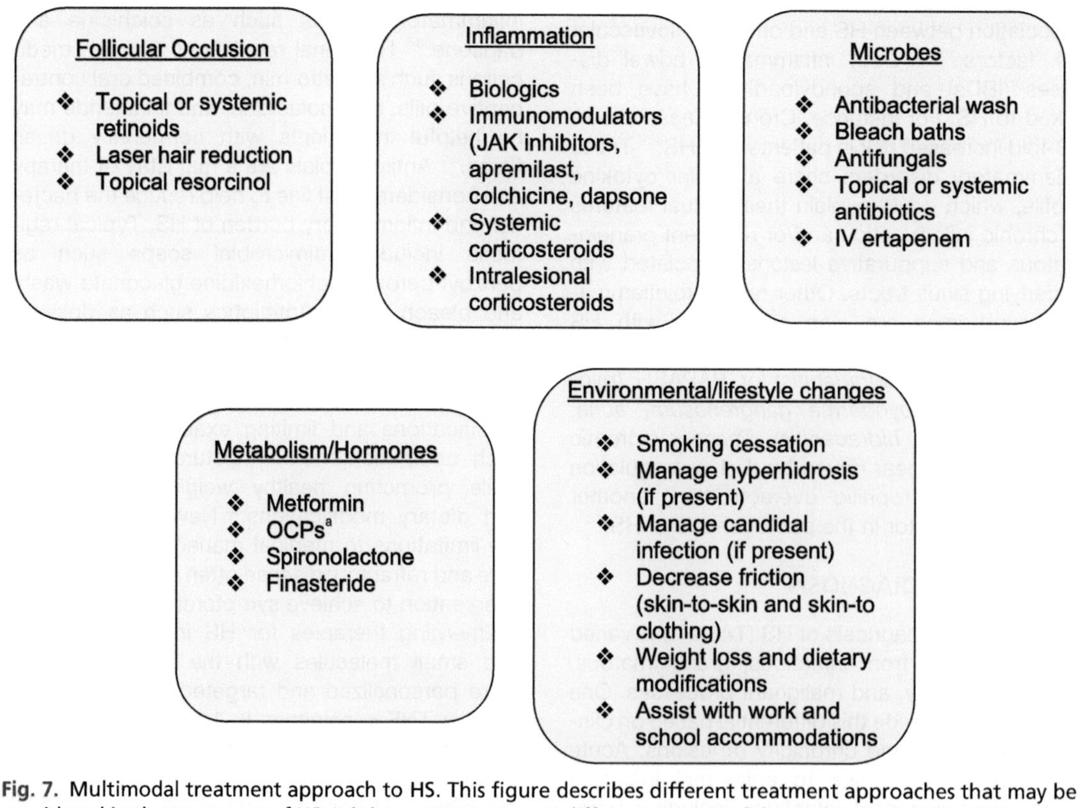

Follicular Occlusion
- ❖ Topical or systemic retinoids
- ❖ Laser hair reduction
- ❖ Topical resorcinol

Inflammation
- ❖ Biologics
- ❖ Immunomodulators (JAK inhibitors, apremilast, colchicine, dapsone
- ❖ Systemic corticosteroids
- ❖ Intralesional corticosteroids

Microbes
- ❖ Antibacterial wash
- ❖ Bleach baths
- ❖ Antifungals
- ❖ Topical or systemic antibiotics
- ❖ IV ertapenem

Metabolism/Hormones
- ❖ Metformin
- ❖ OCPs[a]
- ❖ Spironolactone
- ❖ Finasteride

Environmental/lifestyle changes
- ❖ Smoking cessation
- ❖ Manage hyperhidrosis (if present)
- ❖ Manage candidal infection (if present)
- ❖ Decrease friction (skin-to-skin and skin-to clothing)
- ❖ Weight loss and dietary modifications
- ❖ Assist with work and school accommodations

Fig. 7. Multimodal treatment approach to HS. This figure describes different treatment approaches that may be considered in the treatment of HS. It is important to target different aspects of the pathophysiology of disease as HS is driven by both physiologic and environmental factors. JAK, Janus kinase; OCP, oral contraceptive pills. [a]Combined oral contraceptives pills with low levels of progestins or progesterone analogs are preferred.

must be carefully discussed. Exercise is difficult to perform during painful flares and can even trigger flares in some patients. Additionally, the redundant skin left behind after massive weight loss results in more "intertriginous" areas and can sometime lead to the development of new HS lesions.[51]

Laser and light-based therapies have proven helpful to prevent future outbreaks by reducing the hair follicles and promoting thermal injury of bacteria.[52] It is also helpful in Hurley stages II and III disease to surgically excise or "deroof" chronic sinus tracts (see **Fig. 2**).[45] Patients with advanced disease should also be monitored for potential malignant transformation because cases of SCC have been associated with longstanding HS lesions.[2,28]

SUMMARY

HS is a chronic debilitating disease, which significantly influences patients' quality of life. This disease disproportionally affects populations of color causing undue psychological, financial, and medical burden on these populations. Given the multiple comorbidities associated with HS, a multimodal and multidisciplinary treatment approach is often recommended for patients. Significant efforts have been made to elucidate the pathogenesis and identify novel therapeutic targets for this complex disease. However, more studies including patients with skin of color are warranted to investigate the differences in disease prevalence and severity in this population, to ameliorate differences in access to dermatologic care, and to assess clinical response to emerging therapies.

CLINICS CARE POINTS

- Clinicians should maintain a high index of suspicion for HS in patients with refractory, draining and recurrent boils and abscesses affecting intertriginous regions.

- While assessing patients, it is important to evaluate for other elements of the follicular occlusion tetrad and syndromic forms of HS.[41]

- Screening for comorbidities such as metabolic syndrome, cardiovascular disease, IBD, arthropathy, and mental illness is integral to the care of patients with HS.[39]

- Treatment should be multimodal, targeting different components of the disease pathogenesis including follicular occlusion, inflammation, hormonal or metabolic dysregulation, bacterial overgrowth, and lifestyle or environmental factors.[42–46]

- Clinical outcomes are improved with early diagnosis and multimodal management. Currently, the goal of therapy is to control flares and decelerate disease progression.[49]

DISCLOSURE

G.A. Okoye: Consultant: Unilever; Grants (Janssen, United States, Pfizer, United States); Honoraria for Advisory Boards (Abbvie, United States, Pfizer, UCB, United States, Janssen, Novartis, United States, Lilly, United States); Board member: Hidradenitis Suppurativa Foundation.

REFERENCES

1. Nguyen TV, Damiani G, Orenstein LAV, et al. Hidradenitis suppurativa: an update on epidemiology, phenotypes, diagnosis, pathogenesis, comorbidities and quality of life. J Eur Acad Dermatol Venereol 2020;35(1):50.
2. Fabbrocini G, Ruocco E, De Vita V, et al. Squamous cell carcinoma arising in long-standing hidradenitis suppurativa: An overlooked facet of the immunocompromised district. Clin Dermatol 2017;35(2):225–7.
3. Vellaichamy G, Amin AT, Dimitrion P, et al. Recent advances in hidradenitis suppurativa: Role of race, genetics, and immunology. Front Genet 2022;13:918858.
4. Mortimer PS, Lunniss PJ. Hidradenitis suppurativa. J R Soc Med 2000;93:420–2.
5. Karagiannidis I, Nikolakis G, Sabat R, et al. Hidradenitis suppurativa/Acne inversa: an endocrine skin disorder? Rev Endocr Metab Disord 2016;17(3):335–41.
6. Luck ME, Tao J, Lake EP. The skin and gut microbiome in hidradenitis suppurativa: current understanding and future considerations for research and treatment. Am J Clin Dermatol 2022;23(6):841–52.
7. Jiang SW, Whitley MJ, Mariottoni P, et al. Hidradenitis suppurativa: host-microbe and immune pathogenesis underlie important future directions. JID Innov 2021;1(1):100001.
8. Macklis PC, Tyler K, Kaffenberger J, et al. Lifestyle modifications associated with symptom improvement in hidradenitis suppurativa patients. Arch Dermatol Res 2022;314(3):293–300.
9. Fernandez JM, Marr KD, Hendricks AJ, et al. Alleviating and exacerbating foods in hidradenitis suppurativa. Dermatol Ther 2020;33(6):e14246.
10. Tzellos T, Yang H, Mu F, et al. Impact of hidradenitis suppurativa on work loss, indirect costs and income. Br J Dermatol 2019;181:147–54.

11. Tzellos T. and Zouboulis C.C., Which hidradenitis suppurativa comorbidities should I take into account?, *Exp Dermatol*, 2022;31 Suppl 1:29-32.

12. Quinto RM, Mastroeni S, Sampogna F, et al. Sexuality in persons with hidradenitis suppurativa: Factors associated with sexual desire and functioning impairment. Front Psychiatr 2021;12:729104.

13. Janse IC, Deckers IE, van der Maten AD, et al. Sexual health and quality of life are impaired in hidradenitis suppurativa: a multicentre cross-sectional study. Br J Dermatol 2017;176:1042–7.

14. Frings VG, Bauer B, Glöditzsch M, et al. Assessing the psychological burden of patients with hidradenitis suppurativa. Eur J Dermatol 2019;29(3):294–301.

15. Phan K, Huo YR, Smith SD. Hidradenitis suppurativa and psychiatric comorbidities, suicides and substance abuse: systematic review and meta-analysis. Ann Transl Med 2020;8(13):821.

16. Ortiz-Álvarez J, Hernández-Rodríguez JC, Durán-Romero AJ, et al. Hidradenitis suppurativa and suicide risk: a multivariate analysis in a disease with a high psychological burden. Arch Dermatol Res 2023;315(3):637–42.

17. Garg A, Kirby JS, Lavian J, et al. Sex- and age-adjusted population analysis of prevalence estimates for hidradenitis suppurativa in the United States. JAMA Dermatol 2017;153(8):760–4.

18. Choi ECE, Phan PHC, Oon HH. Hidradenitis suppurativa: racial and socioeconomic considerations in management. Int J Dermatol 2022;61(12):1452–7.

19. Kulkarni V, Okoye GA, Garza LA, et al. Geospatial heterogeneity of hidradenitis suppurativa searches in the United States: infodemiology study of google search data. JMIR Dermatol 2022;5(2):e34594.

20. CDC. Adult Obesity Maps, Available at: https://www.cdc.gov/obesity/data/prevalence-maps.html, Accessed September 28, 2022.

21. Kozera EK, Lowes MA, Hsiao JL, et al. Clinical considerations in the management of hidradenitis suppurativa in women. Int J Womens Dermatol 2021;7(5Part B):664–71.

22. Garg A, Lavian J, Lin G, et al. Incidence of hidradenitis suppurativa in the United States: a sex- and age-adjusted population analysis. J Am Acad Dermatol 2017;77(1):118–22.

23. Liy-Wong C, Kim M, Kirkorian AY, et al. Hidradenitis suppurativa in the pediatric population: an international, multicenter, retrospective, cross-sectional study of 481 pediatric patients. JAMA Dermatol 2021;157(4):385–91.

24. Kilgour JM, Li S, Sarin KY. Hidradenitis suppurativa in patients of color is associated with increased disease severity and healthcare utilization: a retrospective analysis of 2 U.S. cohorts. JAAD international 2021;3:42–52.

25. Khanna R, Whang KA, Huang AH, et al. Inpatient burden of hidradenitis suppurativa in the United States: analysis of the 2016 National inpatient sample. J Dermatolog Treat 2022;33(2):1150–2.

26. Anzaldi L, Perkins JA, Byrd AS, et al. Characterizing inpatient hospitalizations for hidradenitis suppurativa in the United States. J Am Acad Dermatol 2020;82(2):510–3.

27. Navrazhina K, Frew JW, Gilleaudeau P, et al. Epithelialized tunnels are a source of inflammation in hidradenitis suppurativa. J Allergy Clin Immunol 2021;147(6):2213–24.

28. Goldburg SR, Strober BE, Payette MJ. Hidradenitis suppurativa: epidemiology, clinical presentation, and pathogenesis. J Am Acad Dermatol 2020;82:1045–58.

29. Boer J, Jemec GB. Mechanical stress and the development of pseudo-comedones and tunnels in Hidradenitis suppurativa/Acne inversa. Exp Dermatol 2016;25(5):396–7.

30. Kozera EK, Frew JW. The pathogenesis of hidradenitis suppurativa: evolving paradigms in a complex disease. Dermatological Reviews 2022;3:39–49.

31. Jourabchi N, Fischer AH, Cimino-Mathews A, et al. Squamous cell carcinoma complicating a chronic lesion of hidradenitis suppurativa: a case report and review of the literature. Int Wound J 2017;14(2):435–8.

32. Saunte DM, Boer J, Stratigos A, et al. Diagnostic delay in hidradenitis suppurativa is a global problem. Br J Dermatol 2015;173(6):1546–9.

33. Garg A, Neuren E, Cha D, et al. Evaluating patients' unmet needs in hidradenitis suppurativa: Results from the Global Survey Of Impact and Healthcare Needs (VOICE) Project. J Am Acad Dermatol 2020;82(2):366–76.

34. Hurley H. Axillary hyperhidrosis, apocrine bromhidrosis, hidradenitis suppurativa and familial benign pemphigus. Surgical approach. In: Roenigk R, Roenigk H, editors. *Dermatologic surgery, principles and practice*. New York: Marcel Dekker; 1989. p. 623–46.

35. Sartorius K, Emtestam L, Jemec GBE, et al. Objective scoring of hidradenitis suppurativa reflecting the role of tobacco smoking and obesity. Br J Dermatol 2009;161:831–9.

36. Shi VY, Vivian YS, Lowes M, et al. In: Disease Evaluation and Outcome Measures". A Comprehensive guide to hidradenitis suppurativa. Philadelphia, PA: Elsevier; 2022. p. 123–4.

37. Sokumbi O., Hodge D.O., Ederaine S.A., et al., Comorbid diseases of hidradenitis suppurativa: a 15-year population-based study in olmsted county, Minnesota, USA, *Int J Dermatol*, 2022, Available at: https://www.ncbi.nlm.nih.gov/pubmed/35485975. Accessed September 28, 2022.

38. Ergun T. Hidradenitis suppurativa and the metabolic syndrome. Clin Dermatol 2018;36(1):41–7.

39. Garg A, Malviya N, Strunk A, et al. Comorbidity screening in hidradenitis suppurativa: Evidence-

based recommendations from the US and Canadian Hidradenitis Suppurativa Foundations. J Am Acad Dermatol 2022;86(5):1092–101.

40. Egeberg A, Gislason GH, Hansen PR. Risk of major adverse cardiovascular events and all-cause mortality in patients with hidradenitis suppurativa. JAMA Dermatol 2016;152(4):429–34.

41. Garcovich S, Genovese G, Moltrasio C, et al. PASH, PAPASH, PsAPASH, and PASS: the autoinflammatory syndromes of hidradenitis suppurativa. Clin Dermatol 2021;39(2):240–7.

42. Scala E, Cacciapuoti S, Garzorz-Stark N, et al. Hidradenitis suppurativa: where we are and where we are going. Cells 2021;10(8):2094.

43. Saunte DML, Jemec GBE. Hidradenitis suppurativa: advances in diagnosis and treatment. JAMA 2017; 318(20):2019–32.

44. Scheinfeld N. Hidradenitis suppurativa: A practical review of possible medical treatments based on over 350 hidradenitis patients. Dermatol Online J 2013;19(4):1.

45. Alikhan A, Sayed C, Alavi A, et al. North American clinical management guidelines for hidradenitis suppurativa: a publication from the United States and Canadian Hidradenitis Suppurativa Foundations: part I: diagnosis, evaluation, and the use of complementary and procedural management. J Am Acad Dermatol 2019;81(1):76–90.

46. Braunberger TL, Nartker NT, Nicholson CL, et al. Ertapenem - a potent treatment for clinical and quality of life improvement in patients with hidradenitis suppurativa. Int J Dermatol 2018;57(9):1088–93.

47. Lee DE, Clark AK, Shi V, et al. Hidradenitis suppurativa: disease burden and etiology in skin of color. Dermatology 2017;233:456–61.

48. Okeke CAV, Perry JD, Simmonds FC, et al. Clinical trials and skin of color: the example of hidradenitis suppurativa. Dermatology 2022;238:180–4.

49. Wang SC, Wang SC, Sibbald RG, et al. Hidradenitis suppurativa: a frequently missed diagnosis, part 1: a review of pathogenesis, associations, and clinical features. Adv Skin Wound Care 2015;28(7):325–32 [quiz: 333-4].

50. Hua VJ, Kilgour JM, Cho HG, et al. Characterization of comorbidity heterogeneity among 13,667 patients with hidradenitis suppurativa. JCI insight 2021; 6(21):e151872.

51. Sivanand A, Gulliver WP, Josan CK, et al. Weight loss and dietary interventions for hidradenitis suppurativa: a systematic review. J Cutan Med Surg 2020; 24(1):64–72.

52. Hamzavi IH, Griffith JL, Riyaz F, et al. Laser and light-based treatment options for hidradenitis suppurativa. J Am Acad Dermatol 2015;73(5 Suppl 1): S78–81.

53. Lacarrubba F, Musumeci ML, Nasca MR, et al. Double-ended pseudocomedones in hidradenitis suppurativa: clinical, dermoscopic, and histopathological correlation. Acta Derm Venereol 2017;97(6): 763–4.

Skin Cancer in Skin of Color

Ananya Munjal, MS[a], Nkanyezi Ferguson, MD[b],*

KEYWORDS

- Melanoma • Squamous cell cancer • Basal cell cancer • Mycosis fungoides
- Cutaneous T- cell lymphoma • Epidemiology • Disparity • Cutaneous malignancy

KEY POINTS

- The presentation of skin cancer in skin of color patients can vary from that in lighter skinned patients.
- Effective recognition and awareness of these unique skin cancer presentations can lead to more timely diagnosis for skin of color patients.
- There are significant disparities in the diagnosis and surgical management of cutaneous malignancies in skin of color patients.
- There is a need for additional research to further determine risk factors and factors contributing to disparities in outcomes for skin of color patients.

INTRODUCTION

Skin cancer is less common in skin of color patients than in lighter skinned patients but is often associated with greater morbidity and mortality in this population.[1] Most research on skin cancer to date has been predominantly focused on lighter skin types, and medical literature and public health efforts have targeted the white population as the gold standard for the development of prevention and treatment guidelines.[2] However, in today's rapidly evolving demographic landscape, it is crucial that dermatologic providers be able to recognize different presentations of skin cancer in skin of color patients, in an effort to optimize early detection of these tumors and ensure equitable outcomes.

Here we detail the epidemiology, risk factors, clinical features, and disparities in treatment of melanoma, squamous cell carcinoma, basal cell carcinoma, and mycosis fungoides subtype of cutaneous T-cell lymphoma in skin of color patients.

MELANOMA IN SKIN OF COLOR
Epidemiology

During the past decade, the overall incidence of melanoma in the United States has been increasing by an average of 1.4% annually, and the current incidence of melanoma is estimated at 22.8 per 100,000 annually.[3] Non-Hispanic White men have the highest incidence rate with 34.7 per 100,000 and Black women have the lowest incidence rate at 0.9 per 100,000 annually.

Although overall melanoma mortality rates have decreased, racial disparities in melanoma-specific survival have persisted. In a study comparing patients diagnosed with melanoma before the year 2000 to those diagnosed after 2010 in the United States, melanoma survival improved for White patients, whereas skin of color patients continued to have poor overall survival.[3] This contributes to the "minority melanoma paradox," a phenomenon of lower incidence but higher mortality among Black melanoma patients, due in part to more advanced tumors at presentation as compared with White patients.[2] The 5-year survival rate for Black patients with melanoma has been found to be less than 60% compared with more than 80% seen in White patients.[4] In the Hispanic population, studies have reported a 7.3% annual increase in the incidence of invasive melanoma in Hispanic men, and a 3.4% annual increase in the incidence of invasive melanoma from 1990 to 2004 in Hispanic women.[5] Overall, melanomas present at

a University of Iowa Carver College of Medicine, Iowa City, IA, USA; b University of Missouri Department of Dermatology, Missouri, Columbia, MO, USA
* Corresponding author. Dermatology and Skin Surgery Center 1020 Hitt Street, Columbia, MO
E-mail address: fergusonnn@health.missouri.edu

Dermatol Clin 41 (2023) 481–489
https://doi.org/10.1016/j.det.2023.02.013

later stages in Black and Hispanic populations and carry a worse prognosis.

Risk Factors for Cutaneous Melanoma in Skin of Color

Ultraviolet (UV) radiation is not thought to be a major risk factor for melanoma in skin of color because darkly pigmented skin is associated with an increased melanin density and larger, more dispersed melanosomes, and has been shown to be protective against UV penetration of the epidermis, DNA damage, and carcinogenesis.[6] However, some studies on UV-induced DNA damage have demonstrated that all skin types experience some degree of DNA damage following UV exposure.[7]

Trauma has been evaluated and not found to be a risk factor for melanoma in skin of color patients but reported risk factors in this population include albinism, history of radiation therapy, immunosuppression, burn scars, preexisting nevus (especially acral), and congenital nevus.[7]

Melanoma Subtypes in Skin of Color

Earlier studies in Black individuals have found that more than 90% of melanomas in this population are acral lentiginous, mucosal, and ocular melanoma subtypes, with acral lentiginous melanoma being the most common[8] (**Fig. 1**A). Palmoplantar acral lentiginous melanomas in skin of color typically present as dark brown or blue-black irregular pigmented patches or a reddish-pink color if amelanotic, and these lesions commonly progress to large exophytic nodules.[3] These melanoma subtypes are in predominately sun protected locations, reinforcing the fact that UV likely has less to no role in the pathogenesis of melanoma in Black individuals.

Acral lentiginous melanomas on plantar surfaces are associated with mechanical stress points, and a study in Japanese patients found that the majority of these lesions occur on weight-bearing areas of the front or rear plantar surface.[3] Individuals of Asian or Pacific Islander descent are also diagnosed with the highest proportion of mucosal melanoma overall with anorectal mucosal melanoma being the most common among women.[3]

Clinical Features of Melanoma in Skin of Color

Features of melanoma in skin of color patients frequently do not fit into traditional "ABCD" criteria because they often display symmetry and homogeneous uniform pigmentation and are more likely to be thicker and more ulcerated at time of diagnosis.[3] One feature novel to melanoma in situ in skin of color is a hypopigmented "halo," which in one study surrounded 57% of plantar melanoma lesions.[8]

Subungual melanomas commonly present as brownish-gray pigmented lines in the nail plate that can progress to an exophytic nodule and can be difficult to differentiate from physiologic pigmentation or trauma[3] (**Fig. 1**B). Although the overall incidence of subungual melanomas is similar across racial groups, the relative proportion is higher in patients with skin of color. Recent data shows that 38% to 76% of cases of subungual melanoma begin as longitudinal melanonychia, which is a physiologic process common in skin of color patients presenting as single or multiple parallel, evenly spaced, brown to black bands in the nail.[3] Subungual melanoma should be suspected if in the setting of involvement of a single digit (especially the thumb, great toe, or index finger), abrupt development or change, development in the setting of nail dystrophy or periungual

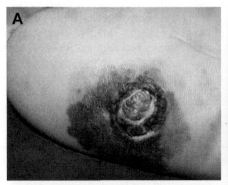
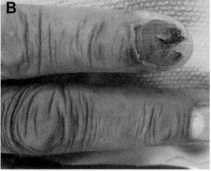

Fig. 1. (*A*) Acral lentiginous melanoma: Ulcerated brown variegated pigmented patch with irregular borders on the plantar foot. (*B*) Subungual acral lentiginous melanoma: Dark brown heterogenous pigmentation on the right second digit nail bed with pigment extension onto the proximal nail fold and nail dystrophy.

extension of pigmentation to the adjacent cuticle and nail fold (Hutchinson sign).[9,10]

Regarding location on the body, melanomas in Black patients commonly occur on skin that is not sun-exposed, where there is less pigment and melanin to protect melanocytes from UV radiation, in contrast to White patients who have melanomas predominantly in sun-exposed areas.[7] Of all melanomas in Blacks, 60% to 75% originate on the palms, soles, mucous membranes, and subungual regions, areas known as acral surfaces.[2] Several studies have identified the foot to be the most common location for melanomas in Black patients. In a retrospective study on melanoma in Asian Americans, the lower extremities were identified as the most common primary site, with fewer truncal, head, and neck melanomas than non-Hispanic White patients.[3] This contrasts with what is observed in White patients, in whom melanoma is commonly truncal.[7]

It is important to be able to appropriately recognize and diagnose melanomas in skin of color patients, as misdiagnosis of melanoma is a barrier to timely care. Melanomas in skin of color patients are often misdiagnosed as other lesions, due in part to underrepresentation of skin of color images in dermatology training, because majority of the images in the largest datasets used to identify skin cancer are of pigmented lesions in white skin.[6] Common misdiagnoses include fungal infection, subungual hematoma, tinea nigra, pigmented basal cell carcinoma, tinea corporis, talon noir, erythema dyschromicum perstans, fixed drug eruption, melasma, localized argyria, exogenous ochronosis, melanotic lupus erythematosus, Berloque dermatitis, and pigmented viral warts.[7] Of note, physiologic pigmentation of the oral mucosal is the most frequent cause of diffuse oral pigmentation and is common in African, Asian, Indian, South American, and Mediterranean population.[10] This pigmentation is due to greater melanocytic activity in skin of color patients, and as oral pigmented lesions are frequently noted on physical examination, they must be adequately differentiated from signs of a malignant process such as melanoma.[10]

Disparities in Diagnosis and Surgical Management in Skin of Color

Skin of color patients with melanoma tend to present late, with delays of up to 5.6 years before diagnosis.[7] In one report, one-third of African American patients were initially seen with stage III or IV disease, whereas only about 12% of the White patients were initially seen at these stages.[4] Black patients with melanoma are also seen with more regional and distant disease at presentation, more than twice as often as their White counterparts.[11]

There are also significant disparities in the management of melanoma in skin of color patients. Individuals with skin of color are more likely to experience significantly longer time from diagnosis to definitive surgery and systemic treatment.[6] In one study, time to definitive surgery for Black patients with melanoma was almost twice as long as compared to non-Hispanic White patients, and time to immunotherapy was more than 20% longer.[6] Additionally, Black, Medicaid, and low-income patients are significantly less likely to receive immunotherapy for the treatment of melanoma.[11]

One study on melanoma-specific survival demonstrated that Hispanic, Black, and Asian/Pacific Islander patients all continue to suffer worse outcomes than their non-Hispanic White counterparts, and that this discrepancy has increased from before the year 2000 as compared with after 2010, despite the introduction of immunotherapy and targeted therapies.[12]

SQUAMOUS CELL CARCINOMA IN SKIN OF COLOR
Epidemiology

Squamous cell cancer is the one of the most common cutaneous malignancies in skin of color patients, representing 30% of skin cancers in Black patients and 65% of skin cancers in Asian Indian patients.[1] Earlier incidences of squamous cell carcinoma in skin of color populations have been reported to be 23 per 100,000 in Japanese Hawaiians, 21 per 100,000 in New Mexican Hispanics, 13.8 to 32.9 per 100,000 in Hispanic residents of Arizona, and 3 per 100,000 in Black individuals.[1] In one review, squamous cell cancer was established as the most common cutaneous malignancy in Black patients overall and found to be 20% more common than basal cell carcinomas.[1] Squamous cell cancer is also the second most common skin cancer in Chinese and Japanese patients, and demographically Hispanic and African American men have the highest rates of penile squamous cell cancer.[1,13]

Clinical Features of Squamous Cell Carcinoma in Skin of Color

Squamous cell carcinomas in Black individuals are often superficial, discrete, and originating from an indurated, rounded, elevated base. Dermatoscopic features of these lesions are similar to those described in White individuals but there is a higher incidence of pigmented variants.[8]

Squamous cell carcinoma in situ in Black patients typically present as a nonspecific scaly, hyperkeratotic, sharply demarcated, brown, or black hyperpigmented plaque, papule, or nodule.[8,14] These lesions are often pigmented and may be velvety, flat, or verrucous, and the perilesional skin may have a dyspigmented or mottled appearance.[8,14]

Regarding location on the body, studies of squamous cell carcinoma in African Americans have shown that these carcinomas occur predominantly in non–sun-exposed areas in contrast to the photodistribution in most Caucasians.[13] Studies in Black Africans and African Americans have shown that the most commonly site affected is the lower limb, which is affected in more than half of cases, followed by the head and neck.[1,13] The anogenital region is also involved in 10% to 23% of total squamous cell carcinoma cases.[13] Although the prevalence of penile squamous cell carcinoma is equal for White and Black patients, Black patients present at a younger age with higher stage of disease and have a shorter survival period.[1]

Risk Factors

The most important predisposing risk factors for the development of squamous cell carcinomas in skin of color are areas of chronic scarring and inflammation, which are noted in 20% to 40% of cases of squamous cell carcinoma in Black patients.[1,13] Earlier studies have shown that squamous cell carcinomas in Black patients have developed within burn scars, in areas of past physical or thermal trauma, in earlier sites of radiation therapy and in areas of chronic inflammation such as ulcers.[1] In one review of squamous cell carcinoma in Nigerian Black patients, the most common predisposing factor was chronic leg ulcers, with most tumors originating from postburn scars.[15] Furthermore, squamous cell carcinomas that develop within a chronic scarring process tend to be aggressive and are associated with up to 40% risk of metastasis, compared with 1% to 4% metastatic rate of UV-induced squamous cell carcinomas in White patients. Other risk factors include history of albinism, human papilloma virus, epidermodysplasia verruciformis, immunosuppression, and exposure to chemical carcinogens including arsenic and tar.[1]

There are also significant risks related to organ transplant because squamous cell carcinoma is the most common skin cancer diagnosed in solid organ transplant recipients and confers significant mortality in this population.[16] Although cutaneous squamous cell cancer develops more frequently in the white transplant population, Black transplant patients are disproportionally affected by genital squamous cell cancer secondary to human papillomavirus.[16] Additionally, among immunocompetent patients, mortality rates of invasive penile squamous cell carcinoma are significantly greater in Black patients.

Although epidemiologic studies have found UV radiation to be a major cause of squamous cell cancer in White patients, ultraviolet radiation (UVR) is not considered an important risk factor in Black patients.[14] Some studies have found positive associations between sun exposure and risk of squamous cell carcinoma in Japanese and Taiwanese populations.[17] Overall, evidence assessing the association of UV exposure with squamous cell carcinomas is limited, and there is a need for further research to evaluate this risk in skin of color populations.

Disparities in Diagnosis and Surgical Management

Focusing on the treatment of squamous cell carcinomas, Mohs micrographic surgery defect sizes were significantly larger among Hispanic and Latino patients compared with non-Hispanic White patients, suggesting that cancers in this population are larger at presentation.[18] Predicted reasons for delays in the treatment of squamous cell carcinomas is the wide range of clinical presentations in skin of color patients, and that they more often occur in non–sun-exposed areas, such as the anogenital region that may be missed on skin examinations.[19]

BASAL CELL CARCINOMA IN SKIN OF COLOR
Epidemiology

Basal cell carcinoma is the most common skin cancer in Caucasian, Hispanic, Chinese, and Japanese populations. In contrast, these carcinomas are the second most common cutaneous malignancy in Black and Asian Indian populations. Basal cell carcinomas represent 65% to 75% of skin cancers in Caucasians, 20% to 30% of skin cancers in Asian Indians, 12% to 35% of skin cancers in American Black individuals and 2% to 8% of skin cancers in African Black individuals. About 1.8% of all basal cell carcinomas occur in Black individuals, and these carcinomas are approximately 19 times more common in White people.[1]

The prevalence of basal cell carcinomas in North American Black patients averages 1% to 2% annually.[1] The incidences of skin of color basal cell carcinoma (BCC) per 100,000 population have been reported in different races as follows: black men (1), black women (2), Kenyan

Africans (0.065), Chinese men (6.4), Chinese women (5.8), Japanese (15–16.5), New Mexican Hispanic women (113), New Mexican Hispanic men (171), Arizona Hispanic women (50), and Arizona Hispanic men (91).[1]

Risk Factors

Previous studies have shown that risks for developing basal cell carcinoma include albinism, previous scarring, ulcers, chronic infections, nevus sebaceous, ingestion of arsenic, immunosuppression, previous radiation treatment, xeroderma pigmentosum, basal cell nevus syndrome and both physical and thermal trauma.[1] Black patients who have a history of basal cell carcinoma are at increased risk of subsequent cancers, hypothesized to be due to elevated skin trans-urocanic acid concentration, which can initiate immune suppression.[13] One study found that 16.5% of Black patients with a basal cell carcinoma also had a second, noncutaneous tumor, 65% of which were lung cancer.[1] Although the incidence of basal cell carcinoma metastasis in the Black population is not well documented because of its low incidence, some studies suggest that Black patients may require closer monitoring after initial basal cell carcinoma diagnosis because they may have increased propensity toward the development of basal cell carcinoma metastasis.[13]

Basal cell carcinoma is primarily related to prolonged UV light exposure in Whites, Blacks, Hispanics, Chinese Asians, Japanese, and Asian Indian patients, and consequently occurs most often in patients after the fifth decade on sun-exposed areas of the head and neck, regardless of the degree of pigmentation of the skin.[1] There is some debate as to whether UV exposure is a risk factor for basal cell carcinoma in Black patients. Some studies suggest that since basal cell cancers in Black patients predominantly occur on the head and neck, UV exposure may be a risk factor in the pathogenesis of this condition.[8] However other studies note that skin of color patients with basal cell nevus syndrome develop fewer basal cell carcinomas due to photoprotection in darker skinned persons, suggesting that UV plays a more significant role in the development of BCC in lighter skin types.[1] Because there is a lack of high-quality research to support evidence on the association of UV exposure and nonmelanoma skin cancer development in skin of color, there is a need for further investigation into this association.[20]

Clinical Features of Basal Cell Carcinoma in Skin of Color

The classic basal cell carcinoma presentation of a pearly papule with rolled borders and telangiectasias may be much more subtle in darker skin tones or in pigmented tumors[1,14] (**Fig. 2**A). Pigmented basal cell carcinomas are very rare overall but are the most prevalent type in Black populations, and earlier studies have demonstrated than 50% of basal cell carcinomas are pigmented in non-White versus only 5% in White individuals[8,14] (**Fig. 2**B). Basal cell carcinomas in Asian patients have been reported clinically to appear brown to glossy black and have a "black pearly" appearance[1] (**Fig. 2**C). Dermatoscopy of these lesions often depicts heavily pigmented lesions with features consistent with pigmented basal cell carcinomas in White patients.[8] Other dermatoscopic findings of pigmented basal cell carcinomas include absence of pigmentary network,

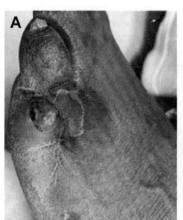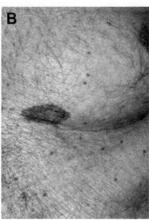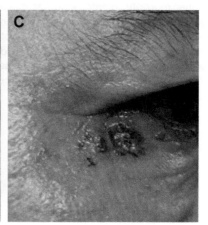

Fig. 2. (*A*) Basal cell carcinoma: Violaceous papule on the left foot. (*B*) Basal cell carcinoma: Dark brown pearly plaque with rolled borders on the left chest. (*C*) Basal cell carcinoma: Brown pearly papule with rolled borders on the right lateral lower eyelid.

peripheral maple leaf–like structures, blue-gray structureless areas, spoke wheel–like structures, blue-white veil, adherent fabric fibers, brown dots, erosions, and adherent and shiny white chrysalis-like structures.[21] Regarding location on the body, earlier studies have shown that about 70% of basal cell cancers in Black patients occur on the head and neck.[8]

Disparities in Diagnosis and Surgical Management

Metastatic basal cell carcinoma is rare, with a reported incidence of less than 1% and poor prognosis, with mean survival of 8 months to 3.6 years after diagnosis. Because there ae limited data on prognosis of locally advanced or metastasis in patents with basal cell carcinoma, analysis of disparities in the management of skin of color patients with basal cell carcinoma is difficult. Earlier studies have not found differences in basal cell carcinoma associated morbidity in Black individuals when compared with White individuals.[14] Previous research has demonstrated that there are no significant differences in preoperative lesion size and the number of Mohs stages required for excisions among white, Hispanic, and Asian patients with basal cell carcinoma.[14]

MYCOSIS FUNGOIDES CUTANEOUS T-CELL LYMPHOMA AND SEZARY SYNDROME IN SKIN OF COLOR
Epidemiology

Mycosis fungoides is a chronic cutaneous T-cell lymphoma that is up to twice as common in Black populations than in Whites, regardless of sex and age.[1] Black patients with this condition are more likely to have an earlier onset, worse prognosis, higher mortality, greater stage at diagnosis, and greater body surface area of involvement than other ethnic groups.[22–24] In one study of skin cancer in Black patients, mycosis fungoides represented 12.1% of all cutaneous neoplasms.[1] It is the fourth most common skin cancer among Japanese patients, representing approximately 5% of all cutaneous malignancies.[1] Cutaneous T-cell lymphoma may follow a more aggressive course in skin of color patients than in Whites, and earlier studies have demonstrated a 44% mortality among Black patients.[1]

Clinical Presentation in Skin of Color

The 3 common presentations of mycosis in skin of color are hypopigmented lesions, hyperpigmented lesions, and pruritus with secondary lichenification and hyperpigmentation.[24] The overall morphology of mycosis fungoides in skin of color patients can vary, and the presentations can be heterogenous.[24,25] Earlier studies have demonstrated the variations of mycosis fungoides presentation and have shown that in skin of color patients, this condition does not present with the classic erythematous patches and plaques found in White patients.[25] Morphologic features of hyperpigmentation, lichenification, and silver hue are present at higher rates in darker skinned patients with mycosis fungoides compared with those with lighter skin, who typically have higher rates of erythema and poikiloderma[25] (Fig. 3A and B). Other distinctive mycosis fungoides features in skin of color patients include polymorphic pigmentation with hypopigmented or hyperpigmented lesions, lesions larger than 5 cm in diameter, wrinkling, scale, and arcuate-annular configuration[24] (Fig. 3C). Regarding location on the body, the most common presentation is a "bathing suit" distribution with breast, buttocks, and intertriginous involvement.[24] The hypopigmented variant of cutaneous T-cell lymphoma presents as ill-defined, pruritic, hypopigmented macules and patches, and occurs almost exclusively in darker skin types, being exceedingly rare in non–skin of color patients.[1,25] Clinical mimickers of mycosis fungoides in skin of color patients include lichen planus pigmentosus inversus digitate dermatosis, pityriasis lichenoides chronica, and actinic reticuloid.[24] Hypopigmented mycosis fungoides is often clinically misdiagnosed and can be easily

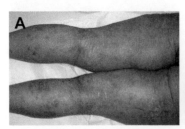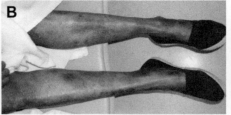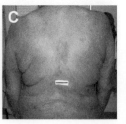

Fig. 3. (A) A Cutaneous T-cell lymphoma: Ill-defined brown plaques and patches with overlying scale on the posterior legs. (B) Cutaneous T-cell lymphoma: Ill-defined brown patches on the bilateral lower legs. (C) Cutaneous T-cell lymphoma: Ill-defined brown patches with overlying scale on the back.

confused with other dermatoses such as vitiligo, pityriasis alba, progressive macular hypomelanosis, tinea versicolor, hypopigmented sarcoid, and postinflammatory hypopigmentation.[1]

The dermatoscopy of mycosis fungoides can also vary in skin of color patients because vessel morphology is often unable to be appreciated due to obscuration by heavy lymphoid infiltrate and significant dermatologic pigment changes.[26] Thus, vessel morphology is not a reliable diagnostic feature in this population. Dermatoscopy of verrucous mycosis fungoides in skin of color patients can mimic seborrheic keratoses, presenting as multicolored amorphous structures with yellow-gray ridges and comedone-like openings.[26] Dermatoscopic features such as rosettes and geometric white lines are unique to mycosis fungoides in SOC patients.[26]

Sezary syndrome, a triad of erythroderma, neoplastic T-cells in the blood, and lymphadenopathy, is also more common in Black patients than in White patients.[27] The erythroderma in this condition is less obvious in darker skin types, and some darker skinned patients with Sezary syndrome may not have any visible erythema.[27] This can make monitoring of skin for treatment response challenging lead to misdiagnosis. Sezary Syndrome in dark skinned patients is often misdiagnosed as erythrodermic psoriasis, erythrodermic atopic dermatitis, generalized allergic drug reaction, or prurigo nodularis.[27] These misdiagnoses can prevent early diagnosis and treatment of this condition in skin of color patients.

Disparities in Diagnosis, Management, Morbidity, and Mortality

Because mycosis fungoides is a rare dermatologic condition, it can be easily misdiagnosed, leading to delays in diagnosis and treatment ranging from 7 months to 10 years from disease onset to diagnosis.[1] It is crucial to adequately diagnose skin of color patients with cutaneous T-cell lymphoma, as early stages are more easily treatable, and later forms of the disease with erythroderma and nodal involvement do not respond as well to therapeutic modalities.[1] Earlier research has demonstrated that hypopigmented mycosis fungoides responds better to phototherapy than the hyperpigmented phenotype because phototherapy has been shown to have decreased efficacy with increasing Fitzpatrick skin types.[25]

Management of mycosis fungoides in skin of color can be compromised by the lack of efficacy of ultraviolet B (UVB) therapy in the majority of patients with darker skin types and the appearance of pigmentary side effects of treatments such as radiation therapy.[24] Additionally, treatments for mycosis fungoides such as oral bexarotene can have side effects specific to skin of color patients, including diffuse hypopigmentation.[24] Studies comparing outcomes for Black and White patients with mycosis fungoides have demonstrated that close monitoring and early consideration of systemic treatments in Black patients may be justified given the earlier presentation and more aggressive course of their disease.[22]

SUMMARY

As we work to better understand manifestations of skin cancer in different skin types, it is crucial that we recognize the variability in presentation among patients with skin of color and acknowledge disparities in diagnosis and treatment in this population. Societal factors greatly contribute to this disparity because earlier studies have shown that minority patients report having significantly less physician performed full-body skin examinations and are less ability to recognize concerning lesions on self-examination.[2] Lack of health education also contributes to this inequity because many skin of color patients view their risk of skin cancer to be minimal, have low awareness of the typical features of skin cancer, and receive inadequate education on UV safety.[6,7]

There is a great need to create metrics that better evaluate skin of color patients for skin cancers. This can be implemented through tailored clinical evaluations that consider the varying presentation of different skin cancers in skin of color, and location-specific skin examinations. It is also necessary to educate providers and bridge the knowledge gap about cutaneous cancer in skin of color, by establishing more research in diverse populations, because minority patients are frequently underrepresented in clinical trials.[12] It is crucial that providers acknowledge individualism of racial identity in dermatology, and not conventionalize all patients of one ethnic group. Additionally, it is essential that dermatologists address misconceptions and educate skin of color patients about the risks of cutaneous malignancies and warning signs that can aid in timely interventions for management of these conditions.

CLINICS CARE POINTS

- When evaluating for skin cancer in skin of color patients, it is crucial to keep in mind the unique presentation patterns specific to this population.

- Unlike presentation of melanoma in white patients, melanoma in Black patients commonly occurs of skin that is not sun-exposed. For this reason it is important that providers pay special attention to these anatomic areas when performing a skin exam.
- It is imperative that dermatologists educate their minority patients on how to recognize concerning lesions on self-examination, and address any misconceptions on the risks of cutaneous malignancy

DISCLOSURE

The authors have nothing to disclose.
  Declaration of Interests
  Authors have no declarations or disclosures.

REFERENCES

1. Gloster HM, Neal K. Skin cancer in skin of color. J Am Acad Dermatol 2006;55(5):741–60.
2. Goldenberg A, Vujic I, Sanlorenzo M, et al. Melanoma risk perception and prevention behavior among African-Americans: the minority melanoma paradox. Clin Cosmet Investig Dermatol 2015;8: 423–9.
3. Brunsgaard E, Wu YP, Grossman D. Melanoma in Skin of Color: Part I. Epidemiology and clinical presentation. J Am Acad Dermatol 2022. https://doi.org/10.1016/J.JAAD.2022.04.056.
4. Byrd KM, Wilson DC, Hoyler SS, et al. Advanced presentation of melanoma in African Americans. J Am Acad Dermatol 2004;50(1):21–4.
5. Clairwood M, Ricketts J, Grant-Kels J, et al. Melanoma in skin of color in Connecticut: an analysis of melanoma incidence and stage at diagnosis in non-Hispanic blacks, non-Hispanic whites, and Hispanics. Int J Dermatol 2014;53(4):425–33.
6. Brunsgaard E, Jensen J, Grossman D. Melanoma in Skin of Color: Part II. Racial disparities, role of UV, and interventions for earlier detection. J Am Acad Dermatol 2022. https://doi.org/10.1016/j.jaad.2022.04.057.
7. Anaba E. Cutaneous malignant melanoma in skin of color individuals. Niger J Med 2021;30(1):1.
8. Manci R, Dauscher M, Marchetti MA, et al. Features of Skin Cancer in Black Individuals: A Single-Institution Retrospective Cohort Study. Dermatol Pract Concept 2022;12(2):e2022075.
9. Baran R, Kechijian P. Hutchinson's sign: A reappraisal. J Am Acad Dermatol 1996;34(1):87–90.
10. Taylor SC, Kelly AP, Lim HW, et al. Anatomy and Diseases of the Oral Mucosa. In: Edmonson KG, Brown RY, editors. Taylor and Kelly's Dermatology for Skin of Color, 2e. New York, NY: McGraw-Hill Education; 2016. 311-332, 381-390.
11. Hu S, Parker DF, Thomas AG, et al. Advanced presentation of melanoma in African Americans: the Miami-Dade County experience. J Am Acad Dermatol 2004;51(6):1031–2.
12. Qian Y, Johannet P, Sawyers A, et al. The ongoing racial disparities in melanoma: An analysis of the Surveillance, Epidemiology, and End Results database (1975-2016). J Am Acad Dermatol 2021; 84(6):1585–93.
13. Higgins S, Nazemi A, Chow M, et al. Review of Nonmelanoma Skin Cancer in African Americans, Hispanics, and Asians. Dermatol Surg 2018;44(7): 903–10.
14. Hogue L, Harvey VM. Basal Cell Carcinoma, Squamous Cell Carcinoma, and Cutaneous Melanoma in Skin of Color Patients. Dermatol Clin 2019;37(4): 519–26.
15. Chuang TY, Reizner GT, Elpern DJ, et al. Nonmelanoma skin cancer in Japanese ethnic Hawaiians in Kauai, Hawaii: an incidence report. J Am Acad Dermatol 1995;33(3):422–6.
16. Nadhan KS, Larijani M, Abbott J, et al. Prevalence and Types of Genital Lesions in Organ Transplant Recipients. JAMA Dermatol 2018;154(3):323.
17. Kolitz E, Lopes FCPS, Arffa M, et al. UV Exposure and the Risk of Keratinocyte Carcinoma in Skin of Color. JAMA Dermatol 2022;158(5):542.
18. Blumenthal LY, Arzeno J, Syder N, et al. Disparities in nonmelanoma skin cancer in Hispanic/Latino patients based on Mohs micrographic surgery defect size: A multicenter retrospective study. J Am Acad Dermatol 2022;86(2):353–8.
19. Shao K, Feng H. Racial and Ethnic Healthcare Disparities in Skin Cancer in the United States: A Review of Existing Inequities, Contributing Factors, and Potential Solutions. J Clin Aesthet Dermatol 2022;15(7):16–22.
20. Kolitz E, Lopes FCPS, Arffa M, et al. UV Exposure and the Risk of Keratinocyte Carcinoma in Skin of Color: A Systematic Review. JAMA Dermatol 2022; 158(5):542–6.
21. Kinnera B, Devi V, Satyanarayana V. The Dermoscopy of Pigmented Basal Cell Carcinoma. J Cutan Aesthet Surg 2020;13(4):365.
22. Huang AH, Kwatra SG, Khanna R, et al. Racial Disparities in the Clinical Presentation and Prognosis of Patients with Mycosis Fungoides. J Natl Med Assoc 2019;111(6):633–9.
23. Sun G, Berthelot C, Li Y, et al. Poor prognosis in non-Caucasian patients with early-onset mycosis fungoides. J Am Acad Dermatol 2009;60(2): 231–5.
24. Hinds GA, Heald P. Cutaneous T-cell lymphoma in skin of color. J Am Acad Dermatol 2009;60(3): 359–75.

25. Espinosa ML, Walker CJ, Guitart J, et al. Morphology of Mycosis Fungoides and Sézary Syndrome in Skin of Color. Cutis 2022;109(3). https://doi.org/10.12788/CUTIS.0484.

26. Nakamura M, Huerta T, Williams K, et al. Dermoscopic Features of Mycosis Fungoides and Its Variants in Patients with Skin of Color: A Retrospective Analysis. Dermatol Pract Concept 2021;11(3): 2021048.

27. Flaum-Dunoyer P, Noor SJ, Myskowski PL. Cutaneous lymphomas in African American/Black patients: pitfalls and presentations. Int J Dermatol 2022. https://doi.org/10.1111/ijd.16374.

Disorders in Children

Elisabeth A. George, MD[a,1], Christy Nwankwo, BA[b,1],
Leslie Castelo-Soccio, MD, PhD[c], Michelle Oboite, MD[d,e,*]

KEYWORDS

- Pediatric dermatoses • Skin of color • Newborn skin • Postinflammatory hyperpigmentation
- Postinflammatory hypopigmentation • Postinflammatory pigment alteration

KEY POINTS

- Anticipatory guidance should be provided to parents to help with the monitoring of birthmarks.
- Birthmarks are vascular or pigmentary in nature with some signifying diagnosis of another syndrome.
- Newborn rashes can pose significant distress to clinicians and parents, and key features can help distinguish benign from more concerning causes.
- Postinflammatory pigment alteration can be a characteristic and prominent feature of inflammatory dermatoses in the skin of color population.
- Hair loss in the pediatric population can cause psychosocial distress but timely diagnosis and management can often help.

INTRODUCTION

Pediatric dermatoses can present at birth or develop over time. When managing dermatology conditions in children, caregiver involvement is important. Patients may have lesions that need to be monitored or need assistance with therapeutic administration. The following section provides a subset of pediatric dermatoses and notable points for presentation in skin of color patients. Providers need to be able to recognize dermatology conditions in patients of varying skin tones and provide therapies that address the condition and any associated pigmentary alterations.

Common Pediatric Birthmarks

Birthmarks are skin changes that appear at or shortly after birth. With a variable spectrum of presentation, they can be best categorized into pigmented or vascular (Box 1)

The most common pigmented birthmarks are dermal melanocytosis, congenital melanocytic nevi (CMN), and café au lait macules (CALMs).[1] Congenital dermal melanocytosis (CDMs) refer to slate gray/blue patches with ill-defined borders usually found on the buttocks or the back. Previously, CDMs were commonly called "Mongolian spots" (Table 1) as a German anthropologist in 1883 assumed they were specific to those of East Asian descent, then referred to as "Mongols."[2] This term has been discontinued. CDMs are more prevalent in infants of African-American, Native American, Hispanic, and Asian descent than Caucasian patients.[1] Oculodermal melanocytosis (ODM) or nevus of Ota presents similar to CDMs, with a gray/blue to brown patch but in the region of the V1/V2 distribution of the trigeminal nerve. Most patients with this condition also have pigmentation in the ipsilateral sclera. There is also an increased prevalence of ODM in those of Asian

[a] Mount Sinai Hospital, 1468 Madison Avenue, New York, NY 100029, USA; [b] University of Missouri, Kansas City School of Medicine, 2411 Holmes Street, Kansas City, MO 64108, USA; [c] National Institute of Arthritis, Musculoskeletal and Skin Diseases, National Institutes of Health, 9000 Rockville Pike, Bethesda, MD 20892, USA; [d] University of Pennsylvania, Perelman School of Medicine, 3400 Civic Center Boulevard, Philadelphia, PA 19104, USA; [e] Children's Hospital of Philadelphia, 3401 Civic Center Boulevard, Philadelphia, PA 19104, USA
[1] Co- first authors.
* Corresponding author. Children's Hospital of Philadelphia, 3401 Civic Center Boulevard, Philadelphia, PA 19104, USA.
E-mail addresses: oboitem@chop.edu; michelle.oboite@pennmedicine.upenn.edu

Dermatol Clin 41 (2023) 491–507
https://doi.org/10.1016/j.det.2023.02.014

and African descent; however, in contrast to CDMs, the lesion tends to persist even as the child ages.

CMN can appear pink/red, black, or variegated in color. Most of the lesions grow proportionally with the child and may develop terminal hair or a raised texture with time. Giant CMNs can be associated with extracutaneous manifestations or malignant melanoma.[3] Generally, small CMNs have a low risk for malignant transformation. CALMs or café au lait spots are flat, brown-pigmented lesions with jagged or smooth borders. In individuals with a lighter skin tone, this appears as a tan/brown drop of coffee in milk, yet in darker skinned individuals, these marks will seem as a darker pigmented macule compared with the rest of the patient's skin color. Multiple or larger spots of CALMs may be a sign of other genetic conditions such as neurofibromatosis type 1 or McCune Albright syndrome.[4]

Birthmarks can also arise due to aberrant blood vessels that form incorrectly. Infantile hemangioma (IH) is a benign tumor that develops in the first few months of life and may grow rapidly for a year. Most patients experience involution of the lesion by age 5 years. Depending on their depth and location, IHs may appear as rubbery bright red nodules if superficial or as a blue patch if deeper,[5] the latter of which may appear subtly in children with skin of color (SOC). Capillary malformations include nevus flammeus and nevus simplex. These lesions can be pink/red or purple in color, have a reticulated or solid pattern, and progress from a flat patch to a darker more textured lesion with increasing age. In darker skin tones, they may look more purple in color in infancy. Multiple genetic syndromes can be associated with capillary malformations such as the finding of port-wine stains in patients with Sturge Weber syndrome.[6] Port-wine stains or nevus flammeus appear on the lateral face versus nevus simplex, which presents more centrally in locations such as the glabella, philtrum, occiput, and sometimes the mid-lower back.

NEWBORN RASHES

Newborn rashes can cause significant distress to caregivers and present a diagnostic challenge to clinicians. In this section, common benign transient dermatoses will be discussed where reassurance can be provided, as well as more concerning eruptions that require urgent evaluation. Clinicians should be aware of key differences in presentation in order to properly diagnose, counsel, and initiate treatment as needed (**Table 2**).

Transient Neonatal Pustular Melanosis

Transient neonatal pustular melanosis (TNPM) is a benign rash that presents at birth, consisting of

Table 1
Terminology of common pediatric birthmarks and examples of associated conditions

Medical Terminology	Other Common Names	Associated Conditions[1]
CDMs	Mongolian spot, slate gray nevi	Hurler syndrome, GM1 gangliosides type 1
ODM	Nevus of Ota, melanosis oculi	Glaucoma, orbital melanocytoma
CMN	Mole	Neurocutaneous melanosis, Leptomeningeal melanoma
Café au lait macule	Café au lait spot	Neurofibromatosis type 1, McCune Albright syndrome
Infantile hemangiomas	Strawberry marks	PHACE syndrome
Nevus flammeus	Port-wine stain	Sturge-Weber syndrome
Nevus simplex	Angel's kiss, stork bite, salmon patches	Beckwith-Wiedemann

Table 2
Key characteristics of common versus concerning newborn rashes

Rash		Lesions	Distribution	Timing	Bedside testing	Treatment
BENIGN cutaneous eruptions	TNPM	Brown macules, collarettes of scale, ± pustules (2–6 mm, larger than ETN)[7] No erythema	Trunk ± face, hands and feet	At birth	Wright stain: neutrophils ± rare eosinophils	None
	ETN	Pink papules +/– pustules (1–3 mm, smaller than TNPM)[7] with surrounding erythema	Trunk	After birth, up to second week of life	Wright stain: eosinophils (see Fig. 3)	None
	NCP	Monomorphic papules and pustules	Face (seborrheic areas)	After birth, up to fifth week of life	Potassium hydroxide (KOH): ± hyphae and spores	None; if severe, clotrimazole
TORCH	CS	Scaly macules, Desquamation, Flat-topped skin-colored or hypopigmented plaques	Hands and feet; perioral, perianal, skin folds	Up to 3 mo[a]	N/A; Skin biopsy may be needed if serum treponemal testing nondiagnostic	IV or IM penicillin G
	HSV	Grouped vesicles or punched out erosions on an erythematous base	Anywhere	Up to 3 mo	Tzanck smear: multinucleated giant cells	IV acyclovir

[a] Rarely can occur up to 2 years of age.

pustules, scale, and hyperpigmented macules. The cause is unknown. Superficial pustules, thought to develop in utero, easily rupture leaving behind white collarettes of scale and hyperpigmented macules.[8] All 3 stages (pustules, scale, and macules) can be present at birth[9]; however, some neonates present only with collarettes of scale and/or hyperpigmented macules[10] (Fig. 1). TNPM may affect any cutaneous surface, including the palms and soles; however, lesions are typically distributed over the chin, neck, upper chest, lower back, and buttocks. TNPM is more commonly observed in newborns of African descent compared with other groups.[11–13] Reassurance is primary management, and caregiver counseling should include anticipatory guidance that while the pustules and scale typically self-resolve within 2 weeks, the hyperpigmented macules may persist for several months.[14]

Erythema Toxicum Neonatorum

Erythema toxicum neonatorum (ETN) is a benign rash that develops after birth, as early as the first 72 hours[8] up to 10 days of life.[15] It is postulated that ETN is an acute innate immune response to penetration of skin-colonizing flora into the hair follicle.[8] Affected infants present with multiple pink macules and papules that may progress into pustules surrounded by blotchy, ill-defined erythema[16] (Fig. 2, Fig. 3). ETN may involve any skin surface; however, the palms and soles are usually spared. ETN more frequently develops in full-term infants with higher birth weight and

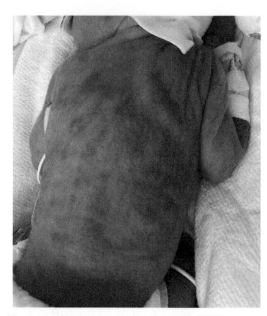

Fig. 2. Erythema toxicum neonatorum (ETN).

greater gestational age, and less commonly in premature infants.[17] ETN is also frequently reported to be more prevalent in infants of European descent[8]; however, this may be reflective of difficulties appreciating erythema in SOC rather than a true demographical characteristic.[18] Interestingly, some authors suggest that TNPM and ETN may be variants of the same condition, and even coexist in rare cases,[19,20] prompting the term sterile transient neonatal pustulosis to describe both entities. Reassurance is the primary management

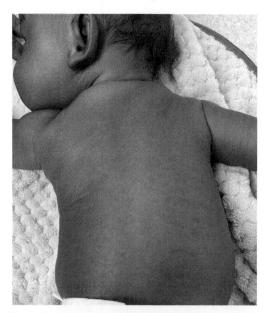

Fig. 1. Transient neonatal pustular melanosis (TNPM).

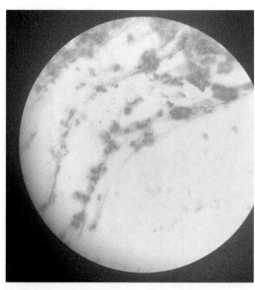

Fig. 3. Eosinophils on Wright stain in ETN.

as the eruption is self-limited, typically resolving within 5 to 7 days without intervention.

Neonatal Cephalic Pustulosis

Neonatal cephalic pustules (NCP) is another benign rash that can develop after birth, between the first and third week of life, presenting as mono-morphic pink papules or pustules on the cheeks, chin, and forehead.[21] The remainder of the body is typically spared. Although the growth of *Malassezia* species on the skin has been observed in infants with NCP, no significant correlation between colonization burden and disease severity has not been established.[22] The mainstay of management is reassurance as most cases spontaneously resolve by 3 to 6 months of age. Caregivers may be counseled to use gentle nonsoap cleansers to wash the affected areas and to avoid occlusive emollients that may exacerbate the eruption.[23] Severe or bothersome cases can improve with topical imidazole therapy or low-potency corticosteroids.

TORCH Infections

TORCH infections refer to a group of infections that may be vertically transmitted from mother to fetus during pregnancy, labor, or in the postnatal period[24] and are among the most concerning conditions in the newborn period. They include infections caused by *Toxoplasma gondii*, *other* pathogens (such as *Treponema pallidum* [syphilis], varicella zoster virus, mumps virus, parvovirus, and human immunodeficiency virus), *rubella* virus, *cytomegalovirus*, and *herpes* simplex virus. TORCH infections can affect fetal organ development, be associated with congenital anomalies, and cause infant death. The dermatologic manifestations of these conditions are varied. Prompt identification is necessary for initiating appropriate treatment to prevent significant infant morbidity and mortality. Two TORCH infections, congenital syphilis (CS) and herpes simplex virus (HSV), will be highlighted in this article given their unique dermatologic and diagnostic characteristics.

In the last decade, the incidence of CS in the United States has increased,[25] and historically, significant disparities exist in the United States with infants of African-American race and Hispanic/Latino ethnicity accounting for the majority of cases.[26] CS can be a diagnostic challenge for clinicians.[27] In the newborn period, CS can present as generalized copper-colored macules and papules involving the palms and soles that desquamate (pemphigus syphiliticus) or moist thin plaques in intertriginous, perineal, and perioral areas (condylomata lata).[28] However, CS has

been reported to mimic other conditions such as neonatal lupus[29] and rarely has even occurred in infants of mothers with adequate prenatal care.[30] As such, there should be a high index of suspicion in infants with atypical papulosquamous eruptions accompanied by rhinorrhea (termed "syphilis snuffles," which may be mucopurulent or blood-tinged)[31] and laboratory abnormalities such as anemia, leukocytosis, thrombocytopenia, transaminitis, or hyperbilirubinemia.[32] Diagnosing neonatal syphilis relies on accurate syphilis diagnosis in the mother, documenting clinical or radiographic signs in the neonate, and obtaining a quantitative nontreponemal test on neonatal and maternal serum.[33,34] Definitive diagnosis is obtained by identifying *T pallidum* spirochetes in infected tissue or fluid. Children at high risk for CS should be treated even if a definitive diagnosis cannot be obtained.[27] Treatment consists of courses of intravenous or intramuscular penicillin G, which can exacerbate cutaneous disease burden as part of the Jarisch-Herxheimer reaction.[35]

Neonatal HSV infection can present on the skin as vesiculopustules or erosions classically grouped on an erythematous base (**Fig. 4**). Definitive diagnosis is confirmed by HSV polymerese chain reaction (PCR) testing of skin lesions. Given the high risk of mortality and morbidity associated with disseminated and neurologic disease, additional workup that includes HSV PCR of serum and cerebrospinal fluid should be performed.[35] Treatment requires hospital admission for IV acyclovir administration and close clinical monitoring. Neonatal HSV infection can be a diagnostic challenge for clinicians in its early stages,[36] and benign transient pustular eruptions discussed in previous sections (TNPM, ETN, NCP) may be considered in the differential diagnosis. Clinical

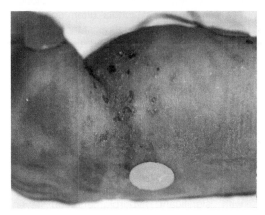

Fig. 4. Neonatal herpes simplex virus (HSV) infection. (Courtesy of P Honig, MD, Philadelphia, PA.)

history and physical examination along with bedside diagnostic testing (ie, Wright stain, potassium hydroxide (KOH) preparations, Tzanck smears) can be helpful to distinguish between the entities.

COMMON INFLAMMATORY DERMATOSES IN CHILDREN WITH SKIN OF COLOR
Acne

Acne is a common pediatric dermatologic condition,[37] and one of the top reasons for children of color to see a dermatologist.[38–40] Pathophysiology involves occlusion, bacterial colonization, and subsequent inflammation of the pilosebaceous unit[41] leading to comedones, pustules, and papules. Areas affected can include the face, upper chest, back, and shoulders. Those with SOC may also present with hyperpigmented macules,[42] and therapies simultaneously targeting acne and hyperpigmentation are preferred. Irritation from topical acne treatments can lead to worsening hyperpigmentation[43] so clinicians should judiciously select more tolerable formulations, particularly in children prone to irritant contact or atopic dermatitis (AD). First-line treatment includes topical retinoids that mediate inflammation, increase cell turnover, suppress tyrosine kinase, and inhibit dermal and epidermal melanosis pathways.[43–45] Adapalene[46,47] and novel lotion formulations of tretinoin[48–50] have proven to be particularly efficacious and well-tolerated in SOC. Azelaic acid can exert anti-inflammatory and antikeratolytic effects for acne as well as antityrosinase activity for hyperpigmentation and has demonstrated efficacy and tolerability for SOC patients.[51] Combination topical retinoid and benzoyl peroxide (BPO) therapy may show greater reductions in both acne and hyperpigmentation; however, these formulations carry increased irritation risks.[52,53] Other effective medications include topical antibiotics such as clindamycin, which is often combined with BPO to prevent bacterial resistance.[54] Combination topical antibiotic-retinoid therapy such as clindamycin-tretinoin gel is tolerable in SOC[55] and can improve adherence in children and adolescents by simplifying regimens to once daily application.[56]

Inflammation can be a prominent feature of acne in Black patients yet, clinically, may present less severe leading to underestimated disease burden[57] and underprescribed systemic therapy for this population.[58] As such, systemic treatment should be considered in children of color presenting with significant hyperpigmentation (even without apparent erythema) or those reporting minimal improvement with topicals. Oral tetracycline antibiotics (doxycycline, minocycline, sarecycline) are generally reserved for children aged older than 8 years due to dental staining and bone development concerns with longer durations of use.[54,59] Younger children can be treated with oral penicillins (amoxicillin), macrolides (azithromycin or erythromycin), cephalosporins (cephalexin), or trimethoprim-sulfamethoxazole.[54] Adolescents with recalcitrant, psychologically distressing, or severe hyperpigmentation-inducing acne may benefit from oral isotretinoin.[44]

Acne may be one of the presenting signs of puberty since androgens increase sebaceous gland activity and can promote comedone formation.[41] In the United States, African-American girls may present with signs of puberty at a younger age than their counterparts; however, structural societal factors such as food insecurity leading to higher rates of obesity, increased environmental exposure to endocrine disrupting chemicals, and early childhood stress have been proposed as potential causes.[60] In general, children presenting with acne between ages 1 to 7 years (some suggest up to age 9 for boys)[61] should be referred to pediatric endocrinology for consideration of hyperandrogenism evaluation.[54,61] Infantile acne (with true comedones as opposed to papulopustules of NCP covered above), although rare, can occur and is often not associated with an underlying endocrinopathy but may be a predictor of severe adolescent acne.[54] Children and adolescents with hormonal-driven acne may present with acne distributed on the chin and jawline, or may report cyclical flaring around menses. Safe and effective treatments include topical clascoterone[62] or, in those eligible, oral spironolactone[63] or combined oral contraceptives (COCs).[64] COCs should not be initiated until a year after menarche.[56]

Personal care products are also an important component of acne management for children with SOC. Pomade acne, characterized by monomorphic acne concentrated on the forehead, hairline, temples, or cheeks, can occur more frequently in children of color who use comedogenic hair greases and oils[65] and smoothing products[66] such as gels and edge controls. Additionally, when prescribing topical acne treatments, proper counseling should be provided to patients and caregivers on using gentle facial cleansers and moisturizers to prevent severe irritation that could worsen hyperpigmentation in SOC.[43,45] Finally, photoprotection with broad-spectrum sunscreen is essential for acne-associated hyperpigmentation.[45] Chemical-based sunscreens that more easily blend into deeper skin tones may increase user satisfaction and adherence. Mineral-based sunscreens may be more suitable for those prone to skin irritation such as younger children or patients with AD.

Atopic Dermatitis

AD, also known as "eczema", is a chronic, relapsing condition characterized by inflamed scaly papules and plaques associated with itch,[67] dryness,[68] and even pain.[69] Affected areas can include the face, trunk, hands, feet, and flexural areas of the arms and legs.[70] AD is an immune-mediated disease frequently associated with other conditions such as allergic rhinitis and asthma, a phenomenon known as atopy.[70,71] AD typically begins in early childhood and can persist through adolescence.[70] The childhood prevalence of AD has increased in the United States[72] and worldwide.[73] In the United States, Black children are more commonly affected than White or Hispanic children.[74] Severe[75] and persistent[76] childhood disease has been associated with non-Hispanic Black race and Hispanic ethnicity. AD itch can lead to poor sleep patterns, daytime fatigue, inattention, and increased risk of anxiety and depression in affected children[77] and their caregivers,[78] and Black and Hispanic children are more likely to miss days of school due to AD.[79] Predisposing societal factors such as increased exposure to environmental triggers, poorer housing quality, and decreased access to health care have been proposed as potential causes for racial and ethnic differences in AD susceptibility and severity in the United States.[80]

Individuals with AD demonstrate strong helper T cell (T_H2) activation; however, immune polarization may vary with race and ethnicity.[81] Earlier studies have demonstrated that African-American patients with AD may have higher IgE serum levels and diminished T_H17 and T_H1 activation compared with European-American and Asian patients.[81,82] Asian patients may have stronger T_H17 and T_H22 activation.[83] Certain genetic defects in the epidermal barrier have been identified as predisposing risk factors for AD; however, most research has focused on loss-of-function mutation of filaggrin, which is an epidermal barrier protein that seems to play a less significant role in disease pathogenesis among African-Americans.[81] In fact, filaggrin mutations are approximately 6 times less likely in African-Americans versus European-Americans with AD.[84] Physical presentation may also differ by race or ethnicity. Papular or annular morphology is more common in African-American children and can be associated with significant itching without apparent redness or significant scaling.[85] Lichenification is also a common feature of AD in SOC.[83,85] Finally, individuals of East Asian descent with AD can present with lesions that have increased scale and demarcation that histologically and phenotypically overlap with psoriasis compared with those of European descent.[83] These characteristics may provide insight into effective targeted treatments[81,86]; however, interpretation should be made on an individualized basis.

Managing acute AD flares typically involves topical corticosteroids.[87] Corticosteroid-sparing topicals (ie, tacrolimus,[88] pimecrolimus,[89] crisaborole[90]) may be indicated for recurrent or prolonged flares. Diffuse or severe flares may necessitate phototherapy or systemic agents, such as dupilumab, oral Janus kinase (JAK) inhibitors, or methotrexate. Secondary bacterial infections commonly occur in pediatric patients and can be managed with antibiotics and dilute bleach baths.[70] Importantly, primary immunodeficiency syndromes should be considered in children with a high burden of bacterial or viral infections and severe recalcitrant atopic disease.[91] Finally, in addition to prescription therapy, emollients are crucial to reducing flare severity and frequency.[68,92] Fragrance-free moisturizing creams or ointments should be used at least once daily to repair the epidermal barrier.

Hidradenitis Suppurativa

Hidradenitis suppurativa (HS) is a chronic disorder in which abnormal follicular keratinization and occlusion induces inflammation within the pilosebaceous unit that leads to painful nodules, malodorous suppurative abscesses, extensive sinus tracts, and hypertrophic band-like scarring in intertriginous regions.[93] The prevalence of HS is increased among SOC populations, particularly among women of African descent.[93] Pediatric HS typically presents in older children or adolescents.[93] Three studies have demonstrated an association between early-onset pediatric HS and longer disease duration but none revealed an association between early-onset HS and objective disease severity.[94–96] Pediatric HS is closely associated with comorbidities such as acne, obesity, inflammatory bowel disease, and psychiatric conditions such as depression and anxiety.[94,97] Pediatric patients are more likely to have a strong family history of HS or underlying hormonal imbalance.[94] There is also an increased prevalence of HS in children and adolescents with Trisomy 21.[98] Genetic autoinflammatory syndromes should be considered in children with severe HS, nodulocystic acne, and systemic symptoms such as joint pain or recurrent fevers.[99,100]

Early diagnosis along with patient and caregiver education may be especially beneficial for pediatric patients with HS. Counseling should include reducing amendable risk factors such as obesity, cigarette smoking, and tight-fitting undergarments.[101,102] Treatment of mild-to-moderate disease includes topical BPO, topical antibiotics, oral antibiotics (tetracyclines in children aged older than 8 years), corticosteroids, and localized surgical procedures.[101] Some data support the use of oral antiandrogen therapy in female children and adolescents.[101,103,104] For severe disease, the use of biologics such as adalimumab or curative surgical excision may be required.[101]

Seborrheic Dermatitis

Seborrheic dermatitis is characterized by ill-defined plaques with scale predominantly involving the scalp, nasolabial folds, ears, glabellar regions, and occasionally intertriginous regions. It is often referred to as "cradle cap" when affecting the scalp of infants. In patients with SOC, seborrheic dermatitis may present as hypopigmented, hyperpigmented, or pink plaques with varying degrees of flaking.[105] Petaloid seborrheic dermatitis refers to a presentation with polycyclic or arcuate lesions and minimal scaling that has been observed in SOC patients.[106] Abnormal sebum production, *Malassezia furfur* colonization, and aberrant immune response all contribute to disease pathogenesis.[105] The condition often waxes and wanes, and often requires chronic therapy. For children with hair that is long, dense, or prone to dryness, scalp treatment regimens should take into account that daily shampooing may not be feasible. In such cases, a leave-in scalp treatment can be as equally effective as a medicated shampoo and is associated with increased user satisfaction and treatment compliance.[107] Olive oil use may worsen flares and should be discouraged.[108] Finally, tinea capitis (TC), a dermatophyte infection of the scalp, should be ruled out in children with scalp flaking that is accompanied by hair breakage, scalp erythema, or cervical lymphadenopathy.

Psoriasis

Psoriasis is a chronic disease of abnormal keratinocyte proliferation that presents as well-demarcated scaly papules and plaques. Different characteristics and variants are more common in children compared with adults.[109,110] Scalp, facial, and intertriginous involvement is more frequently seen in children and can occur concurrently with the extensor elbows and knees, hands and feet, trunk, and the umbilicus involvement seen in adults.[109,110] In infants, the waist and anogenital areas are commonly affected sites due to koebnerization of skin in contact with the diaper.[109,110] Infantile psoriatic plaques usually have less noticeable scale, and lesions in the diaper region typically have no scale.[109,110] Guttate psoriasis presents as smaller, drop-like, round plaques on the trunk and extremities, and has been associated with streptococcal infection (classically pharyngitis, occasionally anogenital) in children and adolescents.[109,111] A rarer variant that is possibly more common in children of color is follicular psoriasis, which presents as hyperkeratotic papules on the trunk and extremities that mimic pityriasis rubra pilaris.[112,113] Similar to adults, psoriatic nail findings such as onycholysis and pitting may also occur in isolation or in tandem with cutaneous lesions. Pediatric psoriasis has also been associated with comorbidities of obesity, hyperlipidemia, metabolic syndrome, insulin resistance, and inflammatory bowel disease.[109] Autoinflammatory syndromes should be considered in infants and children with severe early-onset psoriasis (particularly of the pustular variant), elevated serum inflammatory markers, fevers,[114] or failure to thrive.[100]

The incidence of psoriasis follows a bimodal distribution, first peaking in childhood and later in adulthood. Approximately 20% of adult patients report disease onset in childhood or adolescence.[110] Infantile psoriasis occurs less frequently.[109,110] Pediatric psoriatic arthritis is not uncommon and may have a female predominance.[115] Psoriasis is estimated to be less prevalent in SOC populations compared with Caucasians in all age groups[116,117]; however, SOC patients may present with more extensive and severe disease at the time of diagnosis.[117] The salmon-colored plaques seen in those with lighter skin tones may seem more dark brown or deep purple in those with deeper skin tones, and the micaceous scale more gray or white.[117] Psoriasis may also mimic other conditions such as cutaneous lupus, lichen planus, or sarcoidosis in deeply pigmented skin.[117] Additionally, dyspigmentation may be more prominent and persist for months after psoriatic lesions have resolved, which may be of great concern to patients and caregivers.

Diaper, facial, and intertriginous involvement may be managed with low-potency topical corticosteroids, and clear, detailed counseling to caregivers on appropriate use is important to prevent adverse side effects of skin atrophy.[115,118] Affected areas on the scalp, trunk, and extremities may benefit from mid-to-high-potency corticosteroids. Topical calcineurin inhibitors, vitamin D analogs, and/or topical retinoids can be utilized as corticosteroid-sparing therapy.[115] Phototherapy is a safe, effective, noninvasive treatment of pediatric patients with diffuse or recalcitrant disease[115] but it is important to counsel patients of color and their caregivers that psoriasis-related hyperpigmentation may transiently seem more prominent during treatment.[117] Severe cases can also be treated with systemics such as acitretin, cyclosporin, methotrexate,[117] or pediatric-approved biologics (etanercept, ixekizumab, secukinumab, ustekinumab).[119]

DISORDERS OF PIGMENTATION
Decreased or Absent Pigmentation

Pityriasis alba
Pityriasis alba presents as symmetric, mildly hypopigmented, oval, ill-defined, scaly macules and patches on the face, cheeks, upper trunk, neck, or shoulders, and is more common in children of color.[120] The lesions may be mildly pruritic and the condition is often associated with AD.[120,121] Multiple triggers have been identified including sun exposure, heat, and humidity.[122] The condition can spontaneously resolve without intervention or can be treated with gentle emollients or low-potency topical corticosteroids.

Vitiligo
Vitiligo is an acquired, progressive, autoimmune condition characterized by complete destruction and absence of melanocytes with lesions that are often symmetric and can involve the face, hands, knees, upper chest, and anogenital areas in children.[123] Other variants include generalized disease (affecting >50% of the body surface), segmental (affecting one side of the body and not crossing midline), and poliosis (affecting hair strands). It is often distinguished from other acquired hypopigmentation disorders (such as pityriasis alba discussed above) via Wood lamp examination that is notable for the complete lack of pigment.[120] Approximately 50% of patients have disease onset before 20 years of age.[123] Risk factors for vitiligo include genetic disposition and trauma.[123] Patients with vitiligo are at increased risk of other autoimmune conditions such as Grave disease, Hashimoto thyroiditis, diabetes mellitus type 1, and alopecia areata (AA).[124,125] A retrospective analysis of 922 pediatric patients with AA in the United States found that the prevalence of comorbid vitiligo was approximately 3.1%.[126] The prognosis of vitiligo is variable and there are multiple treatment options.[127] Treatment on the face and anogenital areas in pediatric patients may include daily application of topical tacrolimus 0.03% or 0.1% ointment, which has been demonstrated to promote repigmentation even in cases of facial segmental vitiligo.[128] Topical corticosteroids can be used for areas on the trunk and extremities. Phototherapies such as narrowband ultraviolet B (NBUVB) and excimer lasers are treatments for diffuse and localized disease, respectively. The topical JAK inhibitor ruxolitinib 1.5% cream is the first U.S. Food and Drug Administration (FDA)-approved treatment of nonsegmental vitiligo for children aged 12 years and older.[129]

Mixed

Postinflammatory pigmentation alteration
Among children of color, skin pigmentation alteration is often triggered by the common inflammatory skin conditions discussed above and can present as hypopigmentation or hyperpigmentation. Postinflammatory pigmentation alteration may persist for months to years. Stubborn hyperpigmentation can effectively be treated with hydroquinone, a tyrosinase inhibitor but safety data in the pediatric population has not been established. Additionally, it should be used with caution in children prone to skin irritation or those with AD because it may be a trigger for allergic contact dermatitis.[130] Nonhydroquinone agents include topical azelaic acid, kojic acid, tranexamic acid, licorice extract, niacinamide, and vitamin C[131,132] but require further research on efficacy and safety in children. Sunscreen, particularly tinted formulas with iron oxides, may help alleviate the appearance of hyperpigmentation.[132,133] Finally, ceramide-based sunscreens and moisturizers can provide UV protection and reduce hyperpigmentation, although the exact mechanism for the latter is not completely understood.[134]

Tinea versicolor
Tinea versicolor, also known as pityriasis versicolor, presents as hypopigmented, hyperpigmented, or pink plaques with fine scale on the neck, trunk, arms, and face[135] (Fig. 5). It occurs more frequently in adolescents than younger children.[135] It also predominantly occurs in warmer seasons and climates because the causal yeast organism Malassezia thrives in humid, lipophilic environments.[136] Diagnostic hallmarks of the condition include a "furfuraceous" scale that becomes more apparent with stretching the skin, and a "spaghetti and meatball" appearance of the Malassezia under potassium hydroxide (KOH) prep of scale scrapings.[136] Wood lamp examination may reveal yellowish white or coppery orange lesions.[137] Treatment includes topical therapy with selenium sulfide washes or azole creams for mild cases and systemic therapy with oral azoles for severe cases.[136] Caregivers of children of color should be counseled that pigmentary changes

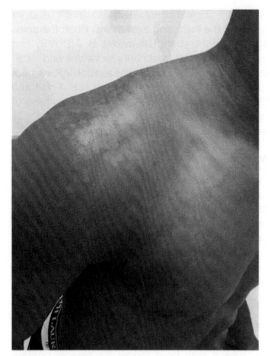

Fig. 5. Tinea versicolor.

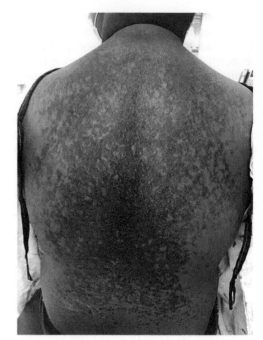

Fig. 6. Confluent and reticulated papillomatosis (CARP).

may persist for a longer duration even after treatment is complete.[136]

Increased Pigmentation

Acanthosis nigricans

Acanthosis nigricans presents as velvety, dark brown plaques on the posterior neck, axillae, flexor surfaces of the extremities, and face.[138] Pathophysiology of the disorder involves overactivation of insulin-like growth factors and tyrosine kinase receptors, which induce overstimulation of keratinocytes and fibroblasts.[139] Thus, acanthosis nigricans is often a marker of insulin resistance.[138] There are multiple disease variants, and in the United States, SOC patients are most commonly diagnosed with the obesity-related subtype.[140,141] Pediatric obesity and insulin resistance are common comorbidities, and baseline screening should be considered, particularly in children of color who are disproportionally affected.[138] Treatment may include ammonium lactate 12% lotion and topical retinoids to promote cell turnover, along with lifestyle modifications such as weight reduction.[138,142] Pediatric patients with diabetes may find that the lesions clinically improve after glycemic control is achieved with oral antidiabetic medications.[139]

Confluent and reticulated papillomatosis

Confluent and reticulated papillomatosis of Gougerot and Carteaud (CARP) consists of verrucous, hyperkeratotic pink to brown papules that may coalesce into a confluent or reticulated pattern with variable peripheral scaling on the chest, back, axillae, and neck[143] (**Fig. 6**). Black adolescents are more commonly affected with a female predominance.[143] Although the pathogenesis remains unknown, various hypotheses exist including abnormal keratinization, insulin resistance, hormonal imbalance, or an abnormal immune response to *Malassezia furfur* or *Cutibacterium acnes* proliferation.[143,144] Treatment with oral antibiotics (minocycline, doxycycline, amoxicillin, or azithromycin)[143,145] can be effective but recurrence is common.[143] Distinguishing CARP from tinea versicolor in children of color may represent a diagnostic challenge; however, negative KOH prep, poor response to antifungal therapy, and superior response to antibiotic therapy confirm the diagnosis.[146] CARP in children can be associated with acanthosis nigricans[143] as well as obesity and insulin resistance.[143,147] In children with moderate-to-severe disease, laboratory screening for insulin resistance should be considered and consists of serum glucose, hemoglobin A1c, and serum insulin, the latter being an earlier predictor for metabolic dysfunction.[147]

RASHES WITH SPECIAL CONSIDERATIONS

Some rashes may present less frequently but should still be considered in pediatric patients under certain circumstances. Pityriasis rosea (PR) is a self-limiting scaly rash. On patients with darker skin tones, PR may seem darker than the rest of the skin, have more conspicuous scaling, and lack the "rosey" appearance or apparent erythema.[148] Additionally, SOC patients are more likely to experience postinflammatory pigmentary changes. Papular PR is a less common form of PR more prevalent in children of African descent.[149] This presents like inverse PR, which occurs in typically spared areas such as the facial, axillary, and groin region.[149]

Childhood granulomatous periorificial dermatitis (CGPD), also called facial Afro-Caribbean childhood eruption, is a subtype of periorificial dermatitis seen in prepubertal SOC children.[150] It appears as micronodular reddish, yellow papules on the central face (Fig. 7). The exact cause of CGPD is unknown but it may be caused by topical or inhaled steroid use, allergens, or irritants.[151]

Finally, childhood-onset systemic lupus erythematosus (cSLE) may have an increased prevalence in Black children.[152] Compared with adult systemic lupus erythematosus (SLE), cSLE has increased morbidity, mortality, and disease severity.[153] Most patients with cSLE will have cutaneous features such as alopecia, Raynaud phenomenon, or oral ulcers.[153] SOC patients may be more likely to have discoid lesions that manifest as pink to purple scaly plaques with scarring and dyspigmentation.[153] Children with discoid lupus erythematosus are also at an increased risk of progression to systemic disease so signs of nephropathy and leukopenia should lead to further testing for SLE.[154]

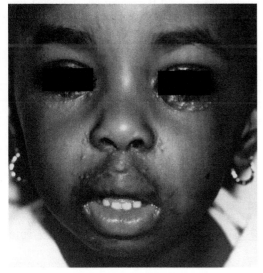

Fig. 7. Granulomatous periorificial dermatitis. (Courtesy of P Honig, MD, Philadelphia, PA.)

HAIR DISORDERS

Hair disorders can significantly affect the psychosocial well-being of pediatric patients due to societal perceptions and the role of hair in self-identity.[155] The most common type of hair loss is AA, which is characterized as a nonscarring autoimmune-mediated process.[156] The spectrum of AA can range from localized hair loss on the scalp, to complete scalp hair loss (alopecia totalis), to total body hair loss (alopecia universalis). More than 40% of patients developed their first patch of hair loss before the age of 20 years.[156] AA has also been shown to have an increased incidence and prevalence in self-identified Black children.[157]

Tinea capitis (TC) can have a similar presentation to AA and is the most common dermatophytosis of childhood.[158] The specific appearance of this condition depends on the degree of inflammation. Individuals affected can present with circular areas of scaling, patches of alopecia with broken hair fibers, or even inflammatory plaques and adjacent lymphadenopathy. African American children have been shown to have a higher incidence of TC.[158]

Scarring alopecias are types of irreversible hair loss as the hair follicle is permanently damaged. Central centrifugal cicatricial alopecia (CCCA) is a type of scarring alopecia that presents as hair loss in the center or the vertex of the scalp. It is typically reported in patients aged older than 30 years but this statistical may be due to delays in care-seeking until hair loss is most severe.[159] Few reports have noted this condition in the pediatric population.[160] However, early recognition of this condition can allow for timely diagnosis and treatment reducing disease progression and severity.

Finally, acquired trichorrhexis nodosa (ATN) is a type of hair loss that occurs in response to external forces on the hair. The affected hair follicle may seem brittle with the presence of spaced-out white nodes. Black patients may be disproportionately affected by ATN due to inherent structure differences in curly hair that increase susceptibility to breakage. Further, the use of hair care practices such as chemical and heat straightening by individuals with textured hair weakens the structure of the hair.[161] This condition should not be confused with traction alopecia (TA), which presents near the hairline due to chronic use of hairstyles or appliances that cause tension.[162] Patients with TA may present with white scales on the hair follicle or tenting of the hair follicle. Children often do not style their own hair so their parent/caregiver can help with the identification and management of hair disorders.[163]

CLINICS CARE POINTS

- Pediatric dermatologists should be familiar with the progression of birthmarks to know when further diagnosis and management are necessary.
- Proper identification of newborn rashes can help determine appropriate counseling and treatment interventions.
- In patients with darker skin tones, inflammatory dermatoses such as AD, psoriasis, and PR may seem hyperpigmented with more apparent scaling and less erythema.
- Pigmentary alterations should be addressed in disease counseling for caregivers and in treatment plan for patients.
- The parent/caregiver will be helpful in helping manage and identify hair disorders in children.

DECLARATION OF INTERESTS

No known competing financial interests or relationships.

FUNDING

Dr Leslie Castelo-Soccio, salary is supported by NIAMS, Intramural Research Program.

DISCLOSURE

The authors have nothing to disclose.

REFERENCES

1. Kanada KN, Merin MR, Munden A, et al. A prospective study of cutaneous findings in newborns in the United States: correlation with race, ethnicity, and gestational status using updated classification and nomenclature. J Pediatr 2012;161(2):240–5.
2. Taylor Robert B. The amazing language of medicine : understanding medical terms and their backstories. Springer; 2017. Available at: https://search.ebscohost.com/login.aspx?direct=true&AuthType=sso&db=edsebk&AN=1462100&site=eds-live&scope=site. Accessed July 3, 2022.
3. Jahnke MN, O'Haver J, Gupta D, et al. Care of Congenital Melanocytic Nevi in Newborns and Infants: Review and Management Recommendations. Pediatrics 2021;148(6). e2021051536.
4. Lalor L, Davies OMT, Basel D, et al. Café au lait spots: When and how to pursue their genetic origins. Clin Dermatol 2020;38(4):421–31.
5. Rodríguez Bandera AI, Sebaratnam DF, Wargon O, et al. Infantile hemangioma. Part 1: Epidemiology, pathogenesis, clinical presentation and assessment. J Am Acad Dermatol 2021;85(6):1379–92.
6. Cho S, Maharathi B, Ball KL, et al. Sturge-Weber Syndrome Patient Registry: Delayed Diagnosis and Poor Seizure Control. J Pediatr 2019;215:158–63.e6.
7. Zhai LL, Hsu S. Diagnosis of Transient Neonatal Pustular Melanosis. Skinmed 2020;18(6):372.
8. Reginatto FP, Muller FM, Peruzzo J, et al. Epidemiology and Predisposing Factors for Erythema Toxicum Neonatorum and Transient Neonatal Pustular: A Multicenter Study. Pediatr Dermatol 2017;34(4):422–6.
9. Merlob P, Metzker A, Reisner SH. Transient neonatal pustular melanosis. Am J Dis Child 1982;136(6):521–2. https://doi.org/10.1001/archpedi.1982.03970420045009.
10. Lucky AW. Transient benign cutaneous lesions in the newborn. Neonatal dermatology 2007;2:85–97.
11. O'Connor NR, McLaughlin MR, Ham P. Newborn skin: Part I. Common rashes. Am Fam Physician 2008;77(1):47–52.
12. Laude TA. Approach to dermatologic disorders in black children. Semin Dermatol 1995;14(1):15–20.
13. Reginatto FP, DeVilla D, Muller FM, et al. Prevalence and characterization of neonatal skin disorders in the first 72h of life. J Pediatr 2017;93(3):238–45.
14. Taieb A, Ezzedine K, Morice-Picard F. Diagnosis of some common and uncommon hyperpigmentation disorders in children. Dermatol Sin 2014;32(4):211–6.
15. Morgan AJ, Steen CJ, Schwartz RA, et al. Erythema toxicum neonatorum revisited. Cutis 2009;83(1):13–6.
16. Roques E, Ward R, Mendez MD. Erythema Toxicum. In: StatPearls [internet]. Treasure Island (FL): StatPearls Publishing; 2022.
17. Liu C, Feng J, Qu R, et al. Epidemiologic study of the predisposing factors in erythema toxicum neonatorum. Dermatology 2005;210(4):269–72.
18. Boccardi D, Menni S, Ferraroni M, et al. Birthmarks and transient skin lesions in newborns and their relationship to maternal factors: a preliminary report from northern Italy. Dermatology 2007;215(1):53–8.
19. Ferrándiz C, Coroleu W, Ribera M, et al. Sterile transient neonatal pustulosis is a precocious form of erythema toxicum neonatorum. Dermatology 1992;185(1):18–22.
20. Fujisawa Y, Miyazono Y, Kawachi Y, et al. A case of sterile transient neonatal pustulosis presenting with large flaccid pustules. Pediatr Dermatol 2013;30(6):e238–9.
21. Reginatto FP, Villa DD, Cestari TF. Benign skin disease with pustules in the newborn. An Bras Dermatol 2016;91(2):124–34.

22. Ayhan M, Sancak B, Karaduman A, et al. Colonization of neonate skin by Malassezia species: relationship with neonatal cephalic pustulosis. J Am Acad Dermatol 2007;57(6):1012–8.

23. Chadha A, Jahnke M. Common Neonatal Rashes. Pediatr Ann 2019;48(1):e16–22.

24. Neu N, Duchon J, Zachariah P. TORCH infections. Clin Perinatol 2015;42(1):77–103, viii.

25. Center for Disease Control and Prevention. Available at: https://www.cdc.gov/std/treatment-guidelines/congenital-syphilis.htm. Accessed September 2022.

26. Center for Disease Control and Prevention. Available at: https://www.cdc.gov/mmwr/preview/mmwrhtml/mm5027a1.htm. Accessed September 2022.

27. Herremans T, Kortbeek L, Notermans DW. A review of diagnostic tests for congenital syphilis in newborns. Eur J Clin Microbiol Infect Dis 2010;29(5): 495–501.

28. Wang EA, Chambers CJ, Silverstein M. A rare presentation of congenital syphilis: Pemphigus syphiliticus in a newborn infant with extensive desquamation of the extremities. Pediatr Dermatol 2018;35(2):e110–3.

29. Spaccarelli N, Wan J, Yan A, et al. Congenital syphilis as a clinical and histopathologic mimic of neonatal lupus. J Cutan Pathol 2018;45(10):791–3.

30. Lugo A, Sanchez S, Sanchez JL. Congenital syphilis. Pediatr Dermatol 2006;23(2):121–3.

31. Keuning MW, Kamp GA, Schonenberg-Meinema D, et al. Congenital syphilis, the great imitator-case report and review. Lancet Infect Dis 2020;20(7):e173–9.

32. Bennett ML, Lynn AW, Klein LE, et al. Congenital syphilis: subtle presentation of fulminant disease. J Am Acad Dermatol 1997;36(2 Pt 2):351–4.

33. Medoro AK, Sánchez PJ. Syphilis in Neonates and Infants. Clin Perinatol 2021;48(2):293–309.

34. O'Connor NP, Gonzalez BE, Esper FP, et al. Congenital syphilis: Missed opportunities and the case for rescreening during pregnancy and at delivery. IDCases 2020;22:e00964.

35. Rac MWF, Stafford IA, Eppes CS. Congenital syphilis: A contemporary update on an ancient disease. Prenat Diagn 2020;40(13):1703–14.

36. Rudnick CM, Hoekzema GS. Neonatal herpes simplex virus infections. Am Fam Physician 2002; 65(6):1138–42.

37. Tan JK, Bhate K. A global perspective on the epidemiology of acne. Br J Dermatol 2015; 172(Suppl 1):3–12.

38. Henderson MD, Abboud J, Cogan CM, et al. Skin-of-color epidemiology: a report of the most common skin conditions by race. Pediatr Dermatol 2012;29(5):584–9.

39. Alexis AF, Sergay AB, Taylor SC. Common dermatologic disorders in skin of color: a comparative practice survey. Cutis 2007;80(5):387–94.

40. Ho T, Taylor MT, Marathe KS, et al. Most common pediatric skin conditions managed in outpatient dermatology clinics in the United States stratified by race and ethnicity. Pediatr Dermatol 2021; 38(Suppl 2):129–31.

41. Kurokawa I, Danby FW, Ju Q, et al. New developments in our understanding of acne pathogenesis and treatment. Exp Dermatol 2009;18(10): 821–32.

42. Taylor SC, Cook-Bolden F, Rahman Z, et al. Acne vulgaris in skin of color. J Am Acad Dermatol 2002;46(2 Suppl Understanding):S98–106.

43. Callender VD, Baldwin H, Cook-Bolden FE, et al. Effects of Topical Retinoids on Acne and Post-inflammatory Hyperpigmentation in Patients with Skin of Color: A Clinical Review and Implications for Practice. Am J Clin Dermatol 2022;23(1):69–81.

44. Chiang C, Ward M, Gooderham M. Dermatology: how to manage acne in skin of colour. Drugs Context 2022;11:2110–9.

45. Yin NC, McMichael AJ. Acne in patients with skin of color: practical management. Am J Clin Dermatol 2014;15(1):7–16.

46. Czernielewski J, Poncet M, Mizzi F. Efficacy and cutaneous safety of adapalene in black patients versus white patients with acne vulgaris. Cutis 2002;70(4):243–8.

47. Jacyk WK. Adapalene in the treatment of African patients. J Eur Acad Dermatol Venereol 2001; 15(Suppl 3):37–42.

48. Bhatia ND, Werschler WP, Cook-Bolden FE, et al. Tolerability of tretinoin lotion 0.05% for moderate to severe acne vulgaris: a post hoc analysis in a black population. Cutis 2020;106(1):45–50.

49. Harper JC, Roberts WE, Zeichner JA, et al. Novel tretinoin 0.05% lotion for the once-daily treatment of moderate-to-severe acne vulgaris: assessment of safety and tolerability in subgroups. J Dermatolog Treat 2020;31(2):160–7.

50. Han G, Armstrong AW, Desai SR, et al. Novel Tretinoin 0.05% Lotion for the Once-Daily Treatment of Moderate-to-Severe Acne Vulgaris in an Asian Population. J Drugs Dermatol 2019;18(9):910–6.

51. Kircik LH. Efficacy and safety of azelaic acid (AzA) gel 15% in the treatment of post-inflammatory hyperpigmentation and acne: a 16-week, baseline-controlled study. J Drugs Dermatol 2011;10(6): 586–90.

52. Alexis AF, Johnson LA, Kerrouche N, et al. A subgroup analysis to evaluate the efficacy and safety of adapalene-benzoyl peroxide topical gel in black subjects with moderate acne. J Drugs Dermatol 2014;13(2):170–4.

53. Kwon HH, Park SY, Yoon JY, et al. Do tutorials on application method enhance adapalene-benzoyl peroxide combination gel tolerability in the treatment of acne? J Dermatol 2015;42(11):1058–65.

54. Eichenfield LF, Krakowski AC, Piggott C, et al, American Acne and Rosacea Society. Evidence-based recommendations for the diagnosis and treatment of pediatric acne. Pediatrics 2013; 131(Suppl 3):S163–86.

55. Callender VD, Young CM, Kindred C, et al. Efficacy and Safety of Clindamycin Phosphate 1.2% and Tretinoin 0.025% Gel for the Treatment of Acne and Acne-induced Post-inflammatory Hyperpigmentation in Patients with Skin of Color. J Clin Aesthet Dermatol 2012;5(7):25–32.

56. Eichenfield L, Hebert A, Desai SR, et al. The New Face of Preadolescent and Adolescent Acne: Beyond the Guidelines. Journal of family practice 2022;71(6):S63–70.

57. Halder RM, Holmes YC, S Bridgeman-Shah AMK. A clinical pathological study of acne vulgaris in black females. J Invest Dermatol 1996;106:888.

58. Barbieri JS, Shin DB, Wang S, et al. Association of Race/Ethnicity and Sex With Differences in Health Care Use and Treatment for Acne. JAMA Dermatol 2020;156(3):312–9.

59. Centers for Disease Control and Prevention. Research on doxycycline and tooth staining. Available at: https://www.cdc.gov/rmsf/doxycycline/index.html#. Accessed November 2022.

60. Osinubi AA, Lewis-de Los Angeles CP, Poitevien P, et al. Are Black Girls Exhibiting Puberty Earlier? Examining Implications of Race-Based Guidelines. Pediatrics 2022;150(2).

61. March C, Witchel S. Acne, Hirsutism, and Other Signs of Increased Androgens. In: Stanley T, Misra M, editors. Endocrine conditions in pediatrics. Cham: Springer; 2021. p. 85–94.

62. Cartwright M, Mazzetti A, Moro L. Clascoterone Topical Cream, 1%, A Novel, Local, Selective Androgen Receptor Inhibitor: Results in Pediatric Subjects with Acne Vulgaris: Section on Advances in Therapeutics and Technology Program. Pediatrics 2020;146(1_MeetingAbstract):594–5.

63. Arowojolu AO, Gallo MF, Lopez LM, et al. Combined oral contraceptive pills for treatment of acne. Cochrane Database Syst Rev 2012;(7): CD004425.

64. Roberts EE, Nowsheen S, Davis DMR, et al. Use of spironolactone to treat acne in adolescent females. Pediatr Dermatol 2021;38(1):72–6.

65. Onwudiwe O, Callender VD. Pomade acne. InAcneiform eruptions in dermatology. New York, NY: Springer; 2014. p. 155–9.

66. Talakoub L, Wesley N. Smooth hair—an acne-causing epidemic. Dermatology News 2016;19:19.

67. Murota H, Katayama I. Exacerbating factors of itch in atopic dermatitis. Allergol Int 2017;66(1):8–13.

68. Szczepanowska J, Reich A, Szepietowski JC. Emollients improve treatment results with topical corticosteroids in childhood atopic dermatitis: a randomized comparative study. Pediatr Allergy Immunol 2008;19(7):614–8.

69. Cheng BT, Paller AS, Griffith JW, et al. Burden and characteristics of skin pain among children with atopic dermatitis. J Allergy Clin Immunol Pract 2022;10(4):1104–6.e1.

70. Ständer S. Atopic Dermatitis. N Engl J Med 2021; 384(12):1136–43.

71. Justiz Vaillant AA, Modi P, Jan A. Atopy. Treasure Island (FL): StatPearls Publishing; 2022 [Updated 2022 Jul 8]. In: StatPearls [Internet].

72. McKenzie C, Silverberg JI. The prevalence and persistence of atopic dermatitis in urban United States children. Ann Allergy Asthma Immunol 2019;123(2):173–8.e1.

73. Asher MI, Montefort S, Björkstén B, et al, ISAAC Phase Three Study Group. Worldwide time trends in the prevalence of symptoms of asthma, allergic rhinoconjunctivitis, and eczema in childhood: ISAAC Phases One and Three repeat multicountry cross-sectional surveys. Lancet 2006;368(9537): 733–43 [Erratum in: Lancet. 2007 Sep 29; 370(9593):1128].

74. Centers for Disease Control and Prevention. Percentage (and standard error) of children aged 0–17 with eczema or skin allergy, by selected demographics: United States. 2014. Available at: https://www.cdc.gov/nchs/data/health_policy/eczema_skin_problems_tables.pdf. Accessed September 2022.

75. Silverberg JI, Simpson EL. Associations of childhood eczema severity: a US population-based study. Dermatitis 2014;25(3):107–14.

76. Kim Y, Blomberg M, Rifas-Shiman SL, et al. Racial/Ethnic Differences in Incidence and Persistence of Childhood Atopic Dermatitis. J Invest Dermatol 2019;139(4):827–34.

77. Fishbein AB, Cheng BT, Tilley CC, et al. Sleep Disturbance in School-Aged Children with Atopic Dermatitis: Prevalence and Severity in a Cross-Sectional Sample. J Allergy Clin Immunol Pract 2021;9(8):3120–9.e3.

78. Su W, Chen H, Gao Y, et al. Anxiety, depression and associated factors among caretakers of children with atopic dermatitis. Ann Gen Psychiatry 2022;21(1):12.

79. Wan J, Margolis DJ, Mitra N, et al. Racial and Ethnic Differences in Atopic Dermatitis-Related School Absences Among US Children. JAMA Dermatol 2019;155(8):973–5.

80. Martinez A, de la Rosa R, Mujahid M, et al. Structural racism and its pathways to asthma and atopic

dermatitis. J Allergy Clin Immunol 2021;148(5): 1112–20.

81. Brunner PM, Guttman-Yassky E. Racial differences in atopic dermatitis. Ann Allergy Asthma Immunol 2019;122(5):449–55.

82. Sanyal RD, Pavel AB, Glickman J, et al. Atopic dermatitis in African American patients is TH2/TH22-skewed with TH1/TH17 attenuation. Ann Allergy Asthma Immunol 2019;122(1):99–110.e6.

83. Noda S, Suárez-Fariñas M, Ungar B, et al. The Asian atopic dermatitis phenotype combines features of atopic dermatitis and psoriasis with increased TH17 polarization. J Allergy Clin Immunol 2015;136(5):1254–64.

84. Margolis DJ, Apter AJ, Gupta J, et al. The persistence of atopic dermatitis and filaggrin (FLG) mutations in a US longitudinal cohort. J Allergy Clin Immunol 2012;130(4):912–7.

85. Vachiramon V, Tey HL, Thompson AE, et al. Atopic dermatitis in African American children: addressing unmet needs of a common disease. Pediatr Dermatol 2012;29(4):395–402.

86. Nomura T, Wu J, Kabashima K, et al. Endophenotypic Variations of Atopic Dermatitis by Age, Race, and Ethnicity. J Allergy Clin Immunol Pract 2020;8(6):1840–52.

87. Lax SJ, Harvey J, Axon E, et al. Strategies for using topical corticosteroids in children and adults with eczema. Cochrane Database Syst Rev 2022;3(3): CD013356.

88. McCollum AD, Paik A, Eichenfield LF. The safety and efficacy of tacrolimus ointment in pediatric patients with atopic dermatitis. Pediatr Dermatol 2010;27(5):425–36.

89. Zuberbier T, Heinzerling L, Bieber T, et al. Steroid-sparing effect of pimecrolimus cream 1% in children with severe atopic dermatitis. Dermatology 2007;215(4):325–30.

90. Luger TA, Hebert AA, Zaenglein AL, et al. Subgroup Analysis of Crisaborole for Mild-to-Moderate Atopic Dermatitis in Children Aged 2 to < 18 Years. Paediatr Drugs 2022;24(2):175–83.

91. Pichard DC, Freeman AF, Cowen EW. Primary immunodeficiency update: Part I. Syndromes associated with eczematous dermatitis. J Am Acad Dermatol 2015;73(3):355–64.

92. Hlela C, Osei-Sekyere B, Senyah AY. Emollients-latest and greatest uses in atopic dermatitis. Current Allergy & Clinical Immunology 2022;35(2):2–5.

93. Alikhan A, Lynch PJ, Eisen DB. Hidradenitis suppurativa: a comprehensive review. J Am Acad Dermatol 2009;60(4):539–61 [quiz 562-3].

94. Deckers IE, van der Zee HH, Boer J, et al. Correlation of early-onset hidradenitis suppurativa with stronger genetic susceptibility and more widespread involvement. J Am Acad Dermatol 2015; 72(3):485–8.

95. Molina-Leyva A, Cuenca-Barrales C. Adolescent-Onset Hidradenitis Suppurativa: Prevalence, Risk Factors and Disease Features. Dermatology 2019;235(1):45–50.

96. Dessinioti C, Tzanetakou V, Zisimou C, et al. A retrospective study of the characteristics of patients with early-onset compared to adult-onset hidradenitis suppurativa. Int J Dermatol 2018;57(6): 687–91.

97. Hallock KK, Mizerak MR, Dempsey A, et al. Differences Between Children and Adults With Hidradenitis Suppurativa. JAMA Dermatol 2021;157(9): 1095–101.

98. Rork JF, McCormack L, Lal K, et al. Dermatologic conditions in Down syndrome: A single-center retrospective chart review. Pediatr Dermatol 2020; 37(5):811–6.

99. Vinkel C, Thomsen SF. Autoinflammatory syndromes associated with hidradenitis suppurativa and/or acne. Int J Dermatol 2017;56(8):811–8.

100. Murthy AS, Leslie K. Autoinflammatory Skin Disease: A Review of Concepts and Applications to General Dermatology. Dermatology 2016;232(5): 534–40.

101. Choi E, Ooi XT, Chandran NS. Hidradenitis suppurativa in pediatric patients. J Am Acad Dermatol 2022;86(1):140–7.

102. Loh TY, Hendricks AJ, Hsiao JL, et al. Undergarment and Fabric Selection in the Management of Hidradenitis Suppurativa. Dermatology 2021; 237(1):119–24.

103. Randhawa HK, Hamilton J, Pope E. Finasteride for the Treatment of Hidradenitis Suppurativa in Children and Adolescents. JAMA Dermatol 2013; 149(6):732–5.

104. Horissian M, Maczuga S, Barbieri JS, et al. Trends in the prescribing pattern of spironolactone for acne and hidradenitis suppurativa in adolescents. J Am Acad Dermatol 2022;87(3):684–6.

105. Elgash M, Dlova N, Ogunleye T, et al. Seborrheic Dermatitis in Skin of Color: Clinical Considerations. J Drugs Dermatol 2019;18(1):24–7.

106. Friedmann DP, Mishra V, Batty T. Progressive Facial Papules in an African-American Patient: An Atypical Presentation of Seborrheic Dermatitis. J Clin Aesthet Dermatol 2018;11(7):44–5. Epub 2018 Jul 1.

107. Chappell J, Mattox A, Simonetta C, et al. Seborrheic dermatitis of the scalp in populations practicing less frequent hair washing: ketoconazole 2% foam versus ketoconazole 2% shampoo. Three-year data. J Am Acad Dermatol 2014;70(5). AB.

108. Siegfried E, Glenn E. Use of Olive Oil for the Treatment of Seborrheic Dermatitis in Children. Arch Pediatr Adolesc Med 2012;166(10):967.

109. Eichenfield LF, Paller AS, Tom WL, et al. Pediatric psoriasis: Evolving perspectives. Pediatr Dermatol 2018;35(2):170–81.

110. Morris A, Rogers M, Fischer G, et al. Childhood psoriasis: a clinical review of 1262 cases. Pediatr Dermatol 2001;18(3):188–98.

111. Abuaf OK, Dogan B. Management of guttate psoriasis in patients with associated streptococcal infection. J Med Dove Press 2012;2:89–94.

112. Sathishkumar D, George R, Daniel D, et al. Clinical profile of childhood-onset psoriasis and prevalence of HLA-Cw6: a hospital-based study from India. Postgrad Med J 2015;91(1076):309–14.

113. Nguyen CV, Farah RS, Maguiness SM, et al. Follicular Psoriasis: Differentiation from Pityriasis Rubra Pilaris—An Illustrative Case and Review of the Literature. Pediatr Dermatol 2017;34(1):e65–8.

114. Santiago F, Torrelo A. Pustular Eruptions in Children as Manifestations of Autoinflammatory Diseases. Journal of the Portuguese Society of Dermatology and Venereology 2019;77(2):145–52.

115. Lewkowicz D, Gottlieb AB. Pediatric psoriasis and psoriatic arthritis. Dermatol Ther 2004;17(5):364–75.

116. Wu JJ, Black MH, Smith N, et al. Low prevalence of psoriasis among children and adolescents in a large multiethnic cohort in southern California. J Am Acad Dermatol 2011;65(5):957–64.

117. Alexis AF, Blackcloud P. Psoriasis in skin of color: epidemiology, genetics, clinical presentation, and treatment nuances. J Clin Aesthet Dermatol 2014;7(11):16–24.

118. Janniger CK, Schwartz RA, Musumeci ML, et al. Infantile psoriasis. Cutis 2005;76(3):173–7.

119. Sun HY, Phan K, Paller AS, et al. Biologics for pediatric psoriasis: A systematic review and meta-analysis. Pediatr Dermatol 2022;39(1):42–8.

120. Miazek N, Michalek I, Pawlowska-Kisiel M, et al. Pityriasis Alba—Common Disease, Enigmatic Entity: Up-to-Date Review of the Literature. Pediatr Dermatol 2015;32(6):786–91.

121. Gawai SR, Asokan N, Narayanan B. Association of Pityriasis Alba with Atopic Dermatitis: A Cross-Sectional Study. Indian J Dermatol 2021;66(5):567–8.

122. Lv Y, Gao Y, Lan N, et al. Analysis of Epidemic Characteristics and Related Pathogenic Factors of 2726 Cases of Pityriasis Alba. Clin Cosmet Investig Dermatol 2022;15:203–9.

123. Nicolaidou E, Mastraftsi S, Tzanetakou V, et al. Childhood Vitiligo. Am J Clin Dermatol 2019;20(4):515–26.

124. Lee H, Lee MH, Lee DY, et al. Prevalence of vitiligo and associated comorbidities in Korea. Yonsei Med J 2015;56(3):719–25.

125. Taïeb A, Seneschal J, Mazereeuw-Hautier J. Special Considerations in Children with Vitiligo. Dermatol Clin 2017;35(2):229–33.

126. Sorrell J, Petukhova L, Reingold R, et al. Shedding Light on Alopecia Areata in Pediatrics: A Retrospective Analysis of Comorbidities in Children in the National Alopecia Areata Registry. Pediatr Dermatol 2017;34(5):e271–2.

127. de Menezes AF, Oliveira de Carvalho F, Barreto RS, et al. Pharmacologic Treatment of Vitiligo in Children and Adolescents: A Systematic Review. Pediatr Dermatol 2017;34(1):13–24.

128. Silverberg NB, Lin P, Travis L, et al. Tacrolimus ointment promotes repigmentation of vitiligo in children: a review of 57 cases. J Am Acad Dermatol 2004;51(5):760–6.

129. Sheikh A, Rafique W, Owais R, et al. FDA approves ruxolitinib (Opzelura) for vitiligo therapy: a breakthrough in the field of dermatology. Annals of Medicine and Surgery 2022;81:104499.

130. Seidenari S, Giusti F, Pepe P, et al. Contact sensitization in 1094 children undergoing patch testing over a 7-year period. Pediatr Dermatol 2005;22(1):1–5.

131. Hollinger JC, Angra K, Halder RM. Are Natural Ingredients Effective in the Management of Hyperpigmentation? A Systematic Review. J Clin Aesthet Dermatol 2018;11(2):28–37.

132. Moolla S, Miller-Monthrope Y. Dermatology: how to manage facial hyperpigmentation in skin of colour. Drugs Context 2022;11.

133. Fatima S, Braunberger T, Mohammad TF, et al. The Role of Sunscreen in Melasma and Postinflammatory Hyperpigmentation. Indian J Dermatol 2020;65(1):5–10.

134. Dumbuya H, Yan X, Chen Y, et al. Efficacy of Ceramide-Containing Formulations on UV-Induced Skin Surface Barrier Alterations. J Drugs Dermatol JDD 2021;20(4):s29–35.

135. Terragni L, Lasagni A, Oriani A, et al. Pityriasis versicolor in the pediatric age. Pediatr Dermatol 1991;8(1):9–12.

136. Renati S, Cukras A, Bigby M. Pityriasis versicolor. BMJ 2015;350:h1394.

137. Ponka D, Baddar F. Wood lamp examination. Can Fam Physician 2012;58(9):976.

138. Sinha S, Schwartz RA. Juvenile acanthosis nigricans. J Am Acad Dermatol 2007;57(3):502–8.

139. Hermanns-Lê T, Scheen A, Piérard GE. Acanthosis nigricans associated with insulin resistance : pathophysiology and management. Am J Clin Dermatol 2004;5(3):199–203.

140. Novotny R, Li F, Fialkowski MK, et al. Prevalence of obesity and acanthosis nigricans among young children in the children's healthy living program in the United States Affiliated Pacific. Medicine (Baltim) 2016;95(37):e4711.

141. Novotny R, Davis J, Butel J, et al. Effect of the Children's Healthy Living Program on Young Child Overweight, Obesity, and Acanthosis Nigricans in the US-Affiliated Pacific Region: A Randomized Clinical Trial. JAMA Netw Open 2018;1(6):e183896.

142. Schwartz RA. Efficacy of topical 0.1% adapalene gel for use in the treatment of childhood acanthosis nigricans: a pilot study. Dermatol Ther 2015;28(4):266.

143. Xiao TL, Duan GY, Stein SL. Retrospective review of confluent and reticulated papillomatosis in pediatric patients. Pediatr Dermatol 2021;38(5):1202–9.

144. Basu P, Cohen PR. Confluent and Reticulated Papillomatosis Associated with Polycystic Ovarian Syndrome. Cureus 2019;11(1):e3956.

145. Mufti A, Sachdeva M, Maliyar K, et al. Treatment outcomes in confluent and reticulated papillomatosis: A systematic review. J Am Acad Dermatol 2021;84(3):825–9.

146. Davis MD, Weenig RH, Camilleri MJ. Confluent and reticulate papillomatosis (Gougerot-Carteaud syndrome): a minocycline-responsive dermatosis without evidence for yeast in pathogenesis. A study of 39 patients and a proposal of diagnostic criteria. Br J Dermatol 2006;154(2):287–93.

147. McKenzie PL, Ogwumike E, Agim NG. Confluent and reticulated papillomatosis in pediatric patients at an urban tertiary care center. Pediatr Dermatol 2022;39(4):574–7.

148. Amer A, Fischer H, Li X. The Natural History of Pityriasis Rosea in Black American Children: How Correct Is the "Classic" Description? Arch Pediatr Adolesc Med 2007;161(5):503–6.

149. Bernardin RM, Ritter SE, Murchland MR. Papular pityriasis rosea. Cutis 2002;70(1):48–51.

150. Lee GL, Zirwas MJ. Granulomatous Rosacea and Periorificial Dermatitis: Controversies and Review of Management and Treatment. Dermatol Clin 2015;33(3):447–55.

151. Kim YJ, Shin JW, Lee JS, et al. Childhood granulomatous periorificial dermatitis. Ann Dermatol 2011;23(3):386–8.

152. Pineles D, Valente A, Warren B, et al. Worldwide incidence and prevalence of pediatric onset systemic lupus erythematosus. Lupus 2011;20(11):1187–92.

153. Ophelia E. Dadzie, Antoine Petit, Andrew F. Alexis. Ethnic Dermatology Principles and practice. Wiley-Blackwell; 2013. Available at: https://search.ebscohost.com/login.aspx?direct=true&AuthType=sso&db=edsebk&AN=531400&site=eds-live&scope=site. Accessed July 3, 2022.

154. Hawat T, Ballouz S, Megarbane H, et al. Pediatric discoid lupus erythematosus: Short report. Dermatol Ther 2022;35(1):e15170.

155. Christensen T, Yang JS, Castelo-Soccio L. Bullying and Quality of Life in Pediatric Alopecia Areata. Skin Appendage Disord 2017;3(3):115–8.

156. Alkhalifah A, Alsantali A, Wang E, et al. Alopecia areata update: part I. Clinical picture, histopathology, and pathogenesis. J Am Acad Dermatol 2010;62(2):177–90.

157. Lee H, Jung SJ, Patel AB, et al. Racial characteristics of alopecia areata in the United States. J Am Acad Dermatol 2020;83(4):1064–70.

158. Mirmirani P, Tucker LY. Epidemiologic trends in pediatric tinea capitis: a population-based study from Kaiser Permanente Northern California. J Am Acad Dermatol 2013;69(6):916–21.

159. Whiting DA, Olsen EA. Central centrifugal cicatricial alopecia. Dermatol Ther 2008;21(4):268–78.

160. Eginli AN, Dlova NC, McMichael A. Central Centrifugal Cicatricial Alopecia in Children: A Case Series and Review of the Literature. Pediatr Dermatol 2017;34(2):133–7.

161. Haskin A, Kwatra SG, Aguh C. Breaking the cycle of hair breakage: pearls for the management of acquired trichorrhexis nodosa. J Dermatolog Treat 2017;28(4):322–6.

162. Khumalo NP, Jessop S, Gumedze F, et al. Determinants of marginal traction alopecia in African girls and women. J Am Acad Dermatol 2008;59(3):432–8.

163. Hollins LC, Butt M, Hong J, et al. Research in Brief: Survey of hair care practices in various ethnic and racial pediatric populations. Pediatr Dermatol 2022. https://doi.org/10.1111/pde.14958. published online ahead of print, 2022 Mar 3.

Keloids and Hypertrophic Scars

Ariel Knowles, MBBS[a], Donald A. Glass II, MD, PhD[a,b],*

KEYWORDS

• Keloids • Hypertrophic scar • Scarring • Fibroblast • Treatment

KEY POINTS

• Keloids are a fibroproliferative inflammatory disorder of the skin where scars grow excessively past the original borders of the inciting agent and invade into normal adjacent tissue.
• At the molecular/genetic level, an autosomal dominant mode of inheritance, a mutation in the protein N-acylsphingosine amidohydrolase 1, single-nucleotide polymorphisms in noncoding regions of the genome, and upregulation of critical fibroproliferative genes have all been linked to patients with keloids.
• Treatment of keloids can be aimed at flattening already formed keloids or at preventing the formation of keloids after trauma/surgery. A postsurgical treatment regimen is necessary to minimize the risk of recurrence after keloid excision.
• More basic/translational research as well as published case-control studies are needed.

INTRODUCTION

Keloids are an exaggerated fibroproliferative response to cutaneous wound healing in which scar tissue grows excessively and invasively beyond the original wound borders. They were first described as early as 3000 BC in the Edwin Smith Papyrus, the first known descriptions of ancient Egyptian medical practice. In the early nineteenth century, the French Dermatologist Jean Louis Alibert termed these scar keloids based on the Greek word for crabs claw "*cheloide*" or "*keloide*," referencing the claw-like extension of the scar beyond the initial wound margins into the surrounding skin.[1] Keloids are raised, firm, fibrotic scars that can develop up to 1 year after injury to the skin, sometimes even beyond 1 year, and they do not tend to regress spontaneously. This contrasts with hypertrophic scars that tend to form within the first few months after injury, stay within the margins of the original wound and may regress spontaneously.[2] The general pathomechanisms that drive fibrotic scars and the biological differences between the formation of keloids and hypertrophic scars are poorly understood, in part due to the lack of suitable animal models to study.[3] Humans are the only species known to develop keloids.

Epidemiology

Race/ethnicity, genetic predisposition, and age may all contribute to keloid predilection. Keloid incidence rates vary greatly between different racial groups.[4] Studies of keloid incidence in the general population report a varying incidence from 4.5 to 6.2 up to 16% in those of African descent while the incidence in the Taiwanese Chinese and Caucasians is reported to be as low as less than 1%.[1] The relative paucity of keloid incidence data in older publications has led some to question the notion of an increased prevalence of keloids in people of color.[5] However, recent studies in head and neck surgical patients and women after caesarian sections show the incidence of keloid scar formation was significantly increased in African Americans (0.8% and 7.1%, respectively) compared with the Caucasian (0.1% and 0.5%, respectively) and Asian

[a] Department of Dermatology, University of Texas Southwestern Medical Center, 5323 Harry Hines Boulevard, Dallas, TX 75390-9069, USA; [b] Eugene McDermott Center for Human Growth and Development, University of Texas Southwestern Medical Center, 5323 Harry Hines Boulevard, Dallas, TX 75390, USA
* Corresponding author. 5323 Harry Hines Boulevard, Mail Code 9069, Dallas, TX 75390, USA.
E-mail address: donald.glass@utsouthwestern.edu

Dermatol Clin 41 (2023) 509–517
https://doi.org/10.1016/j.det.2023.02.010

derm.theclinics.com

populations (0.2% and 5.2%, respectively).[6,7] Despite observed differences in keloid incidence, increased skin pigmentation cannot solely explain the reported racial/ethnic differences in incidence rate. In a study of keloids in Africans with albinism, the prevalence rate of 7.5% was not statistically different from the overall prevalence rate of 8.3% in the general population or the 8.5% observed in the normally pigmented African population.[8,9] In general, it is thought that no gender differences exist in keloid incidence, although some studies report that keloids are more likely to occur in women than men.[10] Although keloids can develop at any age, the incidence is highest between the ages of 10 to 30 years.[6,10,11] A peak in incidence after puberty, exacerbations of keloids during pregnancy, and decreased occurrences postmenopause indicate an endocrinological mechanism underlying keloid pathogenesis.[12]

Comorbidities

Keloids are recognized as an inflammatory skin disorder but evidence supports that the inflammation is not purely cutaneous because keloids are associated with several other medical conditions.[13] Keloids have been associated with hypertension, obesity, atopy, and osteoporosis. Studies show an association between hypertension and keloid formation with hypertension and keloid size and number having a statistically significant positive correlation.[14] Furthermore, individuals aged younger than 30 years with keloids have a higher incidence of hypertension.[15] Evidence suggests that obesity may play a role in the presence of keloids occurring on the ears. A significant difference in obesity prevalence was seen between patients with ear-inclusive versus ear-exclusive keloids.[16] Patients with atopic dermatitis have a higher-than-normal risk of developing keloids; and the coexistence of other allergic diseases further increases the risk.[17,18] There are conflicting reports about an association between keloids and uterine fibroids.[19,20] Keloids and osteoporosis may share a similar pathogenesis through chronic inflammation. Osteoporosis risk is higher in patients with keloids compared with controls, especially in young subjects and subjects without comorbidities.[13] These findings suggest that keloids may be thought of as a cutaneous manifestation of systemic inflammation.

Pathophysiology/Genetics

The mechanisms behind keloid scarring are poorly understood and contribute to our inability to satisfactorily manage this abnormal scarring process.

Genetics—A genetic predisposition for keloid formation is the most relevant patient related factor in the development of keloids. Work in Asian and African-American populations have identified single-nucleotide polymorphisms (SNPs) associated with keloid formation.[21–23] Additional studies have begun to unravel how these SNPs are associated with keloid formation.[24] Having a family member with keloids is associated with increased keloid prevalence.[9–11] Most evidence points to an autosomal dominant pattern of inheritance with incomplete penetration and variable expression. So far, there is one gene that has been identified in a family with multiple generations affected by keloids. A rare variant in the N-acylsphingosine amidohydrolase 1, or ASAH1, segregates within the family. ASAH1 is known to catalyze the degradation of ceramide into sphingosine and free fatty acid but its role in keloid pathogenesis remains unclear.[25] In addition to inherited gene mutations, epigenetic modifications may also play a role in keloid pathogenesis.[12]

Transforming growth factor beta 1—Transforming growth factor beta 1 (TGFβ1) is a secreted cytokine involved in proliferation, differentiation, migration, and apoptosis; it binds to its receptor and signal downstream through small/mothers against decapentaplegic homolog genes (SMADs), which function as intracellular mediators. Overproduction of TGFβ1, which occurs in keloids, has been associated with excessive deposition of scar tissue and fibrosis in the skin as well as in other organs. In contrast, TGFβ3 is present in high levels in embryonic skin—embryonic cutaneous wounds heal without scarring.[26]

Hypoxia—Keloids histologically have large number of microvessels. Partial or total occlusion of these microvessels may contribute to a hypoxic microenvironment. This hypoxia is thought to lead to the upregulation of genes (such as Hypoxia Inducible Factor 1 Subunit Alpha [HIF1A]) and signals that lead to proliferation and fibrosis.

Mechanical stress: Tension and strain on wound edges are important extrinsic factors linked to hypertrophic scar and keloid development. Increased mechanical tension may lead to changes in gene expression within fibroblasts.[27]

Hormones are thought to play a role because there is a higher incidence and tendency for keloids to enlarge after puberty and during pregnancy. Furthermore, tamoxifen is able to downregulate TGFβ1 expression in keloid fibroblasts in vitro.[28] Immunologically, there are increased number of macrophages, mast cells, and epidermal Langerhans cells present. T-lymphocytes and dendritic cells are found in keloids and hypertrophic scars, with evidence of Th2,

Th1, Th17/Th22, and JAK3 signaling in keloidal tissue.[29]

Patient Evaluation and Clinical Findings

When evaluating a patient with keloids, a thorough history should be obtained from the patient. **Box 1** lists pertinent questions applicable to patients with keloids. Baseline photographs of the affected area(s) are important to evaluate the patient's condition at subsequent follow-up visits. Keloid patients will usually present with a history of local trauma or inflammation with subsequent development of a scar extending beyond the original boundary of the wound. The existence of "spontaneous keloids"—keloids that occur without any preceding trauma or inflammation—remains debated. The chest, shoulders, and back are the sites most likely to form keloids per trauma incurred, whereas the ears are the most common site for keloids to be observed. It is extremely rare to find keloids on the hands or feet, or on oral mucosa. Topographic factors that may influence keloid formation in genetically predisposed individuals include areas of increased skin tension during normal movement,[30,31] increased sebaceous glands,[32,33] increased collagen, and decreased macrophage numbers.[34] Keloids can be described as either superficial-spreading (flat) keloids or bulging (raised) keloids.[1] Superficial spreading keloids show irregular subepidermal spread with irregular areas of hyperpigmentation

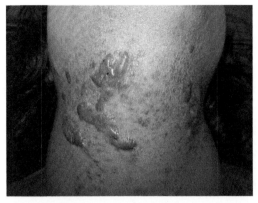

Fig. 1. Superficial spreading keloids on the submental region and neck.

and hypopigmentation (**Fig. 1**).[1] These lesions are often raised at the edges while the central aspect of the keloid is flattened and may represent a quiescent area. The central area may reflect the pigmentation of the surrounding skin, whereas the margins show hyperpigmentation and/or erythema. Bulging keloids are more pendulous or bulbous in shape and may have limited areas of central quiescence (**Fig. 2**). The growth pattern and the resulting shape may be predominately determined by local mechanical factors.[35]

Keloids can be both painful and pruritic. Studies investigating the effect of keloids on patients' quality of life have noted keloids with itch in 66.7% to 95.0% of patients. Keloids were associated with pain in 46% to 53.3% of patients.[36–38] Keloids can also be very sensitive to touch/pressure, making the wearing of a seat belt difficult for patients with chest keloids. Keloids/hypertrophic scars have been shown to affect patients' quality of life as significantly as psoriasis does.[39]

Diagnosis Approach and Differential Diagnosis

Keloid scarring is primarily a clinical diagnosis. Keloids and hypertrophic scars can often be diagnosed by visual inspection and/or palpation. The first step in the Japan Scar Workshop diagnostic algorithm for keloids, hypertrophic scars, or mature scars is to determine which of the scars the lesion is likely to be.[3] Benign skin tumors that resemble keloids and hypertrophic scars include dermatofibromas, neurofibromas and leiomyomas. Sinus histiocytosis with massive lymphadenopathy (Rosai-Dorfman syndrome) may also appear with keloidal-like plaques. Some malignant tumors, such as dermatofibrosarcoma protuberans (DFSP), may present with similar clinical

---

Box 1
Important questions to obtain when evaluating keloids/for keloid susceptibility

When did you first notice your keloid(s)?

Have you experienced itching, pain, burning in your scars?

Does pressure on your scars (eg, seatbelt over the chest) bother your scars?

Is there a family history of similar scars?

What treatment options have you previously tried for your keloids? Did they work at all? Did they work but then the keloids came back after treatments were stopped?

Do you have any of the following medical conditions?

  Hypertension

  Uterine fibroids

  Atherosclerosis

  Atopic Dermatitis

  Osteoporosis

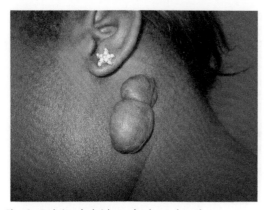

Fig. 2. Bulging keloid on the lateral neck.

features as keloids. Palpation around an atypical appearing keloid revealing focal areas of induration is suspicious for a DFSP and warrants a biopsy for further evaluation. If the patient endorses rapid growth of the lesion, a malignant tumor should be suspected.

Histopathological investigation can differentiate keloids from hypertrophic scars. In both keloids and hypertrophic scars, the epidermis and the papillary dermis can seem normal in structure. Hypertrophic scars are characterized by well-organized, wavy collagen bundles oriented parallel to epidermis surface. In contrast, keloids are characterized by disorganized, large, thick, hyalinized collagen bundles, with poor vascularization and widely scattered small dilated blood vessels.[3,40] Dermoscopy of keloids and hypertrophic scars reveals vascular structures more commonly in keloids than in hypertrophic scars (90% and 27%, respectively). The dermoscopic identification of vascular structures (arborizing, linear irregular or comma-shaped can be a clinically useful tool to differentiate keloids from hypertrophic scars.[41]

Treatment

Prevention is better than cure. Patients with personal history (or family history) are discouraged from piercings, branding, or unnecessary surgeries. It is highly encouraged to pierce earlobes before puberty due to the hormonal contribution to keloid pathogenesis.[42] Tattoos are also discouraged but seem less likely to induce keloids than the other aforementioned procedures. Surgical excision is the most definitive treatment option. However, surgery alone has a high recurrence rate (45%–100%), with the keloid often returning larger than the original scar.[43] Recurrences are also more likely to recur within the first 6 months after the surgical procedure. Therefore, a postsurgical treatment regimen started soon after surgery is necessary to decrease the likelihood for recurrence. These regimens are performed for at least 6 months, if not 1 full year, to minimize the recurrence risk.

Radiation therapy is often used in combination with surgical excision, especially if the keloid being excised is recurrent. Given within 72 hours of excision; 9 Gy to 16 Gy in 2 to 4 different fractions Recurrence rates after excision with adjuvant radiation therapy range from 0% to 8.6%. Mechanism of action is not well known. The main side effects are dyspigmentation, dermatitis, and telangiectasias (**Fig. 3**).[44] A systematic review of 33 studies using radiation therapy (external beam or brachytherapy) as adjuvant

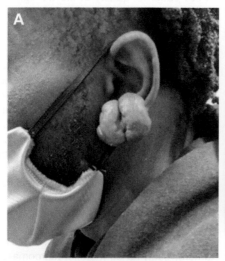
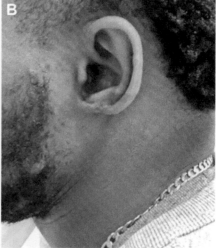

Fig. 3. Keloid before (*A*) and after (*B*) surgery with postoperative radiation therapy.

therapy postexcision of keloids found that the lowest recurrence rates were seen with high-dose radiation brachytherapy, then low-dose radiation brachytherapy and external beam radiation (10.5% vs 21.3% vs 22.2%, respectively). A shorter time interval (<7 hours) between excision and radiation resulted in lower recurrence (compared with >24 hours).[45]

Silicone sheets are Food and Drug Administration (FDA)-approved for the treatment of keloids and hypertrophic scars. They are more effective in the postsurgical setting or on new hypertrophic scars and have minimal efficacy in treating already formed keloids.[46,47] Silicone sheets should be worn over the surgical scar for 8 to 24 h/d for several months. Although the mechanism of action is unclear, it is thought to be secondary to occlusion and hydration.

Intralesional corticosteroids are FDA-approved for the treatment of keloids: they decrease collagen production, increase collagenase expression, and decrease inflammation (Fig. 4). Triamcinolone acetonide (10–40 mg/mL) injections are done every 4 to 6 weeks to treat formed keloids, with a maximum recommended dosage per visit is 80 mg. Response rates: 50% to 100%, with recurrence rates of 9% to 50%.[44] Side effects: pain, dyspigmentation, skin/fat atrophy, and telangiectasias.

Intralesional antineoplastic agents (5-fluorouracil [5-FU], bleomycin, vincristine). 5-FU 50 mg/mL once monthly to three times weekly. Less risk for skin atrophy and telangiectasias than intralesional

steroids; greater risk for hyperpigmentation and wound ulceration. Superior results when combined with corticosteroid injections.[48,49] One combination regimen is a mixture of 1 part triamcinolone (40 mg/mL) to 9 parts 5-FU (50 mg/mL).

Flurandrenolide tape has been shown to flatten hypertrophic scars and thinly raised keloids. They are also effective in the postsurgical setting in the prevention of keloid occurrence.[50] They are worn over the scars for 8 to 24 h/d for 5 d/wk. Expect postinflammatory hypopigmentation of the surrounding normal skin; can also see skin atrophy, telangiectasias.

Cryotherapy works by cellular injury and necrosis of keloidal tissue. Side effects include local pain, blister formation, dyspigmentation, and depigmentation. Intralesional cryotherapy requires fewer treatments and has less risk for depigmentation than spray cryotherapy (Fig. 5).[51]

Mechanical compression has been used primarily to treat earlobe keloids but can be used in other locations. The mechanism of action is unknown but thought to be due to decreased oxygen tension from occlusion of smaller blood vessels or decreased mechanical tension.[52] They can be used after surgery to decrease the chances of keloid formation. They are most effective if worn 24 h/d for several months at a pressure level of at least 24 mm Hg.[53]

Various lasers have been used to treat keloids. Their proposed benefit is via selective photothermolysis, in which direct energy is absorbed by

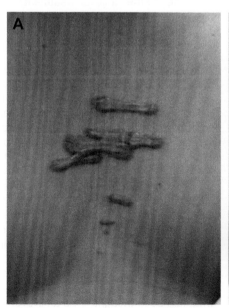 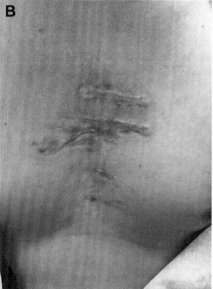

Fig. 4. Keloids before (A) and after (B) intralesional steroids.

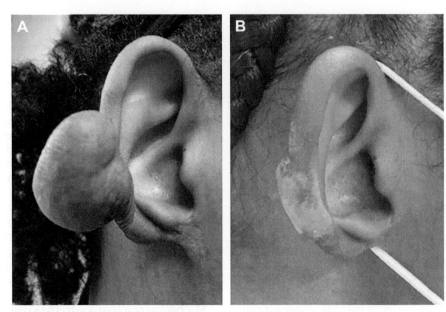

Fig. 5. Keloid before (*A*) and after (*B*) cryosurgery and intralesional steroids.

oxyhemoglobin, leading to thermal injury and reduced collagen. Multiple treatments are required for good outcome, and they may be used in combination with topical applications (steroids, 5-FU). Potential side effects include hyperpigmentation/hypopigmentation, scarring, and purpura. Options are 585 nm PDL, 1064 nm Nd:YAG, and CO_2 lasers.[54]

Pentoxifylline is a xanthine derivative, known to improve erythrocyte flexibility and lower blood viscosity used to treat stroke, claudication, and sickle cell disease. It exerts a dose-dependent inhibition on the in vitro proliferation and collagen synthesis of human fibroblasts derived from normal skin and keloid tissue.[55] Tissue oxygen levels are significantly increased by therapeutic doses of pentoxifylline in patients with peripheral arterial disease. Wong and colleagues reports 3 patients with large keloidal plaques placed on pentoxifylline; they had substantial improvement in their pain and pruritus and lesional growth was halted.[56] A separate study has shown that pentoxifylline decreases the risk of postsurgical keloid recurrence.[57]

Dupilumab has been proposed as a systemic treatment modality for keloids, given evidence for increased interleukin (IL)-4/IL-13 signaling and Th2 inflammation in keloid scars.[58] There are conflicting publications regarding efficacy of dupilumab for keloid growth as well as pain and itch.[58–62] A clinical trial is underway to explore this modality.

Other treatment modalities include intralesional bleomycin, verapamil, hyaluronidase, collagenase, botulinum toxin, radiofrequency ablation, and extracorporeal shockwave therapy.[54]

Long-Term Monitoring

Because of the high rate of recurrence, a follow-up period of at least 1 year is necessary to fully evaluate the effectiveness of therapy. Close follow-up monitoring is vital during immediate and aggressive treatment of subsequent keloid formation. Noncompliant patients who are lost to follow-up care for months often return for further evaluation long after further adjunct treatment would have been most beneficial.

SUMMARY

Keloids remain a condition causing significant morbidity in patients, especially those of skin of color. With identification of its associations with other medical conditions and the inflammatory component to the disease, we are now beginning to understand some of the complexities of this disease process. Future research will hopefully identify more of the causal genes linked to keloids, as well as more of the systemic diseases that we should screen for in our patients diagnosed with CCCA. Future clinical studies should explore possible therapeutic options (local and systemic) that target the inflammatory and the fibroproliferative genes that are upregulated in keloids. As we learn more about keloids, we hope that future treatments will be able to prevent or reverse what has been thought to be an irreversible scarring process.

CLINICS CARE POINTS

- Keloids are an exuberant response to cutaneous wound healing in which scar tissue grows beyond the boundaries of the inciting insult.

- Age, race, location, family history, and personal history of keloids are relevant factors concerning the risk of developing keloids.

- Because keloids are prone to postexcisional recurrence, medical management plays an important role in keloid treatment.

- Many modalities exist to treat keloids/prevent recurrence.

- Multimodal approach is often necessary in difficult cases.

DECLARATION OF INTERESTS

Ariel Knowles has no conflicts of interest to declare. Donald Glass has served on advisory boards for AbbVie, Pfizer and UCB and has received honraria as compensation.

REFERENCES

1. Limandjaja GC, Niessen FB, Scheper RJ, et al. The Keloid Disorder: Heterogeneity, Histopathology, Mechanisms and Models. Front Cell Dev Biol 2020; 8:360.
2. Ud-Din S, Bayat A. New insights on keloids, hypertrophic scars, and striae. Dermatol Clin 2014;32(2):193–209.
3. Ogawa R, Akita S, Akaishi S, et al. Diagnosis and Treatment of Keloids and Hypertrophic Scars-Japan Scar Workshop Consensus Document 2018. Burns Trauma 2019;7:39.
4. Burd A, Huang L. Hypertrophic response and keloid diathesis: two very different forms of scar. Plast Reconstr Surg 2005;116(7):150e–7e.
5. Deyrup A, Graves JL Jr. Racial Biology and Medical Misconceptions. N Engl J Med 2022; 386(6):501–3.
6. Young WG, Worsham MJ, Joseph CL, et al. Incidence of keloid and risk factors following head and neck surgery. JAMA Facial Plast Surg 2014;16(5):379–80.
7. Tulandi T, Al-Sannan B, Akbar G, et al. Prospective study of intraabdominal adhesions among women of different races with or without keloids. Am J Obstet Gynecol 2011;204(2):132 e131–e134.
8. Bran GM, Goessler UR, Hormann K, et al. Keloids: current concepts of pathogenesis (review). Int J Mol Med 2009;24(3):283–93.
9. Kiprono SK, Chaula BM, Masenga JE, et al. Epidemiology of Keloids in Normally Pigmented Africans and African People With Albinism: Population-Based Cross Sectional Survey. Br J Dermatol 2015;173(3):852–4.
10. Bayat A, Arscott G, Ollier WE, et al. Keloid disease: clinical relevance of single versus multiple site scars. Br J Plast Surg 2005;58(1):28–37.
11. Lu WS, Zheng XD, Yao XH, et al. Clinical and epidemiological analysis of keloids in Chinese patients. Arch Dermatol Res 2015;307(2):109–14.
12. Glass DA 2nd. Current Understanding of the Genetic Causes of Keloid Formation. J Investig Dermatol Symp Proc 2017;18(2):S50–3.
13. Lu CC, Qin H, Zhang ZH, et al. The association between keloid and osteoporosis: real-world evidence. BMC Musculoskelet Disord 2021;22(1):39.
14. Arima J, Huang C, Rosner B, et al. Hypertension: a systemic key to understanding local keloid severity. Wound Repair Regen 2015;23(2):213–21.
15. Woolery-Lloyd H, Berman B. A controlled cohort study examining the onset of hypertension in black patients with keloids. Eur J Dermatol 2002;12(6):581–2.
16. Rutherford A, Glass DA 2nd. A case-control study analyzing the association of keloids with hypertension and obesity. Int J Dermatol 2017;56(9):e187–9.
17. Lu YY, Lu CC, Yu WW, et al. Keloid risk in patients with atopic dermatitis: a nationwide retrospective cohort study in Taiwan. BMJ Open 2018;8(7):e022865.
18. Kwon HE, Ahn HJ, Jeong SJ, et al. The increased prevalence of keloids in atopic dermatitis patients with allergic comorbidities: a nationwide retrospective cohort study. Sci Rep 2021;11(1):23669.
19. Sun LM, Wang KH, Lee YC. Keloid incidence in Asian people and its comorbidity with other fibrosis-related diseases: a nationwide population-based study. Arch Dermatol Res 2014;306(9):803–8.
20. Harmon QE, Laughlin SK, Baird DD. Keloids and ultrasound detected fibroids in young African American women. PLoS One 2013;8(12):e84737.
21. Nakashima M, Chung S, Takahashi A, et al. A genome-wide association study identifies four susceptibility loci for keloid in the Japanese population. Nat Genet 2010;42(9):768–71.
22. Zhu F, Wu B, Li P, et al. Association study confirmed susceptibility loci with keloid in the Chinese Han population. PLoS One 2013;8(5):e62377.
23. Velez Edwards DR, Tsosie KS, Williams SM, et al. Admixture mapping identifies a locus at 15q21.2-22.3 associated with keloid formation in African Americans. Hum Genet 2014;133(12):1513–23.
24. Fujita M, Yamamoto Y, Jiang JJ, et al. NEDD4 Is Involved in Inflammation Development during Keloid Formation. J Invest Dermatol 2019;139(2):333–41.

25. Santos-Cortez RLP, Hu Y, Sun F, et al. Identification of ASAH1 as a susceptibility gene for familial keloids. Eur J Hum Genet 2017;25(10):1155–61.

26. Beanes SR, Dang C, Soo C, et al. Skin repair and scar formation: the central role of TGF-beta. Expet Rev Mol Med 2003;5(8):1–22.

27. Harn HI, Ogawa R, Hsu CK, et al. The tension biology of wound healing. Exp Dermatol 2019; 28(4):464–71.

28. Chau D, Mancoll JS, Lee S, et al. Tamoxifen downregulates TGF-beta production in keloid fibroblasts. Ann Plast Surg 1998;40(5):490–3.

29. Wu J, Del Duca E, Espino M, et al. RNA Sequencing Keloid Transcriptome Associates Keloids With Th2, Th1, Th17/Th22, and JAK3-Skewing. Front Immunol 2020;11:597741.

30. Bux S, Madaree A. Involvement of upper torso stress amplification, tissue compression and distortion in the pathogenesis of keloids. Med Hypotheses 2012;78(3):356–63.

31. Ogawa R, Okai K, Tokumura F, et al. The relationship between skin stretching/contraction and pathologic scarring: the important role of mechanical forces in keloid generation. Wound Repair Regen 2012; 20(2):149–57.

32. Al-Attar A, Mess S, Thomassen JM, et al. Keloid pathogenesis and treatment. Plast Reconstr Surg 2006;117(1):286–300.

33. Fong EP, Bay BH. Keloids - the sebum hypothesis revisited. Med Hypotheses 2002;58(4):264–9.

34. Butzelaar L, Niessen FB, Talhout W, et al. Different properties of skin of different body sites: The root of keloid formation? Wound Repair Regen 2017; 25(5):758–66.

35. Huang C, Liu L, You Z, et al. Keloid progression: a stiffness gap hypothesis. Int Wound J 2017;14(5): 764–71.

36. Kouotou EA, Nansseu JR, Omona Guissana E, et al. Epidemiology and clinical features of keloids in Black Africans: a nested case-control study from Yaounde, Cameroon. Int J Dermatol 2019;58(10): 1135–40.

37. Lee SS, Yosipovitch G, Chan YH, et al. Pruritus, pain, and small nerve fiber function in keloids: a controlled study. J Am Acad Dermatol 2004;51(6):1002–6.

38. Kassi K, Kouame K, Kouassi A, et al. Quality of life in black African patients with keloid scars. Dermatol Reports 2020;12(2):8312.

39. Balci DD, Inandi T, Dogramaci CA, et al. DLQI scores in patients with keloids and hypertrophic scars: a prospective case control study. J Dtsch Dermatol Ges 2009;7(8):688–92.

40. Gauglitz GG, Korting HC, Pavicic T, et al. Hypertrophic scarring and keloids: pathomechanisms and current and emerging treatment strategies. Mol Med 2011;17(1–2):113–25.

41. Yoo MG, Kim IH. Keloids and hypertrophic scars: characteristic vascular structures visualized by using dermoscopy. Ann Dermatol 2014;26(5):603–9.

42. Lane JE, Waller JL, Davis LS. Relationship between age of ear piercing and keloid formation. Pediatrics 2005;115(5):1312–4.

43. Butler PD, Longaker MT, Yang GP. Current progress in keloid research and treatment. J Am Coll Surg 2008;206(4):731–41.

44. Berman B, Maderal A, Raphael B. Keloids and Hypertrophic Scars: Pathophysiology, Classification, and Treatment. Dermatol Surg 2017;43(Suppl 1): S3–18.

45. van Leeuwen MC, Stokmans SC, Bulstra AE, et al. Surgical Excision with Adjuvant Irradiation for Treatment of Keloid Scars: A Systematic Review. Plast Reconstr Surg Glob Open 2015;3(7):e440.

46. Dockery GL, Nilson RZ. Treatment of hypertrophic and keloid scars with SILASTIC Gel Sheeting. J Foot Ankle Surg 1994;33(2):110–9.

47. O'Brien L, Jones DJ. Silicone gel sheeting for preventing and treating hypertrophic and keloid scars. Cochrane Database Syst Rev 2013;9: CD003826.

48. Asilian A, Darougheh A, Shariati F. New combination of triamcinolone, 5-Fluorouracil, and pulsed-dye laser for treatment of keloid and hypertrophic scars. Dermatol Surg 2006;32(7):907–15.

49. Srivastava S, Patil AN, Prakash C, et al. Comparison of Intralesional Triamcinolone Acetonide, 5-Fluorouracil, and Their Combination for the Treatment of Keloids. Adv Wound Care 2017;6(11): 393–400.

50. Potter K, Konda S, Ren VZ, et al. Techniques for Optimizing Surgical Scars, Part 2: Hypertrophic Scars and Keloids. Skinmed 2017;15(6):451–6.

51. Mourad B, Elfar N, Elsheikh S. Spray versus intralesional cryotherapy for keloids. J Dermatolog Treat 2016;27(3):264–9.

52. Kelly AP. Medical and surgical therapies for keloids. Dermatol Ther 2004;17(2):212–8.

53. Niessen FB, Spauwen PH, Schalkwijk J, et al. On the nature of hypertrophic scars and keloids: a review. Plast Reconstr Surg 1999;104(5):1435–58.

54. Limmer EE, Glass DA 2nd. A Review of Current Keloid Management: Mainstay Monotherapies and Emerging Approaches. Dermatology and Therapy 2020;10(5):931–48.

55. Berman B, Duncan MR. Pentoxifylline inhibits the proliferation of human fibroblasts derived from keloid, scleroderma and morphoea skin and their production of collagen, glycosaminoglycans and fibronectin. Br J Dermatol 1990;123(3):339–46.

56. Wong TW, Lee JY, Sheu HM, et al. Relief of pain and itch associated with keloids on treatment with oxpentifylline. Br J Dermatol 1999;140(4):771–2.

57. Tan A, Martinez Luna O, Glass DA. 2nd. Pentoxifyl-line for the Prevention of Postsurgical Keloid Recur-rence. Dermatol Surg 2020;46(10):1353–6.

58. Diaz A, Tan K, He H, et al. Keloid lesions show increased IL-4/IL-13 signaling and respond to Th2-targeting dupilumab therapy. J Eur Acad Dermatol Venereol 2019;34(4):e161–4.

59. Wong AJS, Song EJ. Dupilumab as an adjuvant treatment for keloid-associated symptoms. JAAD Case Rep 2021;13:73–4.

60. Tirgan MH, Uitto J. Lack of efficacy of dupilumab in the treatment of keloid disorder. J Eur Acad Derma-tol Venereol 2022;36(2):e120–2.

61. Peterson DM, Damsky WE, Vesely MD. Treatment of lichen sclerosus and hypertrophic scars with dupilu-mab. JAAD Case Rep 2022;23:76–8.

62. Luk K, Fakhoury J, Ozog D. Nonresponse and Pro-gression of Diffuse Keloids to Dupilumab Therapy. J Drugs Dermatol JDD 2022;21(2):197–9.

Scarring Alopecia

Jorge Larrondo, MD, MSc[a,b], Amy J. McMichael, MD[a],*

KEYWORDS

- Cicatricial alopecia • Hair loss • Ethnic hair • Traction alopecia
- Central centrifugal cicatricial alopecia • Discoid lupus erythematosus • Dissecting cellulitis
- Folliculitis decalvans

KEY POINTS

- Although the biochemical composition of human hair is remarkably similar, hair morphology does differ.
- African hair shaft and pigmented scalp have unique features that challenge diagnosis in scarring alopecia.
- The association of 2 or more hair disorders is common in Black patients. Therefore, it is imperative to understand their findings thoroughly to establish a good diagnosis.

BLACK SCALP AND AFRICAN HAIR SHAFT: THEIR DIFFERENCES AND PITFALLS IN DIAGNOSIS

Based on macroscopic characteristics, human hair has traditionally been classified into 3 major groups (African, Asian, and Caucasian).[1] Although the biochemical composition of hair from all 3 groups is remarkably similar; hair morphology does differ.[2] African hair shaft has been described as curlier, drier, and more susceptible to chemical and physical damage.[1,2] There are 4 types of African hair shaft recognized: straight, wavy, helical, and spiral-being the last the most frequent kind of hair. In addition, it seems elliptical in cross-section, with a high degree of irregularity in the diameter along the hair shaft, with frequent twists and random changes in direction.[1–3] It is common to observe knots, longitudinal fissures, and areas of breakage[2,3] (Fig. 1). Overall, hair density in Black people may be less than in other ethnicities. For example, in a 4-mm-diameter punch, African American specimens showed 22 follicles on average, compared with the 36 follicles per 4-mm-diameter in Caucasians.[4] Moreover, studies have shown that African hair grows more slowly than Caucasian and Asian hair.[1,5] In Blacks, the hair follicle is curved and exits the epidermis at an oblique angle relative to the skin (Fig. 2). These factors could favor diseases such as pseudofolliculitis barbae.[3]

Similarly, patients with dark skin phototypes have unique trichoscopic patterns, sometimes challenging the diagnosis. A typical finding is a pigmented network that reflects the rete ridge melanocytes surrounding hypochromic areas of the suprapapillary epidermis.[6] Disruption of the pigmented network can be seen in conditions affecting the interfollicular skin, such as discoid lupus erythematosus, and in secondary scarring alopecias.[7] In addition, some inflammatory scalp disorders can lead to pigment incontinence appearing as blue-gray dots in the skin of color patients. Visualization of the acrosyringeal and follicular openings has been described as the "starry sky" pattern, that is, the presence of multiple small pinpoint white dots (0.2–0.3 mm) regularly distributed on the darker skin background.[6,8] Scarring alopecias can show an irregular distribution of these small pinpoint white dots, interconnected with irregular white patches representing follicular scarring.[7] Erythema is a common finding on the black scalp but vascular patterns are hard to see because of the overlying pigmented skin.

[a] Department of Dermatology, Wake Forest Baptist Health, 4618 Country Club Road, Winston-Salem, NC 27104, USA; [b] Department of Dermatology, Clínica Alemana-Universidad del Desarrollo, Av. Vitacura 5951, Santiago, 7650568, Chile
* Corresponding author.
E-mail address: amcmicha@wakehealth.edu

Dermatol Clin 41 (2023) 519–537
https://doi.org/10.1016/j.det.2023.02.007

derm.theclinics.com

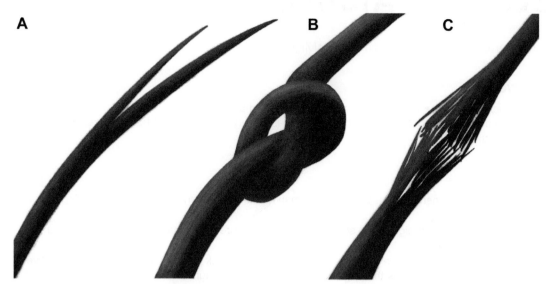

Fig. 1. Black hair shaft illustration showing longitudinal fissures (*A*), knots (*B*), and points of breakage (*C*). (Courtesy of J Larrondo, MD, MSc, Winston-Salem, NC.)

Moreover, clinical assessment could underestimate erythema in black scalp patients when facing inflammatory disorders.[6] Immersion fluid is sometimes helpful to enhance erythema in trichoscopy of skin of color patients (**Fig. 3**). Of note, the association of 2 or more hair disorders is common in Black patients.[2] Therefore, a thorough evaluation will help establish these diagnoses.

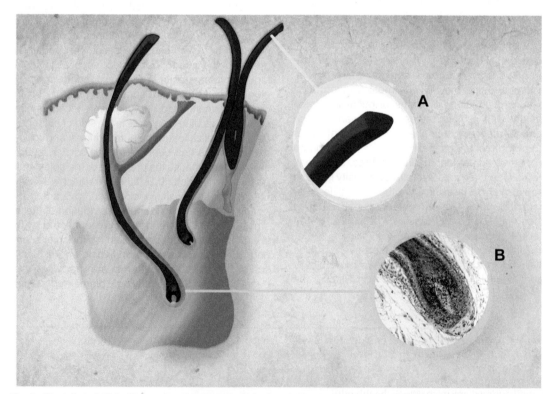

Fig. 2. Black hair follicle illustration showing flattened and elliptical hair shafts (*A*), with a marked hair bulb retrocurvature (*B*). (Courtesy of J Larrondo, MD, MSc, Winston-Salem, NC.)

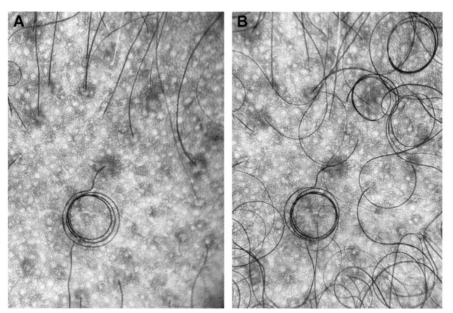

Fig. 3. Trichoscopic evaluation before (*A*) and after immersion fluid (*B*), enhancing erythema in a CCCA case.

TOPOGRAPHIC DIFFERENTIAL DIAGNOSIS IN SCARRING ALOPECIA
Frontal Scalp

Traction alopecia

Traction alopecia (TA) is a mechanical form of hair loss caused by prolonged or repetitive tension on the hair shaft. It has been reported across different ethnicities, affecting men, women, and children.[9,10] Moreover, TA is one of the most prevalent forms of alopecia in patients of color, affecting up to one-third of adult women of African descent.[10] High-tension hairstyling and the concomitant use of chemicals or heat may increase the risk.[11] TA is considered a biphasic form of hair loss, with the early disease being nonscarring and reversible; meanwhile, chronic disease issues scarring alopecia (**Table 1**).[12]

Clinical view

Hair loss may be limited to a minimally decreased hair density in the early stages. Perifollicular papules, erythema, or pustules can be found in areas of highest tension, usually asymptomatic.[11] However, the risk of TA increases with symptomatic traction from hairstyles, including pain, stinging, pustules, or crusting.[10] Hair loss can occur in any area depending on the hairstyle's configuration and the pressure-induced bulk.[13,14] It is also helpful to inquire about nocturnal hair-care practices because various techniques used to maintain hairstyles while sleeping can increase or induce traction.[14] Marginal TA, one of the most common patterns, affects the frontal and temporal scalp

above the ears. It leaves a margin of vellus hairs marking the preexisting hairline, also known as the "fringe sign"[15] (**Fig. 4**A). Nonmarginal TA can occur anywhere throughout the scalp at the site of the installment of the hairstyles with tension. An example would be using volumizers such as volumizing scrunchies or clips in women wearing the hijab.[16] Linear, horseshoe, or stippled hair loss patterns should also alert the clinician about nonmarginal TA. Trichoscopy can show black dots, broken hairs at different levels, and follicular pustules in acute lesions.[11] The presence of hair casts is a sign of ongoing or persistent traction[6,11] (**Fig.5**). In chronic lesions, there is loss of follicular openings, pinpoint white dots irregularly distributed, white patches, and vellus hairs prevailing over terminal hairs[17] (**Fig. 4**B).

Histopathologic findings

In early TA, histopathology shows a usual number of terminal hairs with increased catagen/telogen count, preserved sebaceous glands, trichomalacia (distorted hair shafts), and pigmented casts.[12] Chronic TA shows a decrease in the total number of follicles with follicular dropout. The vellus follicles outnumber the terminal hairs, and sebaceous glands are preserved with minimal inflammation.[13]

Pitfalls and diagnostic clues

Acute forms of TA can mimic alopecia areata or trichotillomania. Chronic marginal TA may be confused with frontal fibrosing alopecia (FFA) or female pattern hair loss. **Table 1** summarizes the clinical characteristics of FFA and TA.

Table 1
Main findings of disorders in the frontal scalp

	Acute Traction Alopecia[11–17]	Chronic Traction Alopecia[11–17]	Frontal Fibrosing Alopecia[17,19–21]
Clinical presentation	Papules, pustules, or erythema in areas of tension. Fringe sign +	Decreased hair density in areas of traction. Increased vellus hairs. Fringe sign +	Pruritus. Hairline recession. Loss of follicular openings. Eyebrow involvement. Lonely hair sign +
Dermatoscopic features	Black dots, broken hairs, and follicular pustules. Hair casts.	Loss of follicular openings, white patches. Vellus > terminal hair. Hair casts.	Loss of follicular openings, absence of vellus, white patches. Perifollicular erythema, peripilar casts.
Histopathology	Normal number of terminal hairs. Increased catagen/telogen. Preserved sebaceous glands. Trichomalacia and pigmented casts.	Decreased number of terminal hairs with follicular dropout. Vellus > terminal hair. Preserved sebaceous glands. Minimal inflammation.	Perifollicular lichenoid lymphocytic infiltrate at the infundibulum and isthmus with concentric fibrosis. Diminished number of sebaceous glands.

Treatment

Education is a fundamental part of therapy. The clinician must be vigilant and proactive in the hair-care practices of patients who may be at risk. Mirmirani and Khumalo proposed 2 important slogans: "Tolerate pain from a hairstyle and risk hair loss" and "No braids or weaves on relaxed hair" as a general rule for patients to avoid high-risk hairstyling.[11] Minimizing chemical and thermal treatment is also recommended.[14] Medical treatment of early cases includes topical and intralesional corticosteroids applied to the affected areas and oral antibiotics for their anti-inflammatory properties.[11] Topical and oral minoxidil can also be considered in the therapeutic arsenal. Advanced stages of TA, characterized by scarring alopecia, are less likely to respond to medical therapy. Therefore, hair restoration surgery may be an ideal option for advanced cases.[12]

Frontal Fibrosing Alopecia

FFA is considered a variant of lichen planopilaris. Most patients are postmenopausal white women.[18] However, FFA can also affect Black patients, even with familial cases being reported, suggesting, among other factors, the possibility of genetic inheritance.[19] One study showed that Black patients with FFA may have higher rates of coexisting entities such as central centrifugal cicatricial alopecia (CCCA), systemic lupus erythematosus, and alopecia areata.[20] In addition, study data have shown that Black patients may present with earlier onset FFA than other ethnicities.[20,21]

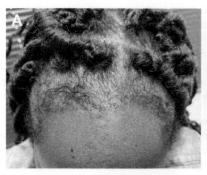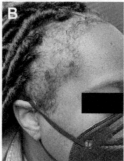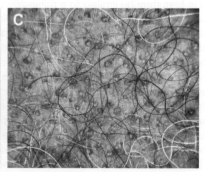

Fig. 4. TA clinical presentation showing the "fringe sign" (*A, B*). Trichoscopy shows loss of follicular openings, pinpoint white dots irregularly distributed, and vellus predominance (*C*).

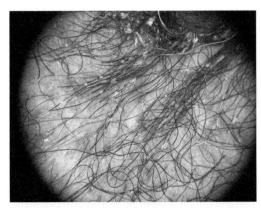

Fig. 5. Dermoscopy in TA. The presence of white to brown cylindrical structures (hair casts) along the hair shaft is a sign of active traction.

Clinical view

Hairline recession is a typical characteristic of FFA and occurs more frequently on the frontotemporal region of the scalp but upper periauricular and occipital localizations are not uncommon.[20,21] The band of alopecia is often readily distinguishable from the sun-damaged skin of the forehead. Alternatively, one may see a lighter band of skin behind where the hairline began that can be highlighted using Wood's light.[22] Black patients are more likely to have vertex/central and occipital scalp involvement.[20] The itch is a common complaint among skin of color patients with FFA; pain or a burning sensation is often reported. Patchy or complete eyebrow involvement and the presence of the "lonely hair sign" are often clues to diagnosis[23] (**Fig. 6**A). Compared with White patients, higher rates of facial hyperpigmentation and less perifollicular hyperkeratosis/scales are found.[20] Trichoscopy typically shows loss of follicular openings, absence of vellus hairs in the hairline, preserved honeycomb pigmentary network, and white patches. Perifollicular erythema and peripilar casts can also be seen[17] (**Fig. 6**B).

Histopathologic findings

Histologic features may be indistinguishable from lichen planopilaris (LPP) on hematoxylin and eosin sections. Typically, lichenoid interface dermatitis affects the infundibulum/isthmus and concentric perifollicular fibrosis with a partial or total absence of sebaceous glands.[24] FFA sometimes can show a more pronounced follicular apoptosis and clefting between the follicular epithelium and the fibrosis zone compared with LPP.[25]

Pitfalls and diagnostic clues

FFA can be misdiagnosed in Black patients due to overlapping features with TA. Literature reports have shown that many black patients with FFA

had a history of hairstyles associated with traction and chemical or heat to straighten the hair.[21] In addition, some of those patients also showed signs of TA, making the diagnosis difficult (see **Table 1**).

Treatment

The goals of treatment are to stop disease progression and provide symptomatic relief. Topical treatments include topical minoxidil, corticosteroids, or topical calcineurin inhibitors. Systemic anti-inflammatory therapies using drugs such as hydroxychloroquine, doxycycline, oral corticosteroids, oral retinoids, and mycophenolate mofetil were reported to be useful.[26,27] 5-alpha reductase inhibitors (finasteride and dutasteride) seem to be effective in stabilizing disease progression,[28] with oral dutasteride being the most effective therapy for patients with FFA compared with other systemic therapies (hydroxychloroquine, doxycycline, and isotretinoin) or no systemic treatment in 224 patients.[29] The most effective regimen was 5 to 7 capsules of dutasteride 0.5 mg/wk.[29] The use of Nd: YAG (1064 nm), nonablative, once a month for 3 months (14 J/cm^2, spot size 5 mm, pulse duration 3 milliseconds) in 5 patients as an adjuvant therapy has also been reported. Four out of five patients reported improvement in at least one symptom (pain, pruritus, burning) and improvement in at least 3 out of 8 clinician-evaluated signs. One patient had worsening of pain. In addition, 2 patients with lichen planus pigmentosus of the face improved after treatment. No major side effects were reported.[30]

MIDDLE SCALP
Central Centrifugal Cicatricial Alopecia

CCCA remains the leading cause of scarring alopecia in women of African descent. It predominantly affects middle-aged women of African ancestry, with a prevalence of 2.7% to 5.7% in that population.[31] Hairstyles and hair-care practices have long been suspected of the development of CCCA but the available evidence is conflicting.[32] Mutations in the PADI3 gene have been identified in women with CCCA,[33] and it is uncommon in men and children (**Table 2**).[34,35]

Clinical view

Symptoms can range from pruritus, tenderness, dysesthesias, or burning.[31] However, many patients are asymptomatic,[36] making a silent and insidious progression and leading to late presentation of the patient for medical care. CCCA commonly presents scarring on the vertex or crown that spreads centrifugally, often symmetrically (**Figs. 7A and 8**A). The severity of central

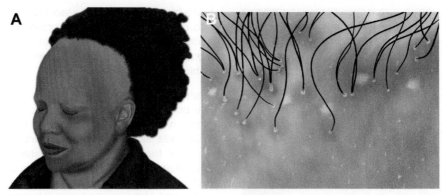

Fig. 6. FFA illustration showing frontotemporal hairline recession and complete eyebrow involvement (*A*). Trichoscopic illustration shows the absence of vellus hairs, peripilar casts, perifollicular erythema, and white patches (*B*). (Courtesy of J Larrondo, MD, MSc, Winston-Salem, NC.)

Table 2
Main features of scarring alopecia in the middle scalp

	Clinical Presentation	Dermatoscopic Features	Histopathology
CCCA[17,31,39]	Pruritus, tenderness, dysesthesias, or burning. Vertex or crown scarring with centrifugal expansion. Hair breakage.	Loss of follicular openings, irregularly distributed pinpoint white dots, white patches, and hair diameter variability. Peripilar gray/white halos.	PDIRS in affected and unaffected follicles. Follicular miniaturization. Varying degrees of perifollicular lymphocytic inflammation, and concentric fibrosis.
Lichen planopilaris[7,17,50,53]	Pruritus, burning, or pain. Focal, multifocal, or diffuse areas of scarring alopecia.	Loss of follicular openings, peripilar casts, small hair tufts, and white patches. Blue-gray dots in a targetoid pattern.	Perifollicular lymphocytic infiltrate around infundibulum and isthmus. Absent/diminished sebaceous glands. Concentric perifollicular fibrosis.
Discoid lupus erythematosus[7,17,55,74]	Burning, pruritus, or tenderness. Central erythema or hypopigmentation and peripheral hyperpigmentation. Follicular plugging.	Loss of follicular openings, perifollicular hyperkeratosis, keratotic plugs, red dots, and large arborizing vessels. Blue-gray dots in a speckled distribution.	Vacuolar interface dermatitis. Superficial and deep perivascular and periadnexal lymphocytic infiltrate. Diffuse deposition of mucin in the dermis and subdermis.
Fibrosing alopecia in a pattern distribution[61,62]	Pruritus, pain, or dysesthesia. Hair loss in a male or female pattern distribution, usually with a slowly progressive course.	Loss of follicular openings, peripilar casts, perifollicular erythema. Hair shaft variability and predominance of single hair follicles.	Lichenoid inflammation affecting single terminal and vellus follicles. Hair follicle miniaturization. Perifollicular lamellar fibrosis.

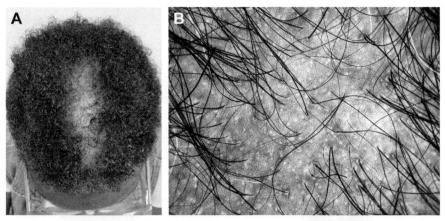

Fig. 7. CCCA clinical presentation (*A*). Trichoscopy shows peripilar gray/white halos, irregularly distributed pinpoint white dots, and hair diameter variation (*B*).

hair loss is graded according to a previously validated photographic scale[37] (Fig. 9). Hair loss can be associated with scaling, crusting, follicular papules, or pustules. In addition, hair breakage has been reported as a possible early clinical presentation.[36] Trichoscopic features include the loss of follicular openings and irregularly distributed pinpoint white dots/white patches. A preserved honeycomb pigmentary network, variation in hair diameter, perifollicular erythema, and occasionally black dots and broken hairs.[17] In addition, the presence of peripilar gray/white halos is a specific and sensitive sign of the diagnosis[38] (Figs. 7B and 8B).

Histopathologic findings

The earliest histologic finding is the premature desquamation of the inner root sheath (PDIRS).[39] However, PDIRS is a nonspecific feature in heavily inflamed follicles in other primary cicatricial alopecias.[40] In CCCA, PDIRS can be detected in affected and unaffected follicles. Variably dense lymphocytic perifollicular inflammation at the infundibulum and isthmus with concentric onion-like follicular fibrosis, fragmented hair shafts in the dermis, follicular miniaturization, and focal preservation of the sebaceous glands are common findings.[39]

Pitfalls and diagnostic clues

Histopathologically, LPP remains the principal differential diagnosis. The absence of follicular apoptosis and only mild/absent lichenoid inflammation favors CCCA over lichen planopilaris.[25] LPP is unlikely to show PDIRS in noninflamed follicles.[39] However, in some cases, the inflammatory infiltrates in CCCA and LPP are not only histologically similar but also immunophenotypically

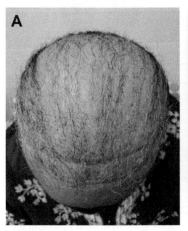
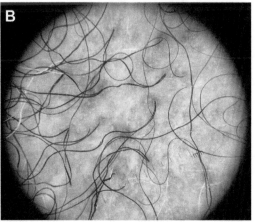

Fig. 8. Severe CCCA with extensive scalp involvement (*A*). Trichoscopy shows loss of follicular openings, peripilar white/gray halos, irregularly distributed pinpoint white dots, and white patches (*B*).

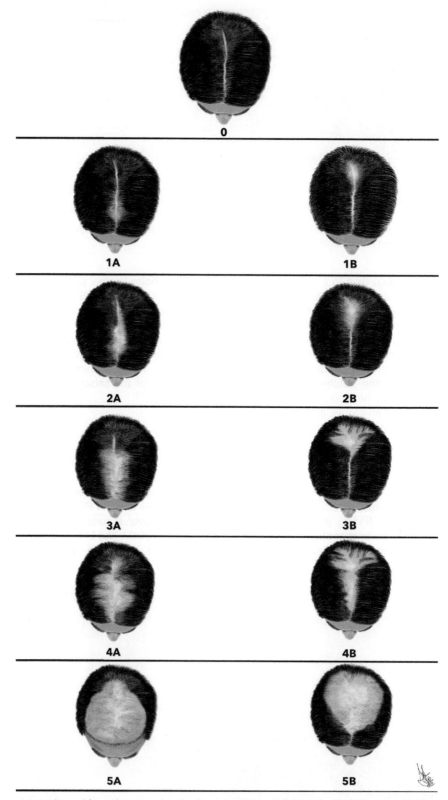

Fig. 9. Illustration adapted from the central scalp alopecia photographic scale in African American women. (*From* Olsen E, Callender V, Sperling L, et al. Central scalp alopecia photographic scale in African American women. Dermatol Ther 2008;21(4):264 to 7.)

indistinguishable.[41] **Table 2** summarizes the main features of scarring alopecia in the middle scalp.

Treatment

The treatment goals in CCCA are to halt the disease progression, control symptoms, and hopefully establish some hair regrowth. Despite the lack of solid evidence directly associating hair-care practices, the removal of potentially harmful hair-care practices is encouraged; minimal trauma and infrequent use of hair chemicals and heat are recommended by some clinicians.[42,43] The use of antiseborrheic shampoos may help decrease pruritus and scaling. Many researchers have reported treating with topical and intralesional corticosteroids, calcineurin inhibitors, and minoxidil.[31] Topical treatments are commonly used daily, with topical corticosteroids usually tapered to 3 days/wk once control of symptoms is achieved.[43] Intralesional corticosteroids ranging in strength from 2.5 to 10 mg/mL may be used every 4 to 8 weeks for at least 6 months.[44,45] The target area of treatment should be at the periphery of areas of hair loss, including normal appearing areas to prevent the progression. Dermoscopy can be a helpful tool to assess clinically unapparent areas of activity.[46] Systemic anti-inflammatory therapies include oral tetracyclines, antimalarials, mycophenolate mofetil, and cyclosporine. The usual regimen is 6 to 9 months for active inflammation or where topical treatment has been unsuccessful. In addition, antiandrogen and 5-alfa-reductase inhibitors have been used with success.[43] Research has highlighted the efficacy of platelet-rich plasma (PRP) therapy in patients with refractory CCCA. However, the investigators also noted a reduction in the follicular density 6 months after treatment, supporting the need for maintenance therapy.[47] Another report of 2 stabilized cases of CCCA found an increase in hair density during the monthly PRP sessions.

Nevertheless, during the 6-month-interval sessions, both patients showed a noticeable decrease in follicular density.[48] An expert opinion states that PRP may be more advantageous in women with concurrent CCCA and androgenetic alopecia.[42] Surgical correction via hair transplantation is a possible option for patients with a stabilized condition for 9 to 12 months and the absence of inflammation histologically.[31]

Lichen planopilaris

A chronic lymphocytic disorder that usually affects the scalp but may also compromise the hair on the face and body. Most patients are caucasian women in their early fifties[49] but it can occur in men and women of all racial groups, including individuals of color.

Clinical view

LPP presents with focal or multifocal patches or diffuse areas of scarring alopecia on the vertex or parietal scalp, often quite symptomatic with pruritus, burning, and tenderness[50] (**Fig. 10**A). Disease can be indolent or slowly progressive but rarely involves the entire scalp. Less typical pigmentary findings in Black patients include hypopigmented macules and patches of varying sizes on the scalp, face, and trunk.[51] Moreover, reticulated hyperpigmentation on the scalp has been reported.[52] Trichoscopic features show loss of follicular openings, peripilar casts, and a preserved honeycomb pattern. Occasionally, there are blue-gray dots in a targetoid pattern corresponding to pigment incontinence.[7] Small, irregularly shaped, whitish areas lacking follicular openings and small hair tufts can be seen[17] (**Fig. 10**B).

Histopathologic findings

LPP shows areas of follicular dropout and an absent/diminished number of sebaceous glands. Perifollicular lichenoid/interface lymphocytic

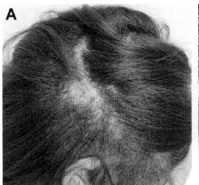
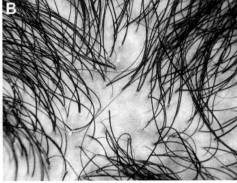

Fig. 10. LPP presenting as a focal patch of scarring alopecia (*A*). Trichoscopy shows loss of follicular openings, peripilar casts, and small hair tufts (*B*).

infiltrate involving the infundibulum and isthmus, and concentric fibrosis involving the permanent portion of the hair follicle may be observed.[53]

Pitfalls and Diagnostic Clues

LPP differs from discoid lupus erythematosus (DLE) by the presence of follicular hypergranulosis, diminished elastic fibers in a wedge shape around the infundibulum, and more frequent colloid bodies.[54]

Treatment

The treatment goals include controlling symptomatology and halting the progression of the disease. High-potency topical corticosteroids, calcineurin inhibitors, and intralesional corticosteroids can be used to target areas of active disease and are the mainstay of treatment of primary symptoms.[55] Additional therapies may be used based on the amount of inflammation and/or involvement, as well as the velocity of progression. These include oral tetracyclines, hydroxychloroquine, mycophenolate mofetil, cyclosporine, azathioprine, dapsone, and isotretinoin.[56] Limited evidence supports the therapeutic potential of Janus kinase (JAK)-1/2 and JAK-1/3 inhibitors for treating recalcitrant LPP.[57,58] Other adjunctive therapy includes low-level light therapy[59] and platelet-rich plasma,[60] awaiting placebo-controlled trials to understand their benefits entirely.

Fibrosing Alopecia in a Pattern Distribution

Fibrosing alopecia in a pattern distribution (FAPD) is a progressive form of scarring alopecia characterized by patterned hair loss similar to androgenetic alopecia but with trichoscopic and histopathologic signs of both lichen planopilaris and androgenetic alopecia.[61] This form of hair loss has been described in Caucasians, patients of African descent, and Hispanics.[62] There are no prevalence data for this form of hair loss in Black patients, which is not well represented in the literature.

Clinical view

FAPD presents with hair loss in a centroparietal distribution, usually with a slowly progressive course. Typically resembles male or female pattern alopecia. A closer look may reveal the pattern of "pink goosebumps" in the patterned area.[63] Some patients may complain of pain, dysesthesia, and scalp pruritus.[61] Trichoscopy is fundamental for suspecting the diagnosis. FAPD shows trichoscopic signs seen in androgenetic alopecia, such as hair diameter variability and predominance of single hair follicles.[61] In addition, features such as loss of follicular openings,

peripilar casts, and perifollicular erythema are seen.[61,63] In higher phototypes, similar features found in CCCA, such as peripilar white halos, a honeycomb pigmented network, and scattered small white patches, have been described, making diagnosis challenging.[61,62]

Histopathologic findings

FAPD shows combined features of both LPP and androgenetic alopecia (AGA). Histopathology shows an increased number of vellus hairs, concentric perifollicular lamellar fibrosis, and a decrease in sebaceous glands. Variably dense, perifollicular lymphocytic infiltrate is also seen, and both terminal and vellus follicles are affected.[61,63]

Pitfalls and diagnostic clues

In the author's opinion, CCCA and FAPD may sometimes be indistinguishable in skin of color. One distinction would be the presence of a lichenoid infiltrate and an interface dermatitis of the follicular epithelium in FAPD.[61] However, although uncommon, CCCA can also show mild follicular lichenoid inflammation and follicular apoptosis in active stages. In addition, early-stage CCCA that presents hair thinning may be mistaken for AGA.[64]

Treatment

FAPD is a chronic and progressive scarring condition, and the treatment goal, as in other scarring alopecias, is to stop the disease progression. Therapy aims to decrease inflammation and block miniaturization. Anti-inflammatory agents include topical, intralesional corticosteroids, and oral hydroxychloroquine.[61] Hair growth promoters such as topical minoxidil 5% or oral minoxidil can be used as adjunctive treatments.[65,66] Antiandrogen therapy and 1 mg daily of oral finasteride have been shown to stabilize the progression of hair loss.[67]

Discoid lupus erythematosus

DLE is a form of chronic lupus erythematosus that commonly affects the scalp, and about one-third of cases are associated with scarring alopecia.[68] DLE has a higher incidence and prevalence in Black individuals.[69] Women are more affected than men, and the disease is more common in adults than children.[70]

Clinical view

Patients may be asymptomatic or describe burning, pruritus, or tenderness in affected areas. In addition, patients may report worsening after ultraviolet (UV) light exposure.[70] Areas of involvement typically include the scalp but it may occur on any other body part, especially in sun-

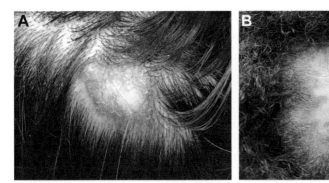

Fig. 11. An active DLE case shows a well-demarcated erythematous patch with scales and peripheral hyperpigmentation (*A*). A well-established patch of alopecia with central hypopigmentation and mild erythema (*B*).

exposed areas. Erythema, scale, and pigmentary changes are more pronounced in DLE than in other forms of cicatricial alopecia.[71] It usually presents as well-demarcated annular lesions with central hypopigmentation and/or erythema, follicular plugging, and peripheral hyperpigmentation (**Fig. 11** A and B). Of note, DLE cases presenting as hyperpigmented patches on the scalp without evident hair loss have also been described.[72] Trichoscopic features include loss of follicular openings, perifollicular hyperkeratosis, interfollicular scales, keratotic plugs, follicular red dots, and large arborizing vessels (**Fig. 12**). In higher phototypes, the loss of pigmentation with disruption of the honeycomb pattern, white patches or a reduction/absence of pinpoint white dots, blue-gray dots distributed in a speckled pattern, and blue-white veil-like features can be appreciated.[7,73]

Histopathologic findings
In DLE, vertical and horizontal sections are helpful for the diagnosis. DLE lesions typically show an interface dermatitis with vacuolar degeneration involving the dermo–epidermal junction, epidermal atrophy with hyperkeratosis, follicular plugging, a diminished number of sebaceous lobules, pigment incontinence, and thickening of the basement membrane.[74] In addition, the presence of mucin in the dermis and subdermis in a diffuse pattern and an infiltrate of plasma cells in a perivascular and periadnexal location are strong pointers to DLE.[75]

Pitfalls and diagnostic clues
Folliculitis decalvans (FD), psoriasis, inflammatory tinea capitis, and especially LPP are differential diagnoses of DLE. In histopathologically inconclusive cases, direct immunofluorescence (DIF) can help establish the diagnosis. In DLE, DIF may show immunoglobulin G (IgG) and complement C3 (C3) along the dermo-epidermal junction in 70% to 95% of cases.[54] Another finding that may help to distinguish alopecic DLE from LPP is the presence of groups of CD123+ plasmacytoid dendritic cells (clusters of at least 5 cells) in discoid lupus, whereas in LPP these are arranged as single interstitial cells.[76]

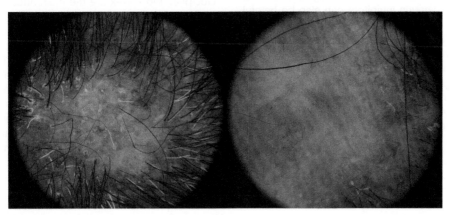

Fig. 12. Trichoscopy of DLE shows loss of follicular openings, pigmentary network disruption, large arborizing vessels, perifollicular hyperkeratosis, and white patches.

Table 3
Main characteristics of disorders in the posterior scalp

	FD[7,55,80]	Dissecting cellulitis[7,55,91]	Acne Keloidalis nuchae[8,55,100]
Clinical presentation	Pain, pruritus, and burning sensation. Purulent folliculitis with scales, erythema, and crusts. Hair tufting.	Pain or tenderness. Multiple boggy scalp nodules, abscesses, and sinus tracts.	Fibrotic papules and pustules. Nodules or plaques of scarring. Hair tufting.
Dermatoscopic features	Loss of follicular openings, peripilar casts, scaling, pustules, and hair tufting.	Black dots, broken hairs, 3D yellow dots, and short regrowing hairs. Milky-red areas and cutaneous clefts.	Broken hairs Ingrown hairs Hair tufting
Histopathology	Mixed inflammatory infiltrate (neutrophils, lymphocytes, histiocytes, and plasma cells). Polytrichia (4–6 follicles), and fragmented hair shafts. Perifollicular concentric fibrosis.	Mixed cell infiltrate affecting the lower follicle. Increased telogen count, trichomalacia. Late-onset disease: Diminished or absent sebaceous glands, follicular dropout, chronic granulomatous infiltrate, fragmented hair shafts and dermal fibrosis.	Dense infiltrate of neutrophils, lymphocytes, and plasma cells distributed around the isthmus and the lower infundibulum. Late-onset disease: Chronic granulomatous inflammation, follicular dropout, fragmented hair shafts, and dense dermal fibrosis without keloidal features.

Treatment

Prompt diagnosis and early therapy are crucial to prevent irreversible hair loss. The general recommendation includes photoprotection and smoking cessation.[72] Early DLE may be managed with topical and intralesional corticosteroids (triamcinolone acetonide 10 mg/mL every 4–6 weeks). Topical calcineurin inhibitors can also be helpful, especially for areas with thinning or atrophy.[77] Systemic agents include oral antimalarial agents, mycophenolate mofetil, methotrexate, retinoids, dapsone, and thalidomide.[3,77] In addition, oral corticosteroids (prednisone 10–20 mg/d, tapering down over time, or dexamethasone as a minipulse of 0.1 mg/kg on 2 consecutive days or the week) can be used as bridging therapy.[1,72]

Posterior Scalp

Folliculitis decalvans

FD is a highly inflammatory neutrophilic cicatricial alopecia characterized by chronic inflammation, hair tufting, and follicular destruction. It is more frequent in young and middle-aged adults.[55]

Cause has not been completely elucidated. An alteration in the host immune response may play a role in the onset of the disease, triggered by a dysbiosis of normal hair microbiota (**Table 3**).[78,79]

Clinical view

Occipital and vertex are the main affected areas. Lesions are often symptomatic with pain, pruritus, and burning sensation. Typical lesions include purulent folliculitis with tufts of hairs, scales, erythema, and perifollicular crusts[80] (**Fig. 13** A and B). Patients may also present concomitant features of LPP, calling this variant FD lichen planopilaris phenotypic spectrum. Some authors consider this a continuum in the evolution from neutrophilic inflammation to chronic lymphoid-plasmacytic inflammation.[81] Trichoscopy typically shows hair tufting—6 or more hairs emerging together—which corresponds to the fused outer root sheaths at the infundibulum level, usually surrounded by a band of yellowish scales.[8] Other findings include focal disruption of the interfollicular pigmentary network, irregular white patches, crusts, scaling,

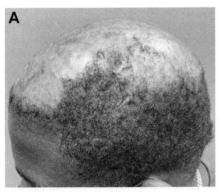
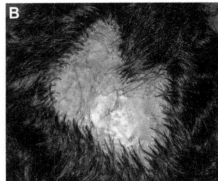

Fig. 13. FD clinical presentation. (*A*) A severe case with extensive scarring, scaling, and erythema. (*B*) Hair tufts, scaling, and perifollicular crusts.

follicular pustules, and elongated loop-like and coiled vessels in a concentric perifollicular arrangement[80,82] (**Fig. 14**).

Histopathologic findings

Histologic findings include intense inflammation around the upper portion of affected follicles, especially at the level of the lower infundibulum.[83] Early lesions include intrafollicular and perifollicular neutrophilic infiltrate, loss of sebaceous glands, and fused outer root sheaths of 4 to 6 follicles at the infundibulum, causing polytrichia. Advanced lesions show a mixed cell inflammatory infiltrate, including neutrophils, lymphocytes, histiocytes, and plasma cells.[80] Hair shaft granulomas with foreign-body giant cells and follicular and interstitial dermal fibrosis can be found.[55]

Pitfalls and diagnostic clues

Very active forms of lymphocytic cicatricial alopecia are in the differential diagnosis and can mimic the FD pattern. A biopsy from a pustular or papular area is less likely to provide useful histopathological information[83] than a sample guided by dermoscopy. A helpful place for biopsy would be a hair tufting area surrounded by thick white, yellowish scales.[84]

Treatment

FD can be an aggressive, resistant, and relapsing disorder making treatment challenging. Due to the host immune response triggered by an altered microbiota, eradicating infectious agents, specifically *Staphylococcus aureus*, has been the mainstay therapy.[55] However, the presence of biofilms could explain, in part, the chronicity and recurrences after appropriate antibiotic treatments. One study isolated gram-negative bacteria in 11 out of 34 FD cases.[79] Therefore, bacterial cultures with antibiotic sensitivities should be obtained in every case. Different regimens have been recommended to reduce the bacterial load of staphylococci effectively. The combination of clindamycin 300 mg and rifampicin 300 mg twice daily systemically for a 10-week course has been commonly used, achieving the most prolonged remission. Other useful treatment regimens include oral doxycycline 100 mg daily for 3 to 6 months, oral minocycline 100 mg daily for 3 to 6 months, and oral azithromycin 500 mg 3 times

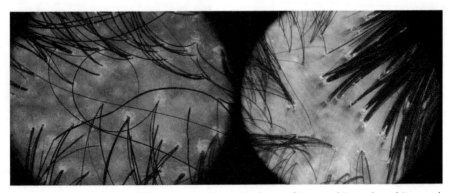

Fig. 14. Trichoscopy in FD shows perifollicular hyperkeratosis, hair tufting, and irregular white patches.

a week for 3 months.[85] Iorizzo M and colleagues reported the successful use of adalimumab in 23 FD refractory cases; 2 patients discontinued the treatment because of insufficient improvement. The regimen was 160 mg at week 0, 80 mg at week 2, and 80 mg every other week.[86] Topical antibiotics and intralesional corticosteroids can be combined with oral regimens. Intralesional triamcinolone acetonide (10 mg/mL) injected into the surrounding hair areas every 4 to 6 weeks can help slow the progression and reduce symptoms.[55] Other therapies include external beam radiation, isotretinoin, human immunoglobulin, infliximab, PRP, and photodynamic therapy.[87–89]

Dissecting cellulitis

Dissecting cellulitis of the scalp (DCS) is a neutrophilic cicatricial alopecia, considered a part of the follicular occlusion disorders that may progressively lead to scarring alopecia and significant morbidity.[55] This occlusion causes a buildup of keratin and other cellular debris, leading to rupture and exposure of the inner follicle and dermis to the environment, with the subsequent inflammatory response. It is more commonly seen in young men of African or Hispanic descent, although it can also occur in Caucasians, women, and children.[55,90]

Clinical view

Occipital and vertex are usually affected. The inflammatory lesions begin as multiple, tender, boggy scalp nodules and sterile abscesses on the occipital scalp. Multifocal lesions can merge to form cerebriform ridges. Lesions often interconnect, forming sinus tracts with overlying permanent alopecia.[55,91] High-frequency ultrasound has been used to characterize inflammatory lesions in DCS[92] (Fig. 15). The lesions are sterile; however, secondary bacterial infection may occur most commonly with coagulase-negative staphylococci.[91] Trichoscopic findings on early stage lesions typically show features of noncicatricial alopecia with regularly distributed pinpoint white dots, enlarged plugged follicular openings (3D yellow dots), black dots, broken hairs, and short regrowing hairs.[17] Inflammatory areas can show erythema, yellow/violaceous structureless areas, arborizing vessels, and giant capillaries. End-stage lesions show loss of follicular openings, confluent ivory-white areas, and cutaneous clefts containing hair shafts.[7,91]

Histopathologic findings

Early lesions show a dense mixed inflammatory infiltrate surrounding the lower half portion of the follicle. The infiltrate may contain individual giant cells or collections of epithelioid cells. There is an increased catagen/telogen hair count, dilated infundibula plugged with keratin and sebum, and trichomalacia. Long-standing lesions can show chronic granulomatous infiltration with sinus tracts and fragmented dermal and subdermal hair shafts in the dermis and subdermis. Partial to complete

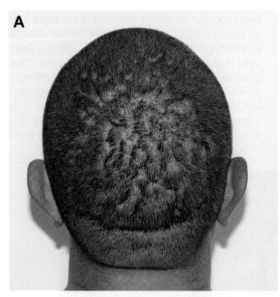
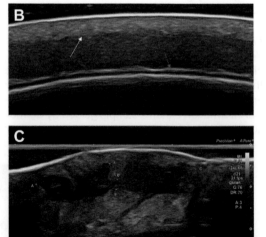

Fig. 15. DCS clinical presentation (A). (B) A healthy scalp ultrasound with typical thickness and echogenicity. The white arrow shows the hypodermal interface; the red arrow indicates epicranial aponeurosis. DCS ultrasound shows thickening of the dermis and subcutaneous planes, with loss of definition of the dermo–hypodermal interface, increased echogenicity of subcutaneous adipose tissue, and presence of confluent cystic lesions with the appearance of merging pseudocysts (C). Courtesy of C Whittle, MD, Santiago, Chile.

loss of sebaceous glands, follicular dropout, and dermal fibrosis may also be present.[91,93]

Pitfalls and diagnostic clues

Early DSC lesions can be patchy emulating alopecia areata in their clinical and trichoscopic findings. Therefore, a scalp biopsy can help establish the diagnosis. A good place for biopsy should include features such as the 3D yellow dots and any areas with black dots.[91] DSC sometimes can clinically and histologically mimic inflammatory tinea capitis. Therefore, a complete workup that includes trichoscopy, histology, and fungal culture should be performed to rule out fungal infections.[94]

Treatment

DCS treatment is often challenging. For limited disease or milder presentation, intralesional corticosteroids and oral antibiotics (tetracyclines, cloxacillin, erythromycin, cephalosporin, and clindamycin) are the standards of care.[55] Incision and drainage is often common step in treating abscesses and fluctuant nodules.[95] In moderate-to-severe cases, oral isotretinoin (0,25–1 mg/kg) has been suggested.[90,96] Secondary line treatments include antitumor necrosis factor α agents, most commonly adalimumab. Oral corticosteroids can be used as adjunctive therapy at low doses or as a bridge to more definitive treatments.[96] For refractory cases, destruction of the hair follicle with CO_2, long-pulse non-Q-switched ruby, and 800-nm pulsed diode have been reported. Other options include oral dapsone, zinc sulfate, colchicine, and photodynamic therapy.[55] Surgical treatment has not been well established. Staged excisions of sinus tracts can help achieve control in refractory patients with draining nodules and sinus tracts without full scalp involvement.[97]

Acne Keloidalis Nuchae

Acne keloidalis nuchae (AKN) is a chronic idiopathic inflammatory scarring condition that mainly occurs in men of African descent.[55] It has been infrequently reported in Caucasians and other ethnic groups.[98] Pathophysiology is not fully understood. Contributing factors involve androgens, autoimmunity, infection, trauma, genetics, and ingrown hairs causing a foreign-body-like immune reaction.[2,55,98] Isolated reports show that AKN can be induced by drugs, such as cyclosporine, diphenylhydantoin, and carbamazepine.[55]

Clinical view

Patients sometimes complain of pruritus and burning sensation.[55] Early lesions are characterized by dome-shaped, fibrotic papules and pustules on the occipital scalp and nape. Secondary infections can result in abscess formation. Hair tufting may also be present.[98,99] In long-term lesions, the papules may coalesce to form hypertrophic scars resembling keloids (**Fig. 16**). Trichoscopy shows broken hairs, tufted hairs,

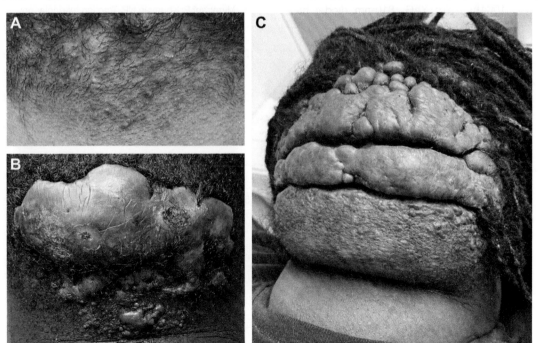

Fig. 16. Clinical spectrum of AKN, starting as fibrotic papules on the occipital scalp (*A*). Papules may coalesce to form hypertrophic scars resembling keloids (*B-C*).

ingrown hairs, and peripilar casts.[8] Late-stage lesions show loss of follicular openings and irregular pinpoint white dots.

Histopathologic findings

Early lesions show a dense infiltrate of neutrophils, lymphocytes, and plasma cells distributed around the isthmus and the lower infundibulum.[100] Complete disappearance of sebaceous glands is associated with inflamed or destroyed follicles. Late lesions show chronic granulomatous inflammation, follicular dropout, fragmented hair shafts, and dense dermal fibrosis without keloidal features.[100,101]

Pitfalls and diagnostic clues

Vertical sections are more appropriate for diagnosis. AKN may be associated with FD, CCCA, or androgenetic alopecia.[98] AKN and FD histologic findings may be identical. Therefore, clinical correlation is advised.[101]

Treatment

AKN is a chronic and recurrent condition; an early treatment may prevent future scarring. Preventive measures include using loose-fitting shirts without occlusive collars and avoiding frequent haircuts with close shaving of the occipital scalp.[2] Early disease is often treated using or combining topical, intralesional corticosteroids, and cryotherapy.[55] When pustules are present, cultures should be obtained to guide the antibiotics regimen. Surgical excision and laser treatment (CO_2, 1064-nm Nd: YAG, 810-nm diode) have been described in refractory cases.[98]

CLINICS CARE POINTS

- African hair shafts have been described as curlier, drier, and more susceptible to chemical and physical damage than other ethnicities.
- Clinical assessment could underestimate erythema in black scalp patients when facing inflammatory disorders.
- The association of two or more hair disorders is common in black patients. Therefore, an excellent clinical-pathological correlation can help us to establish the diagnosis.

DECLARATION OF INTERESTS

J. Larrondo, has no relevant disclosures. Amy J. McMichael, Consulting: Lilly, Janssen, Pfizer, Arcutis, Almirall, Abbvie, Galderma, Bristol Meyers Squibb, Sanofi-Genzyme, UCB, Revian, Johnson & Johnson, L'oreal, and Nutrafol.

REFERENCES

1. Salam A, Aryiku S, Dadzie OE. Hair and scalp disorders in women of African descent: an overview. Br J Dermatol 2013;3:19–32.
2. Lindsey SF, Tosti A. Ethnic hair disorders. Curr Probl Dermatol 2015;47:139–49.
3. Raffi J, Suresh R, Agbai O. Clinical recognition and management of alopecia in women of color. Int J Womens Dermatol 2019;5:314–9.
4. Sperling LC. Hair density in African Americans. Arch Dermatol 1999;135:656–8.
5. Lewallen R, Francis S, Fisher B, et al. Hair care practices and structural evaluation of scalp and hair shaft parameters in African American and Caucasian women. J Cosmet Dermatol 2015;14:216–23.
6. Pirmez R, Tosti A. Trichoscopy Tips. Dermatol Clin 2018;36:413–20.
7. Ocampo-Garza J, Tosti A. Trichoscopy of Dark Scalp. Skin Appendage Disord 2018;5:1–8.
8. Miteva M, Tosti A. Hair and scalp dermatoscopy. J Am Acad Dermatol 2012;67:1040–8.
9. Khumalo NP, Jessop S, Gumedze F, et al. Hairdressing is associated with scalp disease in African schoolchildren. Br J Dermatol 2007;157:106–10.
10. Khumalo NP, Jessop S, Gumedze F, et al. Hairdressing and the prevalence of scalp disease in African adults. Br J Dermatol 2007;157:981–8.
11. Mirmirani P, Khumalo NP. Traction alopecia: how to translate study data for public education–closing the KAP gap? Dermatol Clin 2014;32:153–61.
12. Billero V, Miteva M. Traction alopecia: the root of the problem. Clin Cosmet Investig Dermatol 2018;11:149–59.
13. Goldberg LJ. Cicatricial marginal alopecia: is it all traction? Br J Dermatol 2009;160:62–8.
14. Samrao A, McMichael A, Mirmirani P. Nocturnal Traction: Techniques Used for Hair Style Maintenance while Sleeping May Be a Risk Factor for Traction Alopecia. Skin Appendage Disord 2021;7:220–3.
15. Samrao A, Price VH, Zedek D, et al. The "Fringe Sign" - A useful clinical finding in traction alopecia of the marginal hair line. Dermatol Online J 2011;17:1.
16. Rehman R, Haque M, Ceresnie M, et al. Dermatological considerations and culturally sensitive recommendations for women who wear the hijab. Br J Dermatol 2022. https://doi.org/10.1111/bjd.21795.
17. Yin NC, Tosti A. A systematic approach to Afro-textured hair disorders: dermatoscopy and when to biopsy. Dermatol Clin 2014;32:145–51.

18. Banka N, Mubki T, Bunagan MJ, et al. Frontal fibrosing alopecia: a retrospective clinical review of 62 patients with treatment outcome and long-term follow-up. Int J Dermatol 2014;53:1324–30.

19. Dlova N, Goh CL, Tosti A. Familial frontal fibrosing alopecia. Br J Dermatol 2013;168:220–2.

20. Adotama P, Callender V, Kolla A, et al. Comparing the clinical differences in white and black women with frontal fibrosing alopecia. Br J Dermatol 2021;185:1074–6.

21. Dlova NC, Jordaan HF, Skenjane A, et al. Frontal fibrosing alopecia: a clinical review of 20 black patients from South Africa. Br J Dermatol 2013;169:939–41.

22. Murad A, Bergfeld W. Wood's Light Examination for Assessment in Frontal Fibrosing Alopecia: A Manoeuvre to Enhance the Hairline. J Am Acad Dermatol 2019. S0190-9622(19)33216-33225.

23. Tosti A, Miteva M, Torres F. Lonely hair: a clue to the diagnosis of frontal fibrosing alopecia. Arch Dermatol 2011;147:1240.

24. Miteva M, Whiting D, Harries M, et al. Frontal fibrosing alopecia in black patients. Br J Dermatol 2012;167:208–10.

25. Miteva M., Frontal Fibrosing Alopecia, In: Miteva M., editor. *Hair pathology with trichoscopic correlations*, 2022, CRC Press; Boca Raton, FL, 98–105.

26. Ho A, Shapiro J. Medical therapy for frontal fibrosing alopecia: A review and clinical approach. J Am Acad Dermatol 2019;81:568–80.

27. Samrao A, Chew AL, Price V. Frontal fibrosing alopecia: a clinical review of 36 patients. Br J Dermatol 2010;163:1296–300.

28. Murad A, Bergfeld W. 5-alpha-reductase inhibitor treatment for frontal fibrosing alopecia: an evidence-based treatment update. J Eur Acad Dermatol Venereol 2018;32:1385–90.

29. Pindado-Ortega C, Saceda-Corralo D, Moreno-Arrones ÓM, et al. Effectiveness of dutasteride in a large series of patients with frontal fibrosing alopecia in real clinical practice. J Am Acad Dermatol 2021;84:1285–94.

30. Subash J, Eginli A, Bomar L, et al. Frontal fibrosing alopecia treatment with Nd:YAG (1064 nm) nonablative laser. Int J Womens Dermatol 2020;7:355–6.

31. Dlova NC, Salkey KS, Callender VD, et al. Central Centrifugal Cicatricial Alopecia: New Insights and a Call for Action. J Investig Dermatol Symp Proc 2017;18:S54–6.

32. Shah SK, Alexis AF. Central centrifugal cicatricial alopecia: retrospective chart review. J Cutan Med Surg 2010;14:212–22.

33. Malki L, Sarig O, Romano MT, et al. Variant *PADI3* in Central Centrifugal Cicatricial Alopecia. N Engl J Med 2019;380:833–41.

34. Sperling LC, Skelton HG 3rd, Smith KJ, et al. Follicular degeneration syndrome in men. Arch Dermatol 1994;130:763–9.

35. Eginli AN, Dlova NC, McMichael A. Central Centrifugal Cicatricial Alopecia in Children: A Case Series and Review of the Literature. Pediatr Dermatol 2017;34:133–7.

36. Callender VD, Wright DR, Davis EC, et al. Hair breakage as a presenting sign of early or occult central centrifugal cicatricial alopecia: clinicopathologic findings in 9 patients. Arch Dermatol 2012;148:1047–52.

37. Olsen EA, Callender V, Sperling L, et al. Central scalp alopecia photographic scale in African American women. Dermatol Ther 2008;21:264–7.

38. Miteva M, Tosti A. Dermatoscopic features of central centrifugal cicatricial alopecia. J Am Acad Dermatol 2014;71:443–9.

39. Sperling L. Central centrifugal cicatricial alopecia. In: Sperling L, Cowper S, Knopp E, editors. An atlas of hair pathology with clinical correlations. 2nd edition. New York: Informa Heathcare; 2012. p. 120–5.

40. Sperling LC. Premature desquamation of the inner root sheath is still a useful concept. J Cutan Pathol 2007;34:809–10.

41. Jordan CS, Chapman C, Kolivras A, et al. Clinicopathologic and immunophenotypic characterization of lichen planopilaris and central centrifugal cicatricial alopecia: A comparative study of 51 cases. J Cutan Pathol 2020;47:128–34.

42. Lawson CN, Bakayoko A, Callender VD. Central Centrifugal Cicatricial Alopecia: Challenges and Treatments. Dermatol Clin 2021;39:389–405.

43. Ogunleye TA, McMichael A, Olsen EA. Central centrifugal cicatricial alopecia: what has been achieved, current clues for future research. Dermatol Clin 2014;32:173–81.

44. Gathers RC, Lim HW. Central centrifugal cicatricial alopecia: past, present, and future. J Am Acad Dermatol 2009;60:660–8.

45. Callender VD, McMichael AJ, Cohen GF. Medical and surgical therapies for alopecias in black women. Dermatol Ther 2004;17:164–76.

46. Felix K, De Souza B, Portilla N, et al. Dermatoscopic Evaluation of Central Centrifugal Cicatricial Alopecia Beyond the Vertex Scalp. JAMA Dermatol 2020;156:916–8.

47. Dina Y, Aguh C. Use of Platelet-Rich Plasma in Cicatricial Alopecia. Dermatol Surg 2019;45:979–81.

48. Larrondo J, Petela J, McMichael AJ. Transitory hair growth using platelet-rich plasma therapy in stabilized central centrifugal cicatricial alopecia. Dermatol Ther 2022;35(11):e15798.

49. Chieregato C, Zini A, Barba A, et al. Lichen planopilaris: report of 30 cases and review of the literature. Int J Dermatol 2003;42:342–5.

50. Mirmirani P. Cicatricial Alopecia. In: McMichael AJ, Hordinsky M, editors. *Hair and scalp diseases:*

medical, surgical and cosmetic treatments. New York: Informa Healthcare; 2008. p. 137–48.

51. Arnold D, Hoffman MB, Onajin O, et al. Hypopigmented Macules as Manifestation of Lichen Planus and Lichen Planopilaris. Am J Dermatopathol 2019; 41:514–7.

52. Goldman C, Williams NM, Tosti A, et al. Reticulated Hyperpigmentation as a Sign of Lichen Planopilaris. Skin Appendage Disord 2021;7:397–400.

53. Miteva M. Lichen Planopilaris. In: Miteva M, editor. Hair pathology with trichoscopic correlations. Boca Raton: CRC Press; 2022. p. 89–97.

54. Sperling L. Chronic cutaneous lupus erythematosus. In: Sperling L, Cowper S, Knopp E, editors. An atlas of hair pathology with clinical correlations. 2d edition. New York: Informa Heathcare; 2012. p. 158–65.

55. Otberg N. Primary cicatricial alopecias. Dermatol Clin 2013;31:155–66.

56. Babahosseini H, Tavakolpour S, Mahmoudi H, et al. Lichen planopilaris: retrospective study on the characteristics and treatment of 291 patients. J Dermatolog Treat 2019;30:598–604.

57. Plante J, Eason C, Snyder A, et al. Tofacitinib in the treatment of lichen planopilaris: A retrospective review. J Am Acad Dermatol 2020;83:1487–9.

58. Moussa A, Bhoyrul B, Asfour L, et al. Treatment of lichen planopilaris with baricitinib: A retrospective study. J Am Acad Dermatol 2022;87:663–6.

59. Fonda-Pascual P, Moreno-Arrones OM, Saceda-Corralo D, et al. Effectiveness of low-level laser therapy in lichen planopilaris. J Am Acad Dermatol 2018;78:1020–3.

60. Svigos K, Yin L, Shaw K, et al. Use of platelet-rich plasma in lichen planopilaris and its variants: A retrospective case series demonstrating treatment tolerability without koebnerization. J Am Acad Dermatol 2020;83:1506–9.

61. Griggs J, Trüeb RM, Gavazzoni Dias MFR, et al. Fibrosing alopecia in a pattern distribution. J Am Acad Dermatol 2021;85:1557–64.

62. Teixeira MS, Gavazzoni Dias MFR, Trüeb RM, et al. Fibrosing Alopecia in a Pattern Distribution (FAPD) in 16 African-Descent and Hispanic Female Patients: A Challenging Diagnosis. Skin Appendage Disord 2019;5:211–5.

63. Miteva M. Fibrosing Alopecia in a Pattern Distribution. In: Miteva M, editor. Hair pathology with trichoscopic correlations. Boca Raton: CRC Press; 2022. p. 107–10.

64. Miteva M. Central centrifugal cicatricial alopecia. In: Miteva M, editor. Hair pathology with trichoscopic correlations. Boca Raton: CRC Press; 2022. p. 123–9.

65. Ramanauskaite A, Trüeb RM. Facial Papules in Fibrosing Alopecia in a Pattern Distribution (Cicatricial Pattern Hair Loss). Int J Trichology 2015;7: 119–22.

66. Randolph M, Tosti A. Oral minoxidil treatment for hair loss: A review of efficacy and safety. J Am Acad Dermatol 2021;84:737–46.

67. Chiu HY, Lin SJ. Fibrosing alopecia in a pattern distribution. J Eur Acad Dermatol Venereol 2010;24: 1113–4.

68. Harries MJ, Trueb RM, Tosti A, et al. How not to get scar(r)ed: pointers to the correct diagnosis in patients with suspected primary cicatricial alopecia. Br J Dermatol 2009;160:482–501.

69. Joseph AK, Windsor B, Hynan LS, et al. Discoid lupus erythematosus skin lesion distribution and characteristics in Black patients: a retrospective cohort study. Lupus Sci Med 2021;8(1):e000514.

70. Otberg N, Wu WY, McElwee KJ, et al. Diagnosis and management of primary cicatricial alopecia: part I. Skinmed 2008;7:19–26.

71. Headington JT. Cicatricial alopecia. Dermatol Clin 1996;14:773–82.

72. Desai K, Miteva M. Recent Insight on the Management of Lupus Erythematosus Alopecia. Clin Cosmet Investig Dermatol 2021;14:333–47.

73. Cervantes J, Hafeez F, Miteva M. Blue-White Veil as Novel Dermatoscopic Feature in Discoid Lupus Erythematosus in 2 African-American Patients. Skin Appendage Disord 2017;3:211–4.

74. Miteva M. Lupus Erythematosus of the Scalp. In: Miteva M, editor. Hair pathology with trichoscopic correlations. Boca Raton: CRC Press; 2022. p. 111–8.

75. Restrepo R, Calonje E. Diseases of the hair. In: Calonje E, Brenn T, Lazar A, et al, editors. Mckeés pathology of the skin. 5th edition. Elsevier; 2019. p. 1093–6.

76. Kolivras A, Thompson C. Clusters of CD123+ plasmacytoid dendritic cells help distinguish lupus alopecia from lichen planopilaris. J Am Acad Dermatol 2016;74:1267–9.

77. Udompanich S, Chanprapaph K, Suchonwanit P. Hair and Scalp Changes in Cutaneous and Systemic Lupus Erythematosus. Am J Clin Dermatol 2018;19:679–94.

78. Walker SL, Smith HR, Lun K, et al. Improvement of folliculitis decalvans following shaving of the scalp. Br J Dermatol 2000;142:1245–6.

79. Samrao A, Mirmirani P. Gram-negative infections in patients with folliculitis decalvans: a subset of patients requiring alternative treatment. Dermatol Online J 2020;26. 13030/qt6nw2h5rh.

80. Miteva M. Folliculitis Decalvans. In: Miteva M, editor. Hair pathology with trichoscopic correlations. Boca Raton: CRC Press; 2022. p. 130–4.

81. Yip L, Barrett TH, Harries MJ. Folliculitis decalvans and lichen planopilaris phenotypic spectrum: a case series of biphasic clinical presentation and theories on pathogenesis. Clin Exp Dermatol 2020;45:63–72.

82. Fabris MR, Melo CP, Melo DF. Folliculitis decalvans: the use of dermatoscopy as an auxiliary tool in clinical diagnosis. An Bras Dermatol 2013;88:814–6.

83. Sperling L. Folliculitis decalvans. In: Sperling L, Cowper S, Knopp E, editors. An atlas of hair pathology with clinical correlations. 2nd edition. New York: Informa Heathcare; 2012. p. 131–3.

84. Miteva M, Tosti A. Dermoscopy guided scalp biopsy in cicatricial alopecia. J Eur Acad Dermatol Venereol 2013;27:1299–303.

85. Vañó-Galván S, Molina-Ruiz AM, Fernández-Crehuet P, et al. Folliculitis decalvans: a multicentre review of 82 patients. J Eur Acad Dermatol Venereol 2015;29:1750–7.

86. Iorizzo M, Starace M, Vano-Galvan S, et al. Refractory folliculitis decalvans treated with adalimumab: A case series of 23 patients. J Am Acad Dermatol 2022;87:666–9.

87. Rambhia PH, Conic RRZ, Murad A, et al. Updates in therapeutics for folliculitis decalvans: A systematic review with evidence-based analysis. J Am Acad Dermatol 2019;80:794–801.

88. Suh S, Nguyen C, Zhao L, et al. The role of platelet-rich plasma therapy in refractory folliculitis decalvans. JAAD Case Rep 2021;12:85–7.

89. Miguel-Gomez L, Vano-Galvan S, Perez-Garcia B, et al. Treatment of folliculitis decalvans with photodynamic therapy: Results in 10 patients. J Am Acad Dermatol 2015;72:1085–7.

90. Melo DF, Ramos PM, Machado CJ, et al. Dissecting cellulitis in women: a retrospective multicenter study with 17 patients. Int J Dermatol 2022. https://doi.org/10.1111/ijd.16271. Epub ahead of print.

91. Miteva M. Dissecting Cellulitis of the Scalp. In: Miteva M, editor. Hair pathology with trichoscopic correlations. Boca Raton: CRC Press; 2022. p. 135–41.

92. Cataldo-Cerda K, Wortsman X. Dissecting Cellulitis of the Scalp Early Diagnosed by Color Doppler Ultrasound. Int J Trichology 2017;9:147–8.

93. Sperling L. Dissecting cellulitis of the scalp (perifolliculitis capitis abscedens et suffodiens). In: Sperling L, Cowper S, Knopp E, editors. An atlas of hair pathology with clinical correlations. 2d edition. New York: Informa Heathcare; 2012. p. 166–70.

94. Miletta NR, Schwartz C, Sperling L. Tinea capitis mimicking dissecting cellulitis of the scalp: a histopathologic pitfall when evaluating alopecia in the post-pubertal patient. J Cutan Pathol 2014;41:2–4.

95. Lenzy Y, McMichael A. Cicatricial alopecias. In: Alexis A, Barbosa V, editors. Skin of color. 1 st edition. New York: Springer; 2013. p. p105–22.

96. Thomas J, Aguh C. Approach to treatment of refractory dissecting cellulitis of the scalp: a systematic review. J Dermatolog Treat 2021;32:144–9.

97. Powers MC, Mehta D, Ozog D. Cutting Out the Tracts: Staged Excisions for Dissecting Cellulitis of the Scalp. Dermatol Surg 2017;43:738–40.

98. Ogunbiyi A. Acne keloidalis nuchae: prevalence, impact, and management challenges. Clin Cosmet Investig Dermatol 2016;9:483–9.

99. Alexis A, Heath CR, Halder RM. Folliculitis keloidalis nuchae and pseudofolliculitis barbae: are prevention and effective treatment within reach? Dermatol Clin 2014;32:183–91.

100. Miteva M. Acne/Folliculitis Keloidalis. In: Miteva M, editor. Hair pathology with trichoscopic correlations. Boca Raton: CRC Press; 2022. p. 146–8.

101. Sperling L. Acne keloidalis (folliculitis keloidalis). In: Sperling L, Cowper S, Knopp E, editors. An atlas of hair pathology with clinical correlations. 2d edition. New York: Informa Heathcare; 2012. p. 126–33.

Scalp Infection, Inflammation, and Infestation

Victoria Barbosa, MD, MPH, MBA[a],*, Robert Hight, BS, MS[b,1],
Karina Grullon, BS[b,2]

KEYWORDS

- Tinea capitis • Scalp folliculitis • Seborrheic dermatitis • Pediculosis capitis

KEY POINTS

- Tinea capitis is seen more commonly in patients of African descent and requires treatment with oral antifungal agents.
- *Staphylococcus aureus* is the most common cause of scalp folliculitis.
- Management of seborrheic dermatitis of the scalp in patients with highly textured hair requires medical management that is respectful of cultural hair care and styling practices.
- Pediculosis capitis is seen less frequently in people of African descent than in other populations.

INTRODUCTION

The scalp may be home to several dermatologic conditions, including scarring and non-scarring alopecias, infections, inflammatory skin diseases, and infestations.[1,2] It is also a common site for the development of benign growths and malignant tumors arising in the skin or having metastasized from other organs.[3] Scalp evaluation is an essential part of the dermatologic examination. It is one of the areas that patients cannot see well themselves as part of their skin self-examination, so the clinician is often the only person to visualize the entire scalp. To effectively treat scalp disease in a diverse patient population, one must have knowledge of patients' hair care and hair-styling practices to demonstrate cultural awareness and humility, aid in history taking, normalize the experience of the physical examination, make accurate diagnosis, and to develop a treatment plan to which the patient will adhere. Alopecia is one of the most common reasons that African Americans present to the dermatologist and is addressed elsewhere in this publication.[1,4] Four other common scalp disorders, including tinea capitis, folliculitis, seborrheic dermatitis, and pediculosis capitis, are reviewed here.

TINEA CAPITIS
Overview

Tinea capitis is a common dermatophyte infection seen primarily in children between the ages of 3 and 7 years, but may also be seen in adults. It affects Black and Latinx (Latine) children disproportionately.[5,6] *Trichophyton tonsurans* is the most common cause in the United States, whereas *Microsporum canis* is the most common agent in Europe, Asia, and New Zealand.[6] *M. audouinii* and *Trichophyton soudanense* are common

The authors have no conflicts of interest relevant to this paper. Dr V. Barbosa serves as a consultant and advisory board member for Eli Lilly and Vichy Laboratories and has served on an advisory board for UCB Pharmaceuticals in the last year.

[a] University of Chicago Medicine Section of Dermatology, 5841 South Maryland Avenue, MC5067, L518B, Chicago, IL 60637, USA; [b] University of Chicago Pritzker School of Medicine, 121 West Central Avenue, Maywood, NJ 07607, USA
[1] Present address: 1000 South Clark Street #917, Chicago, IL 60605.
[2] Present address: 810 North Clark Street #605, Chicago, IL 60610.
* Corresponding author.
E-mail address: vbarbosa@uchicago.edu

Dermatol Clin 41 (2023) 539–545
https://doi.org/10.1016/j.det.2023.02.008
0733-8635/23/© 2023 Elsevier Inc. All rights reserved.

culprits in West Africa, and *Trichophyton viola-ceum* and *T soudanense* were commonly found in one study of predominantly African children living in Minnesota.[7–9] Infection due to *Epidermophyton* species is less common.[10]

Clinical Findings and Differential Diagnosis

Tinea capitis may be noninflammatory or inflammatory. Noninflammatory tinea capitis includes both ectothrix and endothrix infections. In ectothrix infection, spores are present on the outside of the hair shaft, and erythematous patches with fine white scales are seen (**Fig. 1**). In some cases, pink patches are present without any scale (**Fig. 2**). "Black dots" representing broken hair shafts may be seen in endothrix infections where the presence of spores inside the hair shaft causes breakage (**Fig. 3**). Tinea infection is often accompanied by alopecia. Inflammatory forms of tinea capitis include kerion which is characterized by inflamed, pus-filled plaques (**Fig. 4**), and favus, which is characterized by thick yellow crusts called scutula.[11]

The differential diagnosis for tinea capitis includes seborrheic dermatitis, psoriasis, alopecia areata, and trichotillomania.[12] The diagnosis is a clinical one. Dermoscopy, potassium hydroxide wet mount, and fungal culture may all be used to aid in diagnosis. Biopsy with microbial staining and tissue culture are rarely needed but remain available for difficult cases.[6,11]

Management

Systemic antifungal medication is needed for the treatment of tinea capitis. Griseofulvin is FDA-approved for adults and children over 2 years of age and remains a first-line treatment of this condition. Per the American Academy of Pediatrics, liver enzyme testing is not required for griseofulvin treatment regimens that are 8 weeks or less, though there is debate in the literature about liver

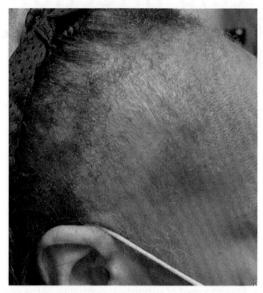

Fig. 2. Tinea capitis with absence of scale in a patient with incidental traction alopecia.

enzyme monitoring necessity and protocol for the other oral antifungal agents.[12] Terbinafine is also a first-line treatment and is FDA-approved for adults and children over 4 years of age. Due to increasing resistance to both griseofulvin and terbenifine, off-label use of fluconazole or itraconazole is used as alternative; both are FDA-approved for use in children but do not have indications for tinea capitis. Topical antifungal shampoos are used by some dermatologists as an adjuvant treatment.[5,6,12]

SCALP FOLLICULITIS
Overview

Folliculitis encompasses a spectrum of diseases distinguished by inflammation of the pilosebaceous

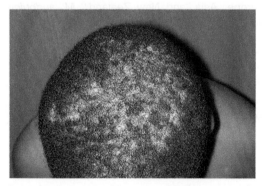

Fig. 1. Tinea capitis. (*Courtesy of* S Stein, MD, Chicago, IL.)

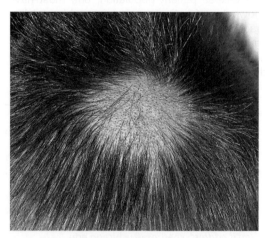

Fig. 3. Tinea capitis with black dots. (*Courtesy of* S Stein, MD, Chicago, IL.)

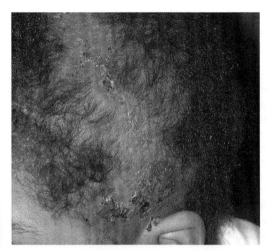

Fig. 4. Kerion. (*Courtesy of* S Stein, MD, Chicago, IL.)

unit.[13] It can occur anywhere on the body except on the palms or soles where there are no hair follicles. There are many types of folliculitis, with common etiologies including both infectious and non-infectious causes. Bacteria, fungi, viruses, and Demodex mites can all cause infectious folliculitis on the body, with *Staphylococcus aureus* being the most frequent causative agent.[14,15] Follicular occlusion, medication, immunosuppression, mechanical trauma, and inflammatory skin diseases may contribute to non-infectious folliculitis.

Although prevalence data are lacking, the scalp is a common location for folliculitis. As with other parts of the body, folliculitis on the scalp is often infectious and most commonly due to *S. aureus*, but may also be caused by *Malassezia* (*Pityrosporum*) species or Demodex mites.[16] Herpes simplex virus type 2 has also been reported as a causative agent on the scalp.[17] Chronic non-scarring scalp folliculitis (CNSF) is another condition that is important to bear in mind. It is less common than infectious folliculitis but should be considered when infectious entities and scarring alopecias have been ruled out. It is considered a neurophilic dermatosis.[13] Finally, eosinophilic pustular folliculitis (EPF) is seen primarily in Japanese women (Ofuji's disease), immunocompromised patients, patients with hematological malignancy, and infants and may occur in the trunk and limbs as well as the scalp.[18]

Clinical Findings and Diagnosis

Follicular papules and pustules are the hallmark of scalp folliculitis. Itching or burning sensations are common symptoms, and scratching may lead to secondary crusting of lesions. Patients may also have associated lymphadenopathy.[13] The differential diagnosis for scalp folliculitis includes several forms of scarring scalp disease, including erosive pustular dermatitis, folliculitis decalvans, lichen planopilaris, and tufted folliculitis.[19]

There are a few studies specifically characterizing non-scarring scalp folliculitis. In a recent retrospective study of 34 patients, all patients were men, with papules and pustules distributed as follows: occipital 80%, vertex 35%, temporal 26%, and parietal 2%. Bacterial cultures were performed on half of the patients, with 70% growing saprophytes and 17.5% showing no growth. The few patients whose cultures were positive grew *S aureus* (one patient) and *S. epidermitis* (one patient). Ten patients received biopsies; all showed neutrophilic folliculitis. Four specimens demonstrated *Malassezia* spores and one showed the presence of *Demodex folliculorum*. Two previous studies showed similar findings, with male sex predominance in 44 out of 48 subjects in one study and men outnumbering women 3:1 in the other. The occipital scalp was the most common area of involvement in all studies.[20]

Differentiation between infectious folliculitis, CNSF, and EPF should be made to help guide treatment. Appropriate diagnostic studies include a bacterial swab for gram stain and culture, a potassium hydroxide (KOH) preparation or fungal culture, and a Tzanck smear, viral culture or viral pcr. CNSF and EPF should be considered when infectious causes have been ruled out. In difficult-to-diagnose or recalcitrant cases, a skin biopsy can be considered.[21]

Management

Mild cases of folliculitis may demonstrate spontaneous resolution without treatment. Topical treatments can be used for mild to moderate infections. Bacterial folliculitis can be treated with mupirocin, topical clindamycin, retapamulin, or fusidic acid. *Malassezia* can be treated with topical azoles or selenium sulfide. Oral therapy is required for moderate to severe cases of infectious folliculitis. Dicloxacillin and cephalexin are utilized for methicillin-sensitive *S. aureus*, and doxycycline, trimethoprim-sulfamethoxazole, or clindamycin are preferred for methicillin-resistant *S. aureus*. Ciprofloxacin is the treatment of choice for pseudomonas. Oral azoles can be used for *Malassezia* and *Candida* folliculitis.[21]

Treatment recommendations for CNSF include oral doxycycline 100 mg twice daily for 3 months. Treatment with clindamycin plus rifampin has also been reported.[13] If relapse occurs after antibiotic therapy, isotretinoin 10 mg daily can be given for 3 months, then tapering to the lowest dose needed to maintain remission for 6 months before discontinuing treatment.[20] There is a case report of treatment success with adalimumab.[13] EPF can be treated with topical tacrolimus, oral indomethacin, or cyclosporin.[18]

SEBORRHEIC DERMATITIS
Overview

Seborrheic dermatitis is a chronic inflammatory skin condition that affects highly sebaceous areas on the scalp, face, and body. The prevalence in the general population is estimated to range from 3% to 12%, and the condition is particularly common in people of African descent, with prevalence estimates of 6.5% in African Americans and 2.9% to 6% in West Africans.[22] It is noted to be one of the most common reasons for Black patients to visit the dermatologist, and these patients tend to have more flaking than patients of other races.[1] The three main factors implicated in the development of seborrheic dermatitis include (1) increased sebum lipid concentration with elevated tryglicerides and cholesterol and decreased free fatty acids and squalenes; (2) increased density of Malassezia species on the skin; and (3) the host's immunologic response.[23] Immunosuppressed patients, such as those with human immunodefieicncy virus (HIV) infection, experience seborrheic dermatitis at rates as high as 83%.[22]

Clinical Findings and Diagnosis

Seborrheic dermatitis has a clinical presentation that consists of erythematous patches with yellow, greasy scales (Fig. 5). The most common areas involved are those with a high density of sebaceous glands. This include the scalp, anterior hairline, eyebrows, glabella, alar grooves, nasolabial folds, beard region, chest, and upper back.[24] It is important to note that in patients with skin of color, hypopigmentation is often appreciated in involved areas. Petaloid seborrheic dermatitis, characterized by coalescing, polycyclic erythematous or hypopigmented patches or plaques with minimal

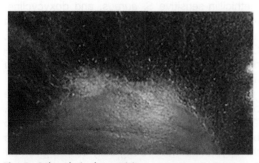

Fig. 5. Seborrheic dermatitis.

scale usually at the anterior hairline or on the face, is another presentation seen in skin of color.[22]

The differential diagnosis for seborrheic dermatitis includes atopic dermatitis, contact dermatitis, nummular dermatitis, psoriasis, tinea capitis, pediculosis, and rosacea. Psoriasis is perhaps the most common of these conditions the clinician must differentiate, and usually features a finer, white or silvery scale in contrast to the thicker yellow scale of seborrheic dermatitis.[23] Diagnosis is usually made clinically and can be assisted by dermoscopy, patch testing, and/or a biopsy. Histopathology demonstrates parakeratosis in the epidermis, spongiosis, and plugged follicular ostia with the presence of neutrophils.[25]

Management

The treatment of seborrheic dermatitis is targeted toward reducing Malassezia and controlling inflammation. There are several treatment options available, and specific medication choice varies based on area of involvement and grooming habits of the patient. The foundation of treatment is the use of an antifungal agent, with addition of either a topical steroid or calcineurin inhibitor for additional benefit. Treatment on the face and body is usually managed by the use of antifungal creams such as ketoconazole, metronidazole, or other azoles, or ciclopirox. These may be used in conjunction with a low-potency topical steroid, pimecrolimus cream, or tacrolimus ointment. Oral antifungal agents may be indicated for particularly severe or resistant cases.[26]

Treatment of seborrheic dermatitis on the scalp utilizes the same medications as the treatment on the face and body, but often with different vehicles and with different frequencies. Patients may try over-the-counter shampoos containing selenium sulfide, zinc pyrithione, or ketoconazole 1%. Shampoos containing ketoconazole 2% or ciclopirox are the mainstays of professional treatment.[26] Ketoconazole may also be used in foam form, as some patients report having a higher rate of satisfaction when compared with the shampoo users.[22] The addition of a topical steroid may occur in the form of a shampoo containing either clobetasol or fluocinolone, or with any topical steroid, with solution, foam, oil, or ointment formulations usually selected for scalp use. Vehicle choice may be offered to the patient for increased compliance.

Caring for patients with highly textured hair, particularly those of African descent, requires an understanding of the patient's normal grooming habits so that treatment can be adjusted to fit within the patient's routine. Shampooing may normally occur once per week, every other week, or less frequently. Patients should be encouraged to shampoo a minimum of every other week to maintain control of seborrheic dermatitis and increasing frequency to once per week may be necessary. Also, antifungal shampoos can be drying to the hair. This is particularly true of ketoconazole shampoo.[1] Patients should be counseled to apply the shampoo to the scalp but not to lather the hair with the product to minimize the drying effect and resulting hair breakage that sometimes results.

PEDICULOSIS CAPITIS
Overview

Pediculus humanus capitus, also known as the head louse, is a wingless insect. An ectoparasite, it feeds on the blood of its human host. Transmission of the head louse is primarily via direct contact, but they can also be spread through sharing of items such as hats, brushes, or combs. Infestation with head lice is common; the Centers for Disease Control estimates that there are 6 to 12 million cases of pediculosis capitis each year in the United States, occurring primarily in children ages 3 to 11 years and their close contact. They also report a higher prevalence in girls and a lower prevalence in African Americans.[27] The worldwide prevalence of head lice is estimated to be 19%.[28] Falagas and colleagues evaluated literature published from 2000 to 2008 to characterize the worldwide rates of the condition; they noted prevalence ranges as follows: Asia 0.7% to 59%; Europe 0.48% to 22.4%; Africa 0% to 58.9%; the Americas 3.6% to 61.4%; Oceania 13%. It is important to note that many of the African studies were from Egypt where people's hair tends to be less curly than in other African countries. In South Africa, cases of head lice were found only among White children but not among Black children.[29] The reason for decreased prevalence in African and African American populations is not known; hypotheses include the shape of the highly curled, elliptical hair shafts impeding lice from attaching or factors relating to styling products such as gels, pomades, or relaxers.[30]

Clinical Findings and Diagnosis

The primary symptom that people with head lice experience is an itch which represents a delayed hypersensitivity reaction.[31] Diagnosis is usually easily made by examining the scalp and hair for eggs (nits), small nymphs, and adult lice. Head lice may be found behind the ears or at the posterior neck in addition to the scalp so these areas should be examined thoroughly. A fine-toothed comb is often used both to aid in the examination

and for nit removal.[32] The American Academy of Pediatrics guidelines note that finding a live insect is the gold standard for diagnosis, however, this can be challenging because they crawl quickly. Nits identified within 1 cm of the scalp are considered viable, are easier to see and are hence quite useful to aid in diagnosis. Nits can remain on the hair shaft for several months, even after successful treatment, so overtreatment should be minimized by recognizing that nits farther from the scalp do not constitute active infestation.[28,33] Because lice and nits are not hard to find, this diagnosis is often made by parents or other caretakers at home. In the dermatology office, a Wood's light may be used to aid in visualization.

It is important to note that other organisms can infest the scalp and should remain on the differential. Pubic lice may be found on the scalp and can be differentiated on microscopic examination by their round body shape. Scabies may also occur on the scalp. Also on the differential are product debris, seborrheic dermatitis, and hair casts (pseudonyms). Dermoscopy can help differentiate these conditions.

Management

Effective treatments for head lice are available over-the-counter (OTC). Permethrin 1% is a synthetic pyrethrin that is sold under several brand names and is perhaps the most frequently used treatment. However, resistance to this medication is a growing concern globally, but fortunately, several other options are available. Topical ivermectin 0.5% offers an additional OTC alternative.[28] OTC product instructions require the use of nit comb; a recent publication points out that nit comb use is not well suited for highly curly hair, and nor is it required after pediculicidal treatment.[30]

Patients have often tried and failed OTC treatments before presenting to the dermatologist. Prescription medications that are FDA-approved and commonly used include abametapir 0.74%, benzyl alcohol 5%, malathione 0.5%, and spinosad 0.9%. It is important to note that although lindane 1% is FDA-approved for the treatment of tinea capitis, it is rarely used due to the risk of neurotoxicity. Dimeticone lotion 4% is an occlusive silicone oil that has demonstrated efficacy in vitro and in vivo but is not currently approved as a pediculicide by the FDA.[28,34]

Permethrin and benzyl alcohol are not ovicidal. Hence, treatment with these agents must be repeated after 7 to 10 days. Malathion is partially ovicidal, hence, repeat treatment is sometimes necessary after 7 to 10 days. All other treatments listed are ovicidal such that one treatment is normally sufficient.

SUMMARY

There are many common scalp diseases that manifest in patients of color. Although diagnosis and management of several common diseases have been discussed here, it is important to reiterate the importance of being knowledgeable about hair care and hair styling practices so that the clinician can gain the patient's trust and obtain a proper history. Journal articles by Roseborogh and colleagues and Bosley and colleagues provide excellent overviews of these hair care practices.[35,36] Grayson and colleagues provide a roadmap to examining the scalp of patients with tightly coiled hair.[37] Combining dermatologic expertise with cultural awareness and humility is the combination needed to successfully treat a diverse population of patients.

CLINICS CARE POINTS

- Tinea capitis requires treatment with systemic antifungal medication; griveofulvin and terbenifine are first line treatments for adults and for children over two and four years of age, respectively.

- It is important to identify the type of scalp folliculitis a patient has, whether infectious, chronic non scarring, or eosinophillic pustular folliculitis, in order to guide treamtent decisions.

- Seborrheic dermatitis is best treated with a combination of an antifungal agent and an anti-inflammatory agent such as a topical steroid or calcineurin inhibitor; vehicle selection varies based on disease location and patient preference.

- Pediculosis capitis is less common in African and African American patients but should remain on the differential for patients with scalp itch; several treatment options are available.

REFERENCES

1. Taylor SC, Barbosa V, Burgess C, et al. Hair and scalp disorders in adult and pediatric patients with skin of color. Cutis 2017 Jul;100(1):31–5. PMID: 28873105.
2. Salam A, Aryiku S, Dadzie OE. Hair and scalp disorders in women of African descent: an overview. Br J Dermatol 2013 Oct;169(Suppl 3):19–32.
3. Richmond HM, Duvic M, Macfarlane DF. Primary and metastatic malignant tumors of the scalp: an update. Am J Clin Dermatol 2010;11(4):233–46.
4. Alexis AF, Sergay AB, Taylor SC. Common dermatologic disorders in skin of color: a comparative practice survey. Cutis 2007 Nov;80(5):387–94. PMID: 18189024.
5. Leung AKC, Hon KL, Leong KF, et al. Tinea Capitis: An Updated Review. Recent Pat Inflamm Allergy Drug Discov 2020;14(1):58–68.
6. Mitchell KN, Tay YK, Heath CR, et al. Review article: Emerging issues in pediatric skin of color, part 1. Pediatr Dermatol 2021 Nov;38(Suppl 2):20–9. Epub 2021 Oct 18. PMID: 34664330.
7. Emele FE, Oyeka CA. Tinea capitis among primary school children in Anambra state of Nigeria. Mycoses 2008 Nov;51(6):536–41. Epub 2008 Apr 16. PMID: 18422917.
8. Fulgence KK, Abibatou K, Vincent D, et al. Tinea capitis in schoolchildren in southern Ivory Coast. Int J Dermatol 2013 Apr;52(4):456–60. PMID: 23432109.
9. Grigoryan KV, Tollefson MM, Olson MA, et al. Pediatric tinea capitis caused by Trichophyton violaceum and Trichophyton soudanense in Rochester, Minnesota, United States. Int J Dermatol 2019 Aug;58(8): 912–5. Epub 2018 Dec 13. PMID: 30548845.
10. Romano C. Case reports. Four paediatric cases of tinea capitis due to unusual agents. Mycoses 1999;42(5–6):421–5.
11. Gupta AK, Hofstader SL, Adam P, et al. Tinea capitis: an overview with emphasis on management. Pediatr Dermatol 1999 May-Jun;16(3):171–89.
12. Gupta AK, Friedlander SF, Simkovich AJ. Tinea capitis: An update. Pediatr Dermatol 2022 Mar;39(2): 167–72. Epub 2022 Jan 24. PMID: 35075666.
13. Soglia S, Maione V, Bugatti M, et al. Adalimumab for interleukin-1β-mediated chronic non-scarring scalp folliculitis: Case report and literature review. J Dermatol 2022 Jan;49(1):157–60. Epub 2021 Sep 2. PMID: 34472127.
14. Herman LE, Harawi SJ, Ghossein RA, et al. Folliculitis. A clinicopathologic review. Pathol Annu 1991; 26 Pt 2:201–46.
15. Jang KA, Kim SH, Choi JH, et al. Viral folliculitis on the face. Br J Dermatol 2000;142(3):555–9. https://doi.org/10.1046/j.1365-2133.2000.03378.x.
16. Sanfilippo AM, English JC 3rd. Resistant scalp folliculitis secondary to Demodex infestation. Cutis 2005 Nov;76(5):321–4. PMID: 16422467.
17. Foti C, Calvario A, d'Ovidio R, et al. Recalcitrant scalp folliculitis: a possible role of herpes simplex virus type 2. New Microbiol 2005;28(2):157–9. PMID: 16035261.
18. Marzano AV, Genovese G. Eosinophilic Dermatoses: Recognition and Management. Am J Clin Dermatol 2020;21(4):525–39.

19. Lugović-Mihić L, Barisić F, Bulat V, et al. Differential diagnosis of the scalp hair folliculitis. Acta Clin Croat 2011 Sep;50(3):395–402. PMID: 22384776.

20. Romero-Maté A, Arias-Palomo D, Hernández-Núñez A, et al. Chronic nonscarring scalp folliculitis: Retrospective case series study of 34 cases. J Am Acad Dermatol 2019 Oct;81(4):1023–4. Epub 2019 Mar 11. PMID: 30872152.

21. Jackson JD. Infectious folliculitis. In: Rosen T, Ofori A, editors. *UpToDate*. Waltham, mass. UpTo-Date; 2022. https://www.uptodate.com/contents/infectious-folliculitis. Accessed November 10, 2022.

22. Elgash M, Dlova N, Ogunleye T, et al. Seborrheic Dermatitis in Skin of Color: Clinical Considerations. J Drugs Dermatol 2019;18(1):24–7.

23. Shamloul G, Khachemoune A. An updated review of the sebaceous gland and its role in health and diseases Part 2: Pathophysiological clinical disorders of sebaceous glands. Dermatol Ther 2021;34(2): e14862. https://doi.org/10.1111/dth.14862.

24. Gupta AK, Batra R, Bluhm R, et al. Skin diseases associated with Malassezia species. J Am Acad Dermatol 2004;51(5):785–98. https://doi.org/10.1016/j.jaad.2003.12.034.

25. Park JH, Park YJ, Kim SK, et al. Histopathological Differential Diagnosis of Psoriasis and Seborrheic Dermatitis of the Scalp. Ann Dermatol 2016;28(4): 427–32. https://doi.org/10.5021/ad.2016.28.4.427.

26. Clark GW, Pope SM, Jaboori KA. Diagnosis and Treatment of Seborrheic Dermatitis. afp 2015;91(3): 185–90.

27. Head lice epidemiology & risk factors. Centers for Disease Control. 2019. Available at: https://www.cdc.gov/parasites/lice/head/epi.html. Acessed November 10, 2022.

28. Ogbuefi N, Kenner-Bell B. Common pediatric infestations: update on diagnosis and treatment of scabies, head lice, and bed bugs. Curr Opin Pediatr 2021;33(4):410–5. PMID: 34074914.

29. Falagas ME, Matthaiou DK, Rafailidis PI, et al. Worldwide prevalence of head lice. Emerg Infect Dis 2008;14(9):1493–4.

30. Shea LA, Lourenço Freitas E, Nguyen T, et al. Over-the-counter Pediculus humanus capitis treatment: The nit comb is not appropriate for all hair types. J Am Pharm Assoc (2003) 2022. S1544-3191(22) 00306-5.

31. Gunning K, Kiraly B, Pippitt K. Lice and Scabies: Treatment Update. Am Fam Physician 2019;99(10): 635–42. PMID: 31083883.

32. Nolt D, Moore S, Yan AC, et al, COMMITTEE ON IN-FECTIOUS DISEASES. Committee on practice and ambulatory medicine, section on dermatology. Head Lice. Pediatrics. 2022;150(4). e2022059282. PMID: 36156158.

33. Frankowski BL. American Academy of Pediatrics guidelines for the prevention and treatment of head lice infestation. Am J Manag Care 2004;10(9 Suppl):S269–72. PMID: 15515631.

34. Woods AD, Porter CL, Feldman SR. Abametapir for the Treatment of Head Lice: A Drug Review. Ann Pharmacother 2022;56(3):352–7. PMID: 34157881.

35. Roseborough IE, McMichael AJ. Hair care practices in African-American patients. Semin Cutan Med Surg 2009;28(2):103–8.

36. Bosley RE, Daveluy S. A primer to natural hair care practices in black patients. Cutis 2015;95(2): 78–80, 106. PMID: 25750968.

37. Grayson C, Heath C. An Approach to Examining Tightly Coiled Hair Among Patients With Hair Loss in Race-Discordant Patient-Physician Interactions. JAMA Dermatol 2021;157(5):505–6. PMID: 33787820.

Cosmetic Enhancement Updates and Pitfalls in Patients of Color

Kamaria Nelson, MHS, MD[a], Janaya Nelson, MS[b], Tiara Bradley, BS[b], Cheryl Burgess, MD[c],*

KEYWORDS

- Patients of color • Cosmetic enhancements • Lasers • Neurotoxins • Body contouring
- Soft tissue augmentation

KEY POINTS

- Patients of color (POC) are seeking out cosmetic enhancements and treatments through utilization of light-based devices, body contouring, skin tightening, neurotoxins, and soft tissue augmentation.
- Adverse events can occur with any cosmetic treatment; therefore, it is important to inform POC of these potential risks.
- Shared decision-making between the patient and dermatologist should be used to determine the desired cosmetic outcomes.
- Minimizing risks of cosmetic procedures involves understanding the skin's structural, functional, and biological differences of patients with different cultural and ethnic backgrounds.

INTRODUCTION

Skin of color (SOC) in dermatology encompasses individuals of various ethnic backgrounds including Black or those of African descent, Hispanic or Latino, Asian, Native American, Pacific Islander, and those of mixed ethnicities.[1] Because these populations continue to expand, more patients of color (POC) are seeking out cosmetic enhancements and treatments. Due to skin structural, functional, and biological differences, POC have unique cosmetic concerns compared with individuals with lighter phenotypes.[2] POC often pursue treatment of pigmentary changes, such as, hyperpigmentation or hypopigmentation, and antiaging remedies. Aside from cosmeceuticals, nonsurgical cosmetic rejuvenation options, such laser and light-based treatments, neurotoxins, soft tissue augmentation, and more recently body contouring and skin tightening, are becoming increasingly popular worldwide,

including in this population. Although these procedures are becoming more common, it is important to understand the risks and benefits associated with each treatment, particularly in patients with darker skin types. In a 2021 review, authors found that POC were at an increased risk for keloid formation, postoperative infections, postinflammatory hyperpigmentation (PIH), and postinflammatory hypopigmentation following cosmetic procedures.[3] This article examines risks of cosmetic enhancement procedures in POC and best practices to prevent adverse events.

Laser and Energy-Based Devices

Light-based devices include ablative, nonablative and resurfacing lasers, flashlamps, including intense pulse light, as well as radiofrequency (RF) and photodynamic therapy. POC are commonly seeking light-based devices for reduction of unwanted hair, disorders of

[a] Department of Dermatology, The George Washington School of Medicine and Health Sciences, 2311 M Street NW, Suite 504 Washington, DC 20037, USA; [b] Meharry Medical College, Nashville, TN, USA; [c] Center for Dermatology and Dermatologic Surgery, Washington, DC, USA
* Corresponding author.
E-mail address: cheryl.burgess@ctr4dermatology.com

Dermatol Clin 41 (2023) 547–555
https://doi.org/10.1016/j.det.2023.02.011
0733-8635/23/© 2023 Elsevier Inc. All rights reserved.

derm.theclinics.com

hyperpigmentation, including melasma and PIH, and acne scars.[2]

When treating disorders of hyperpigmentation with laser, longer wavelengths are typically safer in POC because they penetrate deeper and are more selective to dermal melanocytes.[4–6] Lasers found to be safer in darker skin tones include Q Switched Neodymium:Yttrium Aluminum Garnet-1064 nm (QS Nd:YAG 1064 nm), QS Nd:YAG (532 nm), and QS Alexandrite (755 nm).[4,5] Although the QS Ruby (694 nm) can be used in darker skin tones, there is a higher risk of severe and permanent adverse events due to its excessive absorption by melanin.[5] The QS Nd:YAG is most broadly used in POC with most needing 5 to 10 treatment sessions.[7,8] Common settings are a fluence less than 5 J/cm^2, spot size 6 mm, and frequency of 10 Hz.[5] Additionally, the 650 microsecond 1064 laser can be used to treat melasma, acne, PIH, pseudofolliculitis barbae, acne keloidalis nuchae, and aging in POC.[9] Adverse events include mottled hypopigmentation, erythema, recurrence, and rebound hyperpigmentation.[4,5] To reduce the risk of side effects, it is recommended to extend time between treatments to more than a week and to avoid too many treatment sessions (>6–10). It is also recommended to pretreat and posttreat with a topical lightning agents such as hydroquinone, practice strict sun avoidance, and perform test spots before full treatment to minimize rebound hyperpigmentation.[2,10] Use of cooling devices is also paramount in preventing unwanted side effects.

There are several devices used to remove unwanted hair including long-pulsed Nd:YAG laser, pulsed diode laser, alexandrite laser, and thulium laser. Although other devices can be used for hair removal, long-pulsed Nd:YAG is often the preferred choice in POC given the absorption spectrum of melanin and general tolerability of the procedure. Before treatment with any device, it is recommended to avoid shaving the area 1 week prior, no plucking or waxing, practice sun avoidance, and proper cooling during treatment.[2] After the treatment, again it is important to have proper cooling of the area, sun avoidance, photoprotection, and immediate postprocedural cooling.[2]

Both ablative and nonablative lasers can be used to treat atrophic acne scars. Ablative lasers include the 10,600 nm CO_2 laser and the 2940 nm Er:YAG. PIH is a common complication of the CO_2 laser in darker phototypes; however, the average duration of PIH is 5 weeks and can be treated with hydroquinone.[11] Other side effects include erythema and swelling, which are temporary.[12] Fractional Er:YAG has fewer side effects compared with the CO_2 laser with similar clinical outcomes.[11] PIH can also be seen in darker complexions but occurs less frequently than with CO_2 lasers. Fractional ablative lasers, such as 1550 nm Er-doped laser and 1540 nm Er:glass, have lower side effects and can be used for acne scarring in POC; however, caution is still warranted.

Nonablative nonfractional lasers used in acne scarring include the 1064 nm QS Nd:YAG, 1065 nm-pulsed dye laser (PDL), and the 1320 Nd:YAG nm laser. For POC, the 1064 nm Nd:YAG is most frequently used to treat mild-to-moderate acne scarring with good clinical outcomes.[2,12] Appropriate cooling and strict sun protection should be used to prevent PIH.

Body Contouring

Most body contouring procedures aim to reconstruct an area of the body into a desired shape or size. It may involve procedures to eliminate extra skin, excess fat, or contour a designated area. Body contouring consists of surgical and nonsurgical procedures. The types of body contouring include cryolipolysis, injection lipolysis (deoxycholic acid [DCA]), laser lipolysis, RF, ultrasound lipolysis, abdominoplasty, and liposuction to name a few. These treatments have fewer side effects, quicker recoveries, and can address difficult areas such as the submentum and abdomen compared with surgical options. In cryolipolysis, fat cells are preferentially destroyed by a controlled thermal reduction, which can be used to treat focal fat deposits in the flanks, abdomen, and thighs.[13] Injection lipolysis is a minimally invasive, targeted, fat reduction alternative that can be customized to the patient's level and area of fat accumulation. One example of this uses DCA, an adipocytolytic component of human bile acid.[14] Laser lipolysis is based on a thermal effect and can stimulate the formation of collagen, enhancing skin elasticity and promoting skin contraction in the treated areas.[15] In addition to fat reduction, RF devices can also tighten the overlying skin. The novel combination of RF with epidermal cooling allows for skin tightening without epidermal ablation and prolonged downtime.[16] The abdominoplasty, commonly referred to as a "tummy tuck," is a procedure to reduce excess skin and fat around the abdomen and strengthen the abdominal wall musculature.[17] Liposuction is mainly used to correct deep and superficial fat accumulations and remodel the body contour. It is important to emphasize that liposuction alone cannot eliminate the tendency to accumulate fluids and fat tissue; therefore, it must always be associated with conservative therapies and lymphatic flow regeneration.[18,19]

Although injection lipolysis with the use of DCA mainly affects fat cells, it is relatively nonselective and can lyse muscle and other adjacent nonfatty tissues. DCA treatment is associated with transient side effects such as injection site pain, erythema, ecchymosis, and numbness.[14] High-intensity focused ultrasound (HIFU) has been found to produce nonselective cell necrosis.[14] In rare cases, erythematous papules, papular urticaria, first-degree burns, blisters, and bruising have all been reported with direct contact devices; however, these adverse events, which are generally mild and self-limited, are more likely to be associated with operator error, such as excessively slow movement of the handpiece.[16]

One of the most important methods of preventing pitfalls with body contouring is to take an accurate and extensive medical history to ensure the success of procedures and quality of recovery. If patients are concerned with the adverse outcomes of surgical body contouring, they may pursue nonsurgical body sculpting instead. The advantages of noninvasive body sculpting are decreased procedure time and downtime after treatment, as well as higher safety with minimal adverse events.[20]

Skin Tightening

Skin tightening methods have been used invasively and noninvasively to treat facial, neck, and body skin sagging, laxity, wrinkles, and cellulite. Initially rhytidectomy served as an invasive face-lift procedure; but with advances, subfascial dissection of the anatomic superficial musculoaponeurotic system overtook the technique despite the efficacy of the procedure and excisional nature of the surgery that included visible scars.[21] More recently, noninvasive skin-tightening methods have increased in demand due to faster recovery time and decreased risk. These methods include laser therapy, RF, and microfocused ultrasound (MFUS), which aim to elevate temperatures in the deep layers of the skin.[22] At approximately 65°C, skin tightening occurs by shortening the collagen fibers and preserving heat-stable intermolecular hydrogen bonds, leading to an increase in elastic properties and stimulation of new collagen.[22]

Transcutaneous thermogenesis, which administers RF directly to the dermal and subdermal tissue, includes traditional ablative and fractional ablative laser skin rejuvenation, HIFU, and MFUS. Traditional ablative lasers use CO_2 or erbium to ablate the epidermis off the dermis, forming a partially coagulated area in the dermis and initiating wound healing through neocollagenesis and remodeling. The traditional ablative laser offers a lengthy healing period and the possibility of delayed dyspigmentation; therefore, this method particularly in POC is less frequently used. Fractional ablative laser is an alternative to traditional ablative and generates deeply narrow focal ablations of the dermis and epidermis, allowing for rapid-epithelization and dermal remodeling. In SOC patients, there is a greater risk of dyspigmentation and scarring, requiring careful selection of device and treatment parameters to minimize risks. PIH was observed in up to 40% and 92% of nonablative and ablative fractional laser-treated patients, with the highest incidence in patients with Fitzpatrick skin type V.[23] To prevent unwanted side effects, remaining in the recommended range of energy as well as allowing time for skin cooling in between passes is a preferred strategy.[23]

Introduced in 2009, MFUS offers precision-focused thermal injury zones at therapeutic depths that delivers deep heat energy into the superficial dermis and subdermal connective tissue to induce a greater collagen remodeling.[24] MFU with a high-resolution ultrasound imaging (MFU-V) allows visualization of tissue planes to 8 mm deep and allows users to see where MFU energy will be applied. With MFU-V, one can also customize to meet unique physical characteristics of each patient by adjusting energy and focal depth of the emitted ultrasound (Fig. 1). Adverse effects of MFU treatments for all skin types include brief discomfort during the treatment session, transient erythema, edema, and occasional bruising; it is also best suited for patients with mild-to-moderate skin and soft tissue laxity.[21] Wheals can also appear due to poor treatment technique or use of 3 mm and 1.5 mm transducers.[24] To prevent procedural discomfort, oral acetaminophen or nonsteroidal anti-inflammatory drugs (NSAIDs) such as ibuprofen should be taken and applying treatment with lowest energy setting should be carried out.

RF devices are also used for skin tightening through warming the dermis and subcutaneous tissues to 42°C, which stimulates dermal collagen remodeling and neocollagenesis 4 to 6 weeks after treatment.[22] It also improves skin laxity and wrinkles by long-term stimulation of elastin and can overall improve contours on the face and body. Adverse effects include slight burning sensation and mild erythema that resolved within 1 hour after treatment, hypertrophic scarring, transient PIH, and pain.[22] To prevent, using the lowest energy

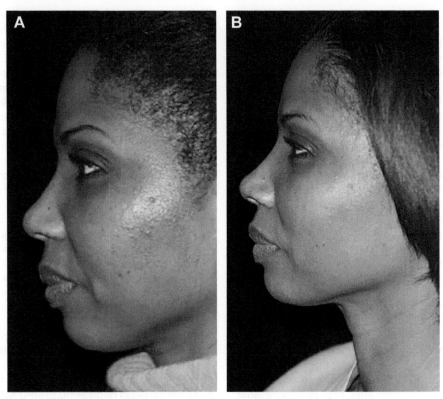

Fig. 1. Before and after microfocused ultrasound. Before 4 months (*A*) and after (*B*).

setting and conducting the procedure in short intervals to reduce pain should be done.

Neurotoxins

Neurotoxins have been commonly used to treat lines of facial expression in POC. Glabellar lines specifically are a sign of aging and can display negative emotions due to the movements of underlying muscles, corrugator superciliaris, and/or procerus muscles.[25] Botulinum toxin type A (BTX-A) has been approved by the US Food and Drug Administration (FDA) to treat frown lines and crow's feet and acts by inhibiting the release of acetylcholine into the synaptic cleft by paralyzing muscle temporarily. There are 4 different FDA-approved neurotoxins that contain the same ingredient, BTX-A: onabotulinumtoxinA, abobotulinumtoxinA, prabotulinumtoxinA, incobotulinumA, and daxibotulinumA. All are approved to treat glabellar lines, yet onabotulinumtoxinA is the only FDA-approved treatment of lateral canthal lines and forehead frontalis lines. Frequent sites of injection include the corrugator, crow's feet, forehead, platysmal neckbands, and the marionette lines (**Fig. 2**). Adverse effects include minor bruising with injection, headache, and injection-site reactions.[26] Less common adverse effects include temporary blepharoptosis and eyebrow ptosis, which are technique-independent.[27] To prevent headache, acetaminophen and/or NSAIDs before treatment and after should be administered. To prevent blepharoptosis and eyebrow ptosis, proper training and technique should be practiced.

SOC patients seek cosmetic procedures for intrinsic and extrinsic aging and dyschromias, scar formation, and hypertrichosis.[28] In POC, the texture and elasticity differ as well as the amount of subcutaneous fat. Asian populations have a greater incidence of masseter hypertrophy and with injections of BoNT-A into the masseters, it lowers facial contouring, producing an improvement in bruxism and reestablishing the triangular-shaped face of youth.[29] Limitations may include smiling and reduced chewing strength. Some studies have shown differences in responses to BTX-A, which include the response rate 30 days after treatment being greater in POC than in White patients.[30] Therefore, there is a more conservative dosing when treating POC, specifically of Asian origin. Identifying the line of convergence (C-line) through bidirectional movement in the forehead is particularly important in Asian populations in order to prevent eyebrow ptosis.[31] Adverse event rates, tolerability, and

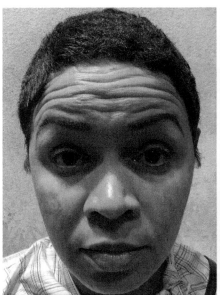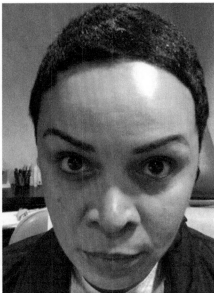

Fig. 2. Before and after botulinum toxin A on the frontalis and glabella in a 41-year-old woman.

effectiveness of treatment were similar in POC and White patients.[30]

Soft Tissue Augmentation/Fillers

Facial anatomy, cultural preferences, ideals of beauty, and characteristics of aging, which vary widely between POC and differ from westernized beauty standards, are primary considerations in the selection and administration of soft tissue fillers in POC and the ultimate satisfaction of POC (Fig. 3). For example, although some anatomic features of the African American face include bimaxillary protrusion, increased midfacial soft tissue, and increased lip prominence, anatomic features of the Asian face include a flatter malar prominence and midface, wider and rounder face, and protuberant lips.[28] Generally, midface aging is a common focal point for soft tissue augmentation, specifically the descent of the malar fat pad, the loss of volume in the oral commissures and lips, the prominence of nasolabial folds, infraorbital hollowing, and temporal fossa hollowing.

The overall structure of the Asian face is wide and short, creating a wider bitemporal, bizygomatic, and bigonial width compared with Caucasians. Although this skeletal width tends to form a more effective scaffolding to support tissue with age, female Asian patients may view a wide lower face as unfavorable.[32] Ideally, an oval-shaped face is preferred for women in both Asian and Western countries. Asian women strive toward an inverted egg-like shape. Facial injectables can assist in creating the "inverted egg" shape while creating a fuller upper half of the face with a narrowing transition from the cheek to the chin.[32] Some of the common facial filler treatment areas in Asian patients include the midface (ie, the nose, medial maxilla, tear trough, nasolabial fold), brow, and chin.[32] Additionally, the midface is often one of the first areas to show signs of aging in African American patients. The smooth transition from periocular skin to malar skin becomes interrupted with age and produces a double convexity. This shape is the result of several factors including the loss of the malar bony eminence, the loss of medial cheek fat, and the sagging of resilient but thick and heavy skin. Practically, this leads to scleral show, infraorbital shadowing, and accentuation of the nasolabial folds. Placement of volumizing filler should be performed with the intent of correcting these changes if present.[32]

It is also important to note that the lower face and neck in African American patients can sag and produce jowls with age. The skin retains its elasticity; however, it can buckle under its weight. Filler injections that globally aid in the support of superior structures may be of assistance for these skin changes.[32] Facial filler use in Latinos also requires addressing the midface. Although variable lip proportions and fewer perioral rhytids have been reported in POC compared with Whites, in African Americans in particular, lip enhancement is still sought after, despite the misconception that these patients have full lips.[28] Similar to African American patients, Latinos often lose the transition of periocular skin to malar skin and exhibit

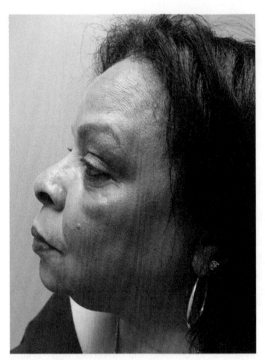

Fig. 3. A 74-year-old woman with cheek festooning and midface volume loss.

double convexity with aging. It may result in infraorbital shadowing and accentuation of the nasolabial folds. Proper placement of facial filler should support any skeletal or facial fat loss in this area.[32]

A variety of filler materials are currently available and have been used for facial soft tissue augmentation. Soft tissue augmentation with dermal fillers have been used in the treatment and correction of fine lines; nasolabial folds; marionette lines; tear trough deformities; lip, cheek, chin, and hand augmentation; volume loss; and acne scars.[1] Hyaluronic acid (HA) derivatives, and biostimulating fillers such calcium hydroxylapatite gel (CaHa) and poly-L-lactic acid (PLLA) are common injectables for facial and body enhancement.[33] Volumizing with an array of dermal fillers with different properties can improve esthetic outcomes in SOC patients (**Fig. 4**). Injectable PLLA and CaHa are both biodegradable and biocompatible fillers. Once injected into the deep dermis, PLLA and CaHa cause collagenesis, producing a gradual fibroblastic scaffold resulting in significant increase in skin thickness while improving the appearance of folds and sunken areas. With proper patient selection and administration techniques, PLLA and CaHa have been used effectively in patients with SOC.[1]

Adverse events to soft tissue augmentation can occur in all patients and include bruising, tenderness, edema, redness, itching, pain, and hyperpigmentation, all with limited duration. In addition, asymmetry because of placement error, contour irregularities, paresthesia, and vascular compromise, including retinal branch artery occlusion ultimately causing vision loss, have been described.[28] In POC, the primary adverse concerns are hyperpigmentation, hypopigmentation, and hemosiderin deposition associated with bruising. As in African American patients, Asian skin is more prone to pigmentation and keloid formation following procedures. Both ethnicities tend to have thicker skin with more pigment, fibroblasts, and collagen relative to Caucasian skin.[32] When particulate HA fillers are inappropriately implanted into the superficial dermis or epidermis, they cause a bluish hue referred to as the "Tyndall effect."[34] The bluish color results from light reflection from particles contained in a clear material (filler). When the light is scattered from these particles, a bluish hue can result. This is most seen in the treatment of the lower eyelid.[1] If not corrected, superficial product has been commonly observed to last for very long periods, even years. The rate of dyschromia was found to be similar between Caucasian and non-Caucasian patients, with no pigmentary changes being observed in patients treated with CaHa.[1] Acute infections, which seem as acute inflammation or abscesses at the site of injection, are typically due to common pathogens present on the skin such as *Staphylococcus aureus* or *Streptococcus pyogenes*.[34]

Bruising can persist for 10 to 14 days. It may be treated with, arnica, aloe vera, or vitamin K creams and light and energy devices such as PDL and 660-nm red light. The risk of bruising may be reduced by injecting the filler slowly. If bruising appears, it can be reduced by pressing with a compress (**Fig. 5**).[34] To achieve pain reduction, calcium hydroxyapatite is mixed with additional 2% lidocaine before injection. This is done by drawing the lidocaine into a 3-mL syringe. This syringe is then attached to the syringe containing the calcium hydroxyapatite by using a leak-proof lock connector. Approximately 10 mixing strokes are performed to adequately combine the 2 ingredients before injection.[1] In addition to bruising and pain, patients may also experience swelling or edema, which can be prevented using anti-inflammatory enzymes. Treatment of the edema may consist of NSAIDs or the use of streptokinase. Any procedure that breaks the surface of the skin carries with it a risk of infection, and injecting dermal fillers is no exception.[34] Although skin infections with dermal filler injections are unusual, a skin assessment before treatment of any active bacterial or viral infection, makeup removal, skin

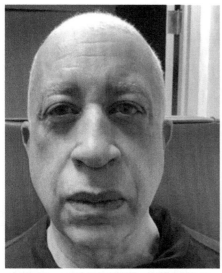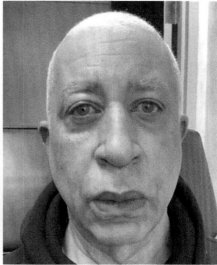

Fig. 4. A 70-year-old man with midface volume loss following treatment with hyaluronic acid filler.

preparation with antibacterial soap (eg, chlorhexidine) or alcohol, or both, and proper attention to clean/sterile technique will further help minimize secondary infections.[35] The "Tyndall effect" can be corrected by injecting hyaluronidase. Hyaluronidase is an enzyme that dissolves HA quickly and efficiently. It should be noted that although effective, hyaluronidase carries its own risks including allergic reactions in patients allergic to bee stings. Minimizing the risks associated with the injection of fillers should include using the linear threading technique, avoiding serial punctures, fanning mid-deep dermal placement, and postinjection topical application of a corticosteroid to decrease inflammation.[1] Avoiding serial puncture techniques with filler placement and being mindful of areas of the face prone to keloids such as the jawline can be helpful.[32] Additionally, using a linear threading or "fanning" technique reduces the risk of

dyspigmentation as well as local adverse events including swelling, tenderness, redness, bruising, and pain.[36]

SUMMARY

POC have unique cosmetic concerns that may differ from other patient populations. These include treatments for pigmentary changes as well as skin rejuvenation and antiaging. Dermatologists should be aware of side effects associated with different cosmetic procedures including laser and light-based therapies, neurotoxins, body contouring, skin tightening, and soft tissue augmentation. Through use of appropriate safety measures, dermatologists can help their POC achieve their desired cosmetic outcomes.

CLINICS CARE POINTS

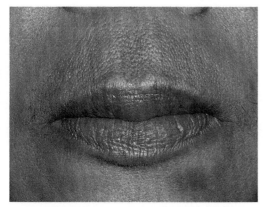

Fig. 5. Bruising following hyaluronic acid filler.

- It is important to counsel patients on appropriate cosmetic procedures.
- Patient selection is important for the desired cosmetic outcomes.
- Adjustments of treatment parameters are often necessary in accounting for the safety of each unique patient.
- Utilizing "test spots" before the full treatment may be warranted to determine potential adverse events.
- The desired cosmetic outcome may require multiple sessions with conservative measures.

FUNDING SOURCE

None.

DECLARATION OF INTERESTS

Financial disclosures and not conflict of interest. Declaration of Interests can be used as well.

REFERENCES

1. Kelly AP, Taylor SC, Lim HW, et al. Taylor and kelly's dermatology for skin of color. 2nd edition. New York, N.Y: McGraw-Hill Education LLC; 2016. Available at: https://dermatology.mhmedical.com/book.aspx?bookid=2585.
2. Quiñonez RL, Agbai ON, Burgess CM, et al. An update on cosmetic procedures in people of color. part 2: Neuromodulators, soft tissue augmentation, chemexfoliating agents, and laser hair reduction. J Am Acad Dermatol 2022;86(4):729–39.
3. Adotama P, Papac N, Alexis A, et al. Common dermatologic procedures and the associated complications unique to skin of color. Dermatol Surg 2021;47(3):355–9.
4. Deshpande A. Efficacy & safety of intense pulsed light therapy for unwanted facial hair: A retrospective analysis in skin of color. J Cosmet Laser Ther 2021;23(5–6):116–21.
5. Dorgham NA, Dorgham DA. Lasers for reduction of unwanted hair in skin of colour: A systematic review and meta-analysis. J Eur Acad Dermatol Venereol 2020;34(5):948–55.
6. Levin MK, Ng E, Bae YC, et al. Treatment of pigmentary disorders in patients with skin of color with a novel 755 nm picosecond, Q-switched ruby, and Q-switched nd:YAG nanosecond lasers: A retrospective photographic review. Lasers Surg Med 2016;48(2):181–7.
7. Davis EC, Callender VD. Postinflammatory hyperpigmentation: A review of the epidemiology, clinical features, and treatment options in skin of color. J Clin Aesthet Dermatol 2010;3(7):20–31.
8. Ogbechie-Godec OA, Melasma EN. An up-to-date comprehensive review. Dermatol Ther 2017;7(3):305–18.
9. Roberts WE, Henry M, Burgess C, et al. Laser treatment of skin of color for medical and aesthetic uses with a new 650-microsecond nd:YAG 1064nm laser. J Drugs Dermatol 2019;18(4):135.
10. Lawson CN, Hollinger J, Sethi S, et al. Updates in the understanding and treatments of skin & hair disorders in women of color. International Journal of Women's Dermatology 2015;1(2):59–75.
11. Gupta A, Kaur M, Patra S, et al. Evidence-based surgical management of post-acne scarring in skin of color. J Cutan Aesthet Surg 2020;13(2):124–41.
12. Bogdan Allemann I, Kaufman J. Fractional photothermolysis—an update. Laser Med Sci 2010;25(1):137–44.
13. Derrick CD, Shridharani SM, Broyles JM. The safety and efficacy of cryolipolysis: a systematic review of available literature. Aesthet Surg J. 2015;35(7):830–6.
14. Goodman GJ, Ho WWS, Chang KJ, et al. Efficacy of a novel injection lipolysis to induce targeted adipocyte apoptosis: a randomized, phase IIa study of CBL-514 injection on abdominal subcutaneous fat reduction. Aesthet Surg J 2022;42(11):NP662–74.
15. Mordon S, Plot E. Laser lipolysis versus traditional liposuction for fat removal. Expert Rev Med Devices 2009;6(6):677–88.
16. Murgia RD, Noell C, Weiss M, et al. Body contouring for fat and muscle in aesthetics: Review and debate. Clin Dermatol 2022;40(1):29–34.
17. Regan J.P. and Casaubon J.T., Abdominoplasty, In: StatPearls., 2022, StatPearls Publishing LLC, Treasure Island, FL, NBK431058, [bookaccession].
18. Bellini E, Grieco MP, Raposio E. A journey through liposuction and liposculture: Review. Ann Med Surg (Lond). 2017;24:53–60.
19. Shermak MA. Body contouring. Plast Reconstr Surg 2012;129(6):963e–78e.
20. Juhász M, Korta D, Mesinkovska NA. A review of the use of ultrasound for skin tightening, body contouring, and cellulite reduction in dermatology. Dermatol Surg 2018;44(7):949–63.
21. Fabi SG. Noninvasive skin tightening: Focus on new ultrasound techniques. Clin Cosmet Investig Dermatol 2015;8:47–52.
22. Kwan KR, Kolansky Z, Abittan BJ, et al. Skin tightening. Cutis 2020;106(3):134–7, 139;E1.
23. Alexis AF. Lasers and light-based therapies in ethnic skin: Treatment options and recommendations for fitzpatrick skin types V and VI. Br J Dermatol 2013;169:91–7.
24. Gutowski KA MD. Microfocused ultrasound for skin tightening. Clin Plast Surg 2016;43(3):577–82.
25. Frampton JE, Easthope SE. Botulinum toxin A (botox cosmetic): A review of its use in the treatment of glabellar frown lines. Am J Clin Dermatol 2003;4(10):709–25.
26. Dessy LA, Fallico N, Mazzocchi M, et al. Botulinum toxin for glabellar lines: A review of the efficacy and safety of currently available products. Am J Clin Dermatol 2012;12(6):377–88.
27. Small R. Botulinum toxin injection for facial wrinkles. Am Fam Physician 2014;90(3):168–75.
28. Quiñonez RL, Agbai ON, Burgess CM, et al. An update on cosmetic procedures in people of color. part 1: Scientific background, assessment, preprocedure preparation. J Am Acad Dermatol 2022;86(4):715–25.
29. Nestor MS, Arnold D, Fischer D. The mechanisms of action and use of botulinum neurotoxin type A in

aesthetics: Key clinical postulates II. J Cosmet Dermatol 2020;19(11):2785–804.

30. Taylor SC, Callender VD, Albright CD, et al. AbobotulinumtoxinA for reduction of glabellar lines in patients with skin of color: Post hoc analysis of pooled clinical trial data. Dermatol Surg 2012; 38(11):1804–11.

31. Cotofana S, Freytag DL, Frank K, et al. The bidirectional movement of the frontalis muscle: Introducing the line of convergence and its potential clinical relevance. Plast Reconstr Surg 2020;145(5):1155–62.

32. Aguilera SB. Ethnic and gender considerations in the use of facial fillers. New York, NY: McGraw Hill; 2018.

33. Humphrey CD, Arkins JP, Dayan SH. Soft tissue fillers in the nose. Aesthet Surg J. 2009;29(6): 477–84.

34. Urdiales-Gálvez F, Delgado NE, Figueiredo V, et al. Treatment of soft tissue filler complications: Expert consensus recommendations. Aesth Plast Surg 2018;42(2):498–510.

35. Sherman RN MD. Avoiding dermal filler complications. Clin Dermatol 2009;27(3):S23–32.

36. Taylor SC, Burgess CM, Callender VD. Safety of nonanimal stabilized hyaluronic acid dermal fillers in patients with skin of color: A randomized, evaluator-blinded comparative trial. Dermatol Surg 2009;35(Suppl 2):1653–60.

Moving?

Make sure your subscription moves with you!

To notify us of your new address, find your **Clinics Account Number** (located on your mailing label above your name), and contact customer service at:

Email: **journalscustomerservice-usa@elsevier.com**

800-654-2452 (subscribers in the U.S. & Canada)
314-447-8871 (subscribers outside of the U.S. & Canada)

Fax number: 314-447-8029

Elsevier Health Sciences Division
Subscription Customer Service
3251 Riverport Lane
Maryland Heights, MO 63043

*To ensure uninterrupted delivery of your subscription, please notify us at least 4 weeks in advance of move.

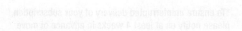

Printed and bound by CPI Group (UK) Ltd, Croydon, CR0 4YY

08/05/2025

01864717-0013